Outcomes in Critical Care

Saxon Ridley MD FRCA

*Consultant in Anaesthesia and Intensive Care, Norfolk and
Norwich University Hospital NHS Trust, Norwich, UK*

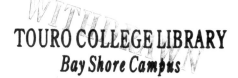
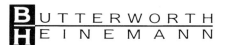

BUTTERWORTH
HEINEMANN

OXFORD   AUCKLAND   BOSTON   JOHANNESBURG   MELBOURNE   NEW DELHI

Butterworth-Heinemann
Linacre House, Jordan Hill, Oxford OX2 8DP
225 Wildwood Avenue, Woburn, MA 01801-2041
A division of Reed Educational and Professional Publishing Ltd

 A member of the Reed Elsevier plc group

First published 2002

British Library Cataloguing in Publication Data
Outcomes in critical care
   1. Critical care medicine   2. Critical care medicine –
   Evaluation   3. Outcome assessment (Medical care)
   I. Ridley, Saxon
   616'.028

Library of Congress Cataloguing in Publication Data
A catalogue record for this book is available from the Library of Congress

ISBN 0 7506 4982 8

For information on all Butterworth-Heinemann publications
visit our website at www.bh.com

Composition by Genesis Typesetting, Rochester, Kent
Printed and bound in Great Britain by MPG Books, Bodmin, Cornwall

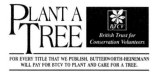

FOR EVERY TITLE THAT WE PUBLISH, BUTTERWORTH-HEINEMANN
WILL PAY FOR BTCV TO PLANT AND CARE FOR A TREE.

4/29/04

Outcomes in Critical Care

Commissioning editor: Melanie Tait
Desk editor: Claire Hutchins
Production Controller: Chris Jarvis
Development editor: Zoë A. Youd
Cover designer: Greg Harris

Contents

Contributors

Dieter Beck, MD, DEAA, EDIC, DA (Lond), DTM&H (Lond)
Consultant in Anaesthesia and Intensive Care, Department of Anaesthesiology and Intensive Care, Charité, Humboldt University Berlin, Berlin, Germany

Malcolm Booth, MBChB, FRCA, MPhil
Consultant in Anaesthesia and Intensive Care, Glasgow Royal Infirmary, Glasgow, Scotland

Owen Boyd, MRCP, FRCA
Consultant in Intensive Care Medicine, The General Intensive Care Unit, The Royal Sussex County Hospital, Brighton, UK

Dave Edbrooke, MBBS, FRCA
Consultant in Intensive Care, Medical and Economics Research Centre, Royal Hallamshire Hospital, Sheffield, UK

Richard Griffiths, BSc, MD, FRCP
Reader in Medicine (Intensive Care), Intensive Care Research Group, Department of Medicine, University of Liverpool, Liverpool, UK

Clare Hibbert, BA (Hons)
Senior Researcher, Medical and Economics Research Centre, Royal Hallamshire Hospital, Sheffield, UK

Christina Jones, BSc (Applied Chem), BSc (Nursing), MPhil
Research Fellow, Intensive Care Unit, Whiston Hospital, Prescot, Merseyside, UK

D. Jim Kutsogiannis, MD, MHS, FRCPC
Assistant Professor, Division of Critical Care and the Department of Public Health Sciences, Royal Alexandra Hospital, Edmonton, Alberta, Canada

Tom Noseworthy, MD, MSc, MPH, FRCPC, FACP, FCCP, FCCM, CHE
Professor and Chair of the Department of Public Health Sciences, Faculty of
Medicine and Dentistry, University of Alberta, Edmonton, Alberta, Canada

Daliana Peres-Bota, MD
Fellow in the Department of Intensive Care, Hôpital Universitaire Erasme,
Bruxelles, Belgium

Dinis Reis Miranda, MD, PhD
Professor of Surgical Intensive Care, Director of Health Services Research Unit,
Groningen University Hospital, The Netherlands

Saxon Ridley, MD, FRCA
Consultant in Anaesthesia and Intensive Care, Norfolk and Norwich University
Hospital NHS Trust, Norwich, UK

Jean-Louis Vincent, MD, PhD, FCCM, FCCP
Professor of Intensive Care, Head of the Department of Intensive Care, Hôpital
Universitaire Erasme, Bruxelles, Belgium

Duncan Young, BM, DM, FRCA
Clinical Reader in Anaesthetics, Nuffield Department of Anaesthetics, Radcliffe
Infirmary, Oxford, UK

Preface

Outcome measurement of healthcare is becoming increasingly important. Healthcare workers are encouraged to practice evidence-based medicine so that only those therapies proven to be effective and efficient are employed. However, the value of such evidence-based therapy can only be properly assessed if the outcome following therapy is also effectively and efficiently measured. Outcome measurement is thus an integral part of evidence-based medicine.

Critical care is a relatively modern specialty, having developed over the last 50 years. However, as critical care involves applying many interdependent therapeutic pathways, it has been difficult to isolate a single, yet clearly recognizable way to demonstrate its value. Furthermore, because of the life-sustaining nature of critical care, alternative forms of care are not really feasible. There is no viable alternative to some of the organ support measures applied in intensive care. Proving the benefits of critical care by rigorous scientific means has thus been difficult. Partly because of the lack of an alternative, patients and healthcare providers have assumed that critical care is effective and, hence, vital to the delivery of a comprehensive hospital service. The lack of a single, clearly defined and satisfactory end-point has meant that on occasion outcome measurement following critical care has not been approached in a systematic fashion. This has resulted in outcomes following critical care being loosely and inappropriately measured.

The aim of this book is to draw upon the experience and knowledge of a wide range of experts to define clearly the numerous aspects of outcome following critical illness. Their critical analysis of the facets of outcome should enable the reader to assess other published works with greater clarity of thought. Hopefully, this book will improve the understanding of outcomes and their measurement to interested parties outside medicine and to this end, a glossary has been included. Perhaps, armed with the knowledge contained within these pages, future researchers will be guided to measure outcomes in a more effective and, hence, worthwhile manner. The book has been written because, at present, no other publication covers all aspects of outcome following critical illness. Textbooks of intensive care medicine correctly concentrate on the pathophysiological processes that render patients critically ill and detail explanations of therapeutic options presently available. Individual scientific papers and review articles investigate or summarize the individual facets of outcome, but no publication endeavours to draw all these concepts together. None the less, this book is not entirely comprehensive. Critical care covers all ages and all medical specialities. The book concentrates on adult general critical care and does not attempt to describe outcome measures following paediatric intensive care. Paediatric medicine is a separate specialty and the outcome goals and measurements following paediatric intensive care are different from those of adult practice. Similarly, the specialized subgroups of cardiac, neurosurgical and hepatological critical care have their own organ specific emphasis. All of these specialist areas will focus on particular outcomes, but the principles of outcome measurement described in this book could be applied in these areas.

The ability to measure effectively outcomes following critical illness allows the opportunity for all practitioners to start comparing performance. Many institutions and agencies are involved in quality assurance and performance measurement. Such activities are much more meaningful if the outcome measures are widely applied and comprehensively understood. Being able to describe properly and measure the outcomes of patients who develop critical illness will enable practitioners of critical care to demonstrate their value to the hospital in particular and society in general. As critical care is so expensive, the resources invested must be wisely and effectively used. Since most healthcare systems have fixed or limited budgets, this is vital for not only maintaining, but also improving the service. If outcomes following critical care are not properly measured, we may not be able to defend critical care in the face of competing healthcare programmes. As professionals our wide experience and understanding of critical illness means we are ideally placed to become involved in outcome measurement. The purpose of this book is to raise awareness of outcomes and to offer advice and guidance on how to apply and measure them.

Glossary

Abdominal compartment syndrome The normal intra-abdominal pressure is around 0 mmHg. Small increases in intra-abdominal pressure (≥ 10 mmHg) disturb blood circulation inside the abdomen. Further increases in intra-abdominal pressure develop following both intra-abdominal (e.g. bowel, kidney) and extra-abdominal (e.g. cardiovascular, pulmonary) organ failure. Pathology of the intra-abdominal space (e.g. oedema, haemorrhage, infection), and therapeutic procedures (e.g. intra-abdominal surgical packing) are frequent causes of increased intra-abdominal pressure. Because of adaptation to gradual increase in intra-abdominal pressure, chronic increases are better tolerated than acute changes.

Acute Physiology And Chronic Health Evaluation (APACHE) is a measure of severity of disease. This system has been developed over 20 years as APACHE (Knaus, W. A., Zimmerman, J. E., Wagner, D. P., Draper, E. A., Lawrence, D. E. (1981). APACHE – Acute Physiology And Chronic Health Evaluation: a physiologically based classification system. *Crit. Care Med.*, **9**, 591–597), APACHE II (Knaus, W. A., Draper, E. A., Wagner, D. P., Zimmerman, J. E. (1985). APACHE II: A severity of disease classification system. *Crit. Care Med.*, **13**, 818–829) and APACHE III (Knaus, W. A., Wagner, D. P., Draper, E. A. *et al.* (1991). The APACHE III prognostic system: risk prediction of hospital mortality for critically ill hospitalized adults. *Chest*, **100**, 1619–1636). It has been used as a technique for case-mix adjustment when comparing hospital mortality rates between ICUs. A score is computed using physiological variables collected in the first 24 h of admission, chronic health status, reason for admission and age. By averaging the predicted mortality over a large number of patients a predicted group mortality can be determined and compared with the observed group mortality to give a standardized mortality ratio (SMR). Any difference from unity may reflect different efficacy of care between the ICU under study and those used to derive the APACHE score. It can never be 100% accurate and is more appropriately used for population risk rather than individual risk.

Adults with Incapacity (Scotland) Bill 2000 This bill was passed by the Scottish Parliament and received royal assent in May 2000. Among other provisions for the medical care of incapacitated adults, it includes a provision for the appointment of a proxy decision-maker who could act on behalf of the incapacitated person. The proxy may be the next of kin or 'nearest and dearest'. The proxy's usefulness will depend upon his or her knowledge of the person's wishes. The Act became law in spring 2001. You may read the bill on the Scottish Parliament website at:

www.scottish.parliament.uk/parl_bus/bill-final.htm#5.

Alveolar-arterial oxygen difference (A-a DO$_2$) is the difference in oxygen partial pressure between the lungs (alveolar space) and the blood in arterial vessels. In healthy persons breathing room air, this difference is small (10–15 mmHg). Lung disease can impair the diffusion of oxygen from the alveolar space into the blood thereby increasing the alveolar-arterial oxygen gradient.

American Medical Association's Education for Physicians on End-of-Life Care This is a training project for physicians in the USA to improve competency in end-of-life care. It consists of a core curriculum incorporating the basic knowledge and skills needed to care for a dying patient. In a series of plenary modules and workshops it covers communication skills, ethical decision making, psychosocial considerations and the management of pain and other symptoms. The full curriculum and other information are available on the Association's website at: www.ama-assn.org/ama/pub/category/2719.html then choose 'The EPEC Project'.

Anxiety describes a chronic state with irritability, distractibility, sleep disturbance, headaches and a feeling of poor memory and concentration.

Audit is the methodical examination and analysis of the practice and outcomes of a health care service.

Autocorrelation Most standard statistical techniques, such as ordinary least squares regression, assume that each observation within a data set is independent of all of the others. This assumption is often inappropriate if repeated observations over time are performed on the same individual because observations within an individual tend to be correlated with one another. Autocorrelation implies that two observations taken at random from the same individual are likely to be more similar (or correlated) than two random observations from two different individuals. As an example, two random measurements of forced expiratory volume in one second (FEV$_1$) divided by forced vital capacity (FVC) (FEV$_1$/FVC ratio) in a patient with chronic obstructive airways disease are more likely to correlate and be low whereas two random measurements of FEV$_1$/FVC from two individuals picked at random from a general population are not likely to correlate.

Benchmarking is the process by which a standard of current practice or conditions is defined. Different ICUs or the same ICU over time can be compared to this 'benchmark'.

Bottom-up method of costing assigns a cost to individual patients based on their use of healthcare resources. The individual resources can be grouped together (e.g. the resources used to treat pneumonia) to produce a profile of cost for individual patients with certain diseases.

Calibration is the process of correlating a new measure with the accepted standard. For predictive models, it is the evaluation of the degree of accuracy concerning the model's predictive ability. It is particularly relevant to identify failures of prediction in a particular range of risk.

Case-mix ICU workload varies in different types of hospital serving differing populations. The case-mix of an ICU recognizes this by describing the different types of patients found in differing proportions in different ICUs. The description is often based on diagnostic or demographic background.

Clinical ethics committee has a remit is to assist patients and healthcare workers to resolve ethics issues or disputes. They also have a role in policy development, case review and education. While common in almost every medical institution in the USA such bodies are still relatively rare in the UK. Such committees are usually led by a trained ethicist who can guide discussions.

Confidence intervals present a range of values derived from sample (study) data, within which a population value for the same parameter is likely to lie. As such it can be used for descriptive or comparative statistics.

Cost-benefit analysis reviews the costs and benefits of alternative treatments, and produces results in monetary units. Any intervention where the benefit is greater than the costs is considered to be worthwhile.

Cost block method is a retrospective top-down method for determining the annual expenditure of a critical care unit that produces average costs per patient and per patient-day by dividing expenditure by the unit's throughput.

Cost-effectiveness analysis examines both the costs and the consequences of varying healthcare treatments to produce a ratio displaying the cost per unit of effect for competing interventions.

Cost-minimization analysis compares the costs of alternative forms of treatment that are assumed to have an equivalent medical effect, with the aim of finding the cheapest way of achieving the same outcome.

Cost-utility analysis compares healthcare interventions that produce different results with regard to both quantity and quality of life. The results are expressed as utilities (i.e. measures that capture both length of life and subjective levels of well-being, for example, quality-adjusted-life-years or QALYs). Competing interventions are compared in terms of cost per utility, in order to relate cost to a measure of usefulness or outcome.

Delphi method uses questionnaires to arrive at a consensus. The method consists of several rounds whereby participants are invited to rank their agreement with a number of statements; the rankings are then summarized and included in the questionnaire, and the participants asked to rank again. They are able to change their opinion after viewing the group rankings. The rankings are then summarized again and assessed for the degree of consensus. If insufficient consensus, participants are asked to complete the questionnaires a third time.

Delta The delta score represents the difference between the score on admission and the maximum score achieved during the selected period, e.g. a 24-h period of ICU stay.

Deontology is the philosophical theory that focuses on the rightness or wrongness of an act rather than its consequences. Based on the teachings of Kant who stressed that every person must be treated as an end in themselves and not as a means to an end.

Depression is an affective disorder characterized by low mood or loss of enjoyment of previously pleasurable activities, sleep disturbance (difficulty falling asleep or early waking), impaired concentration, lack of energy, reduced or increased appetite with resultant loss or gain of weight and suicidal intent.

Diagnosis related groups (DRGs) is a methodology, developed in the USA, for stratifying hospital patients according to the use of resources (e.g. hours of direct professional care, therapeutic interventions, diagnostic procedures, hotel services and social services). The use of five variables: primary diagnosis, secondary diagnosis, primary surgical procedure, secondary surgical procedure and age, enabled the meaningful stratification of hospital admissions into about 80 groups and 400 subgroups according to their use of hospital resources.

Diffusing capacity is the volume of gas (usually carbon monoxide) transferred across the alveoli per minute per unit of alveolar partial pressure. It has a normal value of 17–25 ml/min/mmHg. Its value will be reduced if the alveolar membrane is thickened, if there are areas of ventilation/perfusion mismatch or reduced alveolar membrane.

Direct costs are all the goods, services and other resources consumed in the provision of a health intervention, or in dealing with side effects or other current or future aspects linked to it. These costs can be medical and non-medical.

Discrimination is the ability of a test to distinguish between two outcomes, often survivors and non-survivors. It is frequently tested by the area under the receiver operating characteristic curve.

Effectiveness measures the extent to which medical interventions are beneficial, i.e. the treatment does more good than harm when applied in the specific clinical circumstance appropriate to a particular patient or group of patients.

Efficiency describes the efficacy of an intervention in relation to input, i.e. the best possible use of available resources.

Evidence-based medicine is the conscientious, explicit and careful use of the best current evidence in decision-making concerning individual patients. It is a method of finding the appropriate evidence from the exponentially expanding database; there are almost 1 000 000 randomized controlled trials published. The practice of evidence-based medicine allows the available information to be critically appraised for its applicability to the patient actually under the clinician's care who may, or may not be, similar to those in the published study(ies).

Fixed costs are those costs that will remain a constant (within a short period of time) regardless of the quantity of production.

Forced expiratory volume is the volume of gas forcibly expired from full inspiration in a set time, usually one second. Normally it has a value of about

80% of forced vital capacity but this will be reduced in obstructive pulmonary disease.

Forced vital capacity is measured when expiration is forced and has a normal value for adults of about 4.5 litres. Closure of some smaller airways may occur when the intrathoracic pressures are high and as a result forced vital capacity may be less than true vital capacity. Forced vital capacity is reduced in restrictive pulmonary disease, supine position, elderly patients and with muscle weakness.

General estimating equations extend general linear models including ordinary least squares linear regression and incorporate random effects. When considering a set of data on individuals which is repeated over time (such as the measurement of health related quality of life by the SF–36), a general estimating equation model measures the correlation of the outcome measure (SF–36 in this instance) within an individual and uses this estimate to estimate better the regression coefficient and its variance. General estimating equation models also permit the determination of robust estimates of the variance about a regression coefficient even if the strength of the correlation within individuals varies from individual to individual.

Glasgow Coma Scale is a system developed to grade the degree of coma according to three types of responses (i.e. eye opening, verbal response and motor response). The scoring ranges from 1 (no response) to a normal score of 4 for eye opening, 5 for verbal response and 6 for motor response. The lower the score, the greater the degree of coma. (Teasdale, G., Jennett, B. (1974). Assessment of coma and impaired consciousness, a practical scale. *Lancet*, **ii**, 81–84).

Goodness of fit is a combination of calibration and discrimination.

Gross national product describes the total market value of the absolute goods and services generated by a nation's economy within a specific time period (usually a year) calculated without reference to the depreciation or consumption of capital used during the production process.

High dependency unit (HDU) is a designated area in a hospital providing a level of care intermediate between ICU care and ward care, usually providing monitoring and support for patients with single organ failure.

Hillsborough disaster In April 1989 overcrowding in Hillsborough football stadium resulted in a number of football fans being crushed. Many of them died either at the scene or soon afterwards. The families of victims have since, unsuccessfully, sued senior police officers in charge of crowd control for damages. Most famous victim was Anthony Bland who entered a permanent vegetative state and whose family won the right to have all forms of feeding and hydration stopped to allow his eventual death in 1993.

Hosmer-Lemeshow C Statistic is a chi-squared statistic used to test the calibration of predictive ability by dividing the observations into deciles for comparison purposes (Lemeshow, S., Hosmer, D. W. Jr. (1982). A review of goodness of fit statistics for use in the development of logistic regression models. *Am. J. Epidemiol.*, **115**, 92–106). The lower the number and the higher the P value, the better the calibration, as the observed and expected outcomes are more similar. A second statistic, the H statistic, also proposed by Hosmer and Lemeshow uses fixed deciles rather than natural deciles.

Incremental analysis is the examination of added costs and clinical outcomes that result from different treatments. Incremental cost-effectiveness ratios reveal the cost per unit of benefit changing practice to introduce a new treatment, i.e. the benefit gained in relation to the extra expense.

Indirect costs refer to the lost productivity suffered by the national economy as a result of an individual's illness. For example, absence from the workplace, the effect any ailment has on individual productivity or more extremely, the loss resulting from an early death.

Intensive Care National Audit and Research Centre (ICNARC) Case Mix Programme Database The Case Mix Programme is the national, comparative audit of patient outcomes coordinated by ICNARC. These analyses are based on data for 46 587 admissions to 91 adult ICUs based in NHS hospitals geographically spread across England, Wales and Northern Ireland. For more information on the representativeness and quality of these data, please contact ICNARC, Tavistock House, Tavistock Square, London, WC1H 9HR, UK.

Intensive care outreach teams are part of a multidisciplinary approach to the identification of patients at risk of developing critical illness and those patients following a period of critical illness, to enable early intervention or transfer (if appropriate) to an area more suited to care for that patient's individual needs. Outreach is a collaboration and partnership between the critical care department and other departments to ensure a continuum of care for patients regardless of location and will enhance the skills and understanding of all staff in the delivery of critical care.

Kaplan-Meier survival curve is a technique to calculate a survival curve when there are differing follow-up periods for different patients. It is used to estimate the proportion of a population that will survive for a given time in a similar set of circumstances.

Kappa statistic is an expression of how much better (or worse) the agreement between two observers was than chance alone. Kappa has a maximum value of 1 when agreement is perfect, zero when agreement is no better than chance and negative values indicate worse than chance agreement. For further details see Altman, D. G. (1991). *Practical Statistics for Medical Research*. Chapman and Hall.

Lead-time bias is the time that a patient has been under treatment prior to the collection of data variables used in a scoring system. Some variables (e.g. age) will not change, but others (e.g. temperature or blood pressure) might be expected to change during this time as they respond to treatment.

Local research ethics committee (LREC) is the committee that assesses proposed research protocols for ethical acceptability. Its function is to ensure that rigid ethical standards are maintained in order to protect the subjects of medical research, to prevent abuses and to protect the quality of research. Separate assessors examine the scientific quality of the proposed research on behalf of the committee. Poor quality science is unethical. Such committees are normally based at NHS trust level and have lay, theological and professional members. The committee has no function in resolving ethical problems outside the area of research. Multicentre research ethics committees (MREC) oversee multicentre research. Local or multicentre research ethics committee approval is mandatory before a research project can commence.

Logistic regression is a mathematical technique for estimating the association of several explanatory (predictor) variables on binary outcome events. A logistic transformation is applied to generate probabilities. By definition, the probabilities range from zero to one, or expressed as a percentage, from 0–100%. Logistic regression allows estimation of the effect of each variable on outcome, while simultaneously controlling for the effects of all other variables included in the regression equation.

Logrank test is a technique to determine if two samples of patients have similar survival curves. The technique uses data from the whole survival curve to provide an overall answer, rather than examining each time point individually.

Marginal costs are the costs of producing an extra unit of service.

Medicaid is publicly funded healthcare in the USA available only to those who cannot afford private insurance.

Medical emergency teams see Intensive care outreach teams.

Mortality Prediction Model is a technique for case-mix adjustment when comparing hospital mortality rates between ICUs. It uses age, three physiological variables, three chronic diseases, five acute diagnoses, the type of admission and the use of cardiopulmonary resuscitation and mechanical ventilation to produce a predicted mortality. The current version is MPM II. Variants can be used to predict mortality on admission and after 24 and 72 h (MPM_0, MPM_{24} and MPM_{72}). (Lemeshow, S., Teres, D., Pastides, H., Avrunin, J. S., Steingrub, J. S. (1985). A method for predicting survival and mortality of ICU patients using objectively derived weights. *Crit. Care Med.*, **13**, 519–525; Lemeshow, S., Teres, D., Klar, J., Avrunin, J. S., Gehbach, S. H., Rapoport, J. (1993). Mortality Probability Models (MPM II) based on an international cohort of intensive care unit patients. *JAMA*, **270**, 2478–2486).

Multiple logistic regression is a statistical technique that produces a formula that predicts the probability of the occurrence as a function of the independent variables.

Multiple Organ Dysfunction Score (MODS) is a score of the severity of dysfunction of seven organ systems developed as an objective measure of severity of illness. The MODS has been evaluated against ICU mortality to establish criterion validity (i.e. does an increasing severity of illness measured using the MODS score correlate with increased ICU mortality?). (Marshall, J. C., Cook, D. J., Christou, N. V. *et al.* (1995). Multiple Organ Dysfunction Score: a reliable descriptor of a complex clinical outcome. *Crit. Care Med.*, **23**, 1638–1652).

National Institute of Clinical Excellence is a special Health Authority within the NHS established in 1999 to provide patients, health professionals and the public with authoritative, robust and reliable guidance of 'best practice'. Its remit is to set clear national standards (for England and Wales) of what patients can expect to receive from the NHS. It will help to promote clinical and cost effectiveness through guidance and audit. It has been accused of rationing health services and some of its decisions have been controversial such as the recommendations against routine use of Relenza for 'flu prevention and the use of interferon beta in multiple sclerosis. More information is available at: www.nice.org.uk/nice-web/Cat.asp?c=20.

Nosocomial infection The incidence and severity of infections in the hospital is much higher than in the community outside the hospital. To control infections in hospital it is important to identify and study those acquired inside the hospital. Nosocomial infection is the infection that is identified in a patient at least 48 h after admission to hospital.

Occult hypoperfusion describes the subclinical reduction of oxygen transport to the tissues. Occult hypoperfusion is measured by the proportional increase in lactic acid in the serum. The increase of lactic acid above 2.4 mmol/l is significantly associated with increased morbidity and mortality in patients after trauma.

Odds ratio is an estimate of the relative risk. In a prospective study, the odds ratio is defined as the odds of exposed persons to the odds of non-exposed persons to experience an outcome event (e.g. death or disease). If the exposure is not related to the outcome, the odds ratio equals one. If there is a positive association between the exposure and the outcome, the odds ratio is > 1 (increased risk); if there is a negative association, the odds ratio is < 1 (reduced risk).

Office for National Statistics (ONS) (web site at: www.statistics.gov.uk) is the Government body charged with collecting and disseminating data on a wide range of health care and other issues.

Opportunity cost can be considered as the value of the best alternative use of resources; that is the value relinquished by the investment in a particular programme over other options. Therefore, the value of resources consumed are defined in relation to the benefit that an alternative use of the resources would have generated and is expressed as the value of the next alternative for using these resources.

Organ Dysfunction and/or Infection (ODIN) score is a technique to score the severity of dysfunction of six organ systems in the first 24 h of ICU admission. The presence or absence of each organ failure is assigned a weight and the sum of the weighted values is used to predict ICU mortality. As ODIN was developed and validated in one ICU and on one data set it may not be transferable to other situations. See Fagon, J. Y., Chastre, J., Novara, A. *et al.* (1993). Characterization of intensive care unit patients using a model based on the presence or absence of Organ Dysfunction and/or Infection: the ODIN model. *Intensive Care Med.*, **19,** 137–144.

Organisation for Economic Cooperation and Development (OECD) is an international organization whose members include several European countries and also Mexico, Canada, the USA and Japan. The group is a mainly consultative body whose primary purpose is the achievement of the highest possible economic growth and employment and the elevation of living standards within member states, while simultaneously striving for the maintenance of financial stability.

Organophosphates are a group of widely used pesticides. Organophosphate poisoning causes muscle weakness and respiratory failure.

Panic attack describes an acute anxiety state, often with an obvious precipitant. The patient may experience palpitations, dry mouth, sweating, diarrhoea, hyperventilation, muscle tension resulting in aches and pains, may feel terror or in immediate danger of dying.

Patient at risk teams see Intensive care outreach teams.

Patient Self Determination Act 1991 is legislation in USA requiring hospitals to inform patients of their right to make an advance directive and to honour it subject to state law

Pediatric Risk of Mortality (PRISM) is a technique for case-mix adjustment when comparing intensive care unit mortality rates between paediatric ICUs. It was derived from the physiological stability index (PSI). A score is computed using 14 physiological variables collected in the first 24 h of admission, the type of admission and age, and used to derive a predicted hospital mortality. It is used in a similar way to APACHE scores (see Pollack, M. M., Ruttimann, U. E., Getson, P. R. (1988). Pediatric Risk of Mortality (PRISM) score. *Crit. Care Med.*, **16,** 1110–1116).

Perseveration is the persistent repetition of words or actions despite the individual's efforts to say or do something else.

Post-traumatic stress disorder is characterized by intrusive memories of the original accident (i.e. flash-backs), recurrent nightmares, emotional numbing, autonomic hyperarousal and avoidance of stimuli reminiscent of the original trauma. It occurs frequently after serious road traffic accidents, life-threatening burns and terrorist incidents.

Prevalence is defined as the proportion of affected persons (e.g. diseased or dead) in the population at a given point in time.

Psychometric properties Psychometrics is the science of using standardized tests to measure attributes of an individual or object, in this case health status attributes. Psychometric theory and methods are used to translate a person's ratings and reports into scales to measure health attributes.

Quality Adjusted Life Years (QALY) is a method of assigning economic value to healthcare interventions based on the cost of the intervention, its effectiveness and the life expectancy of the patient. QALYs describe the years of life saved by a technology, service, or treatment, adjusted by the quality of those lives. This is calculated by estimating the total life-years gained and weighting each year with a quality-of-life score (from 0, representing worst health, to 1 or 100, representing best). This allows very different treatments to be compared by the numbers of QALYs gained. In some ways it promotes equality as treatments with the same QALY value are equally merited. However, the old and the chronically disabled or ill have a smaller health gain compared to the healthy young and therefore their QALYs are always lower for the same intervention. Thus QALYs actively discriminate against the elderly and disabled.

Random effects (coefficient) regression Ordinary least squares regression models estimate population average effects. When within-individual observations are correlated (such as when forced expiratory volume in one second (FEV_1) divided by forced vital capacity (FVC) (FEV_1/FVC ratio) in a patient with chronic obstructive airways disease are consistently low over time as compared with a normal subject's FEV_1/FVC measurements) ordinary least squares models do not properly estimate the mean and variance of the estimated regression parameters. Under random coefficient regression models, observations within individuals are assumed to be correlated and each individual's effect deviates from a group mean effect. Random coefficient variance models better approximate the true variance structure of the population and provide more efficient estimates of effects and their variances than ordinary least squares models.

Receiver operating characteristic (ROC) represents the overall discrimination across a complete range of risks. It is a plot of sensitivity versus 1-specificity, where a value of 0.5 is discrimination no better than chance and a value of 1.0 represents perfect discrimination. (McNeil, B. J., Hanley, J. A. (1984). Statistical approaches to the analysis of receiver operating characteristic (ROC) curves. *Med. Decis. Making,* **4,** 137–150).

Regression analysis (R^2) Regression is a statistical analysis that examines the dependence of the *dependent* variable on one or more *explanatory* variables, with the aim of estimating and/or predicting the mean or average of the dependent variable in relation to the values of the explanatory variables. The R^2 symbol, the coefficient of determination, is used in the regression analysis of multiple variables to provide a summary of how well the sample regression line fits the data under consideration. It measures the percentage of variation in dependent variable as explained by the regression analysis.

Reproducibility A reproducible measure is one that yields the same results, no matter how many times the test is repeated.

Riyadh Intensive Care Program is a computerized analysis of APACHE II scores corrected for the presence and duration of major organ failure and can be used to predict death among a population of intensive care patients. Patients are grouped as 'predicted to die' or 'outcome unknown'. It was developed in Riyadh with apparently a high degree of accuracy for identifying non-survivors. However, it appears to be less accurate when applied to other population groups with some false positive predictions (patients predicted to die but who do not). For greater detail see Chang, R. W. S., Lee, B., Jacobs, S., Lee, B. (1989). Accuracy of decisions to withdraw therapy in critically ill patients: clinical judgement versus a computer model. *Crit. Care Med.,* **17,** 1091–1097).

Sequential Organ Failure Score (SOFA) aims to quantify daily organ system dysfunction/failure, using measurement of 14 physiological variables. Three of the variables measure respiratory function, six cardiovascular, two renal, one liver, one neurological, and one haematological functions. SOFA is also called *'Sepsis-related Organ Failure Assessment'*. (Vincent, J. L., Mendonca, A., Cantraine, F. *et al.* (1998). Use of the SOFA score to assess the incidence of organ dysfunction/failure in intensive care units: results of a multicenter, prospective study. *Crit. Care Med.,* **26,** 1793–1800).

Simplified Acute Physiology Score (SAPS-II) SAPS-II is a scoring system that stratifies severity of illness (physiological derangement) within the first 24 h after admission in the ICU. The score is based on weights attributed to 16 physiological variables, together with the Glasgow Coma Score. The comparison of the severity of illness of groups of patients is therefore possible in one ICU, or between ICUs. Moreover, the use of coefficients attributed to the variables (by means of logistic regression analysis in large samples of patients, having mortality as the dependent variable) allows for the prediction of mortality (at hospital discharge) in relation to severity of illness. Because of the large confidence intervals at patient level, the reliability of the prediction depends on a minimum number of 200 patients (Le Gall, J. R., Lemeshow, S., Saulnier, F. (1993). A new Simplified Acute Physiology Score (SAPS II) based on a European/North American multicenter study. *JAMA*, **270**, 2957–2963).

Spearman rank correlation (r$_s$) is a statistical test that quantifies the degree of association between two variables that have been measured on a nominal or ordinal scale. The r$_s$ symbol represents the correlation coefficient, i.e. the level of association between the variables at the same level of significance.

Standardized mortality ratio (SMR) is the ratio of the frequency of observed deaths to expected frequency of deaths. In most epidemiological studies the expected death rate is calculated from age-specific national death rates, but in intensive care outcome studies the expected deaths are often calculated with a scoring system.

Systemic Inflammatory Response Syndrome (SIRS) represents a non-infectious 'septic condition' associated with endothelium damage; SIRS is frequently associated with infection. The early diagnosis of the infection determining the systemic inflammatory response is important. Often, however, no infectious vector is isolated in the blood. Several definitions of septic syndrome tried to accommodate the systemic response to infection, in the absence of its evidence in the laboratory. The SIRS concept hypothesizes that the mediators of the systemic response can be released by triggers other than infection (e.g. shock, trauma).

Terence Higgins Trust is a leading HIV/AIDS charity offering support and advice to sufferers and their families. More information is available at: www.tht.org.uk/advice.htm.

Therapeutic Intervention Scoring System (TISS) is an activity scoring system assessing severity of illness according to the number of interventions required to support the critically ill patient. The original version contained over 70 interventions which were scored from 1 (e.g. hourly vital signs) to 4 (e.g. pulmonary artery catheterization) depending upon the complexity and invasiveness of the procedure. Recent modifications have reduced the number of scored interventions to less than 30. Although widely used for a number of different purposes, the score is very dependent upon the practices of physicians and the protocols used in individual institutions. Further details of the score can be found in Cullen, D. J., Keene, R., Waternaux, C., Peterson, H. (1984). Objective, quantitative measurement of severity of illness in critically ill patients. *Crit. Care Med.*, **12**, 155–160, and Cullen, D. J., Nemeskal, A. R.,

Zaslavsky, A. M. (1994). Intermediate TISS: a new Therapeutic Intervention Scoring System for non-ICU patients. *Crit. Care Med.*, **22**, 1406–1411.

Top-down method of costing involves apportioning of the total annual cost to the critical care unit by the number of admissions, number of patient-days or number of beds to produce an average cost per patient, an average cost per patient-day or an average cost per bed.

Total lung capacity is the volume of gas in the lungs after maximal inspiration and has a normal value of about 6 litres in adults. It can be measured by helium dilution or whole body plethysmography.

Transportability A transportable measure is one that yields the same results when repeated in a different population, regardless of geographic or time boundaries.

Trauma and Injury Severity Score is a measure of severity of disease applied to trauma patients. It combines the trauma score, the Injury Severity Score, the patient's age and the injury type to predict outcome (Champion, H. R., Sacco, W. J., Hunt, T. K. (1983). Trauma severity scoring to predict mortality. *World J. Surg.*, **7**, 4–11).

Utilitarianism Classically the test of an action's moral value is the extent to which it promotes good or bad consequences. More modern utilitarian thinking acknowledges the importance of moral goals so that the happiness of the majority does not overshadow the rights of the few.

Utility is a concept applied in healthcare as a measure of the preference for, or desirability of, a certain level of health status or health outcome. Utility is measured as an absolute quantity and it can describe how much outcome X is preferred to outcome Y.

Validation set is the population in whom the variable (scoring system in this case) is tested to ensure that it does indeed measure what it claims to measure.

Voluntary Euthanasia Society was established in 1935 as the world's first voluntary euthanasia society. Its stated aims are to campaign for adults to have the right to receive medical help to die if suffering unbearably from an incurable disease. The Society campaigns to increase public awareness and debate of these issues. They publish a living will form on their website at: www.ves.org.uk/DpFS_LivW.html.

Whole-time equivalents is a term used to describe total employment activity. The staffing provided in any workplace is dependent upon the level of work, and the hours completed by those employed. For example, if there are five full-time nurses working in a critical care unit, this is the equal to five whole time equivalents. However, it is possible to achieve these five whole-time equivalents in different ways, for example, with ten part-time nurses, or, with three full-time nurses and four part-time nurses.

Wilcoxon rank sum test is a statistical test used to determine whether or not two independent groups have been drawn from the same population. It is a useful test because it has few assumptions, especially with regard to data that are not normally distributed. The test is sometimes also called Mann-Whitney U test. Further details can be found in Myles, P. S., Gin, T. (2000). *Statistical Methods for Anaesthesia and Intensive Care*. Butterworth-Heinnemann.

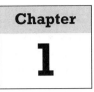
Critical care – modality, metamorphosis and measurement

Saxon Ridley

History and development

Intensive care medicine originated in response to an epidemic of poliomyelitis in Copenhagen 50 years ago. From these humble beginnings, intensive care developed into a specialty at the forefront of organ support and other advances in medicine and surgery. However, this makes critical care a relatively modern specialty; for example intensive care medicine did not gain specialty status in the UK until June 1999. Unfortunately, the development of intensive care in most countries has not been coordinated by a long-term national or even regional strategic plan. Nearly every aspect of intensive care developed as a reactive response to local clinical pressures rather than as a logical expansion or extension of a service following estimates of future need or changing workload. For example, this lack has ranged from planning a hospital's requirement for critical care beds to training programmes for physicians wishing to undertake a career in intensive care medicine. Furthermore, intensive care development has been influenced by the prevailing national medical systems that determine policies, medical training, legal and financial arrangements. This has resulted in different national structures and processes to look after the most seriously ill patients. Consequently, outcomes may vary between countries for reasons which are not solely patient related.

The concept of progressive patient care describes a system in which patients are grouped together depending upon their need for care as determined by their degree of illness, rather than by traditional factors, such as medical or surgical specialty (Becker *et al.*, 1989). This completely reasonable but pragmatic approach to modern healthcare grouped all patients of similar severity of sickness in one location and led to the development of critical care units. The sickest patients were those who required mechanical ventilation and once they had been congregated in one area, physicians looking after them sought to understand the nature of critical illness. This drive to understand critical illness through science and research has led to better appreciation of the pathophysiological processes involved in multiple organ dysfunction. As a result, intensive care medicine evolved from the application of individual treatment modalities, such as respiratory support, into an entire process involving input from a wide variety of healthcare professionals. Critical care is truly a multidisciplinary specialty and it is therefore very important that outcome data are useful to all personnel looking after seriously ill patients.

Medical and surgical advances have been supported by developments in technology and equipment; this has provided critical care staff with the means to treat patients more effectively. While practitioners of intensive care can be duly proud of their achievements, the relatively disorganized, yet pragmatic, development of critical care, together with concurrent improvements in equipment, has meant that single outcome measures may no longer be appropriate. The pressure to treat and save the sickest patients has emphasized the importance of short-term outcome measures, such as intensive care unit (ICU) or hospital mortality. This is reinforced by the end points produced by the commonly used severity of illness measuring systems. Longer-term sequelae of critical illness, such as alterations in quality of life and functional outcome, have been previously ignored, perhaps because of their perceived distance from organ supporting activities on ICU. However, it is now appreciated that what is inflicted on patients on the ICU may indeed directly and seriously affect their long-term outcome. This, together with the realization that critical care is a process of care rather than a single entity, means that many more types of outcome are now pertinent and valid. Practitioners of critical care need to learn how to interpret and apply these new outcome measures.

Current status of critical care

Marked national differences in healthcare systems, health policies, financial arrangements and cost recovery and differing roles assumed by ICU professionals produce contrasting perspectives and emphases worldwide. As a result, it is unlikely that outcome figures will be similar between countries. Unfortunately, reliable, unbiased and, most importantly, comparable data concerning critical care outcomes in different countries are lacking. From the available data, it is clear that there are marked national differences between critical care services; however, because of the problems relating to definitions and different elements of critical care organization, direct and unqualified comparison of outcome figures between countries may be unwise.

Critical care in the UK

While several surveys of critical care facilities available in the UK have been undertaken, the most recent and extensive was performed by the Audit

Commission (1999). This survey was undertaken between May and August 1998 in all acute hospital trusts in England and Wales. The Audit Commission asked about the number of critical care units within a trust; and in more detail about the provision of general adult critical care beds. Their results represent the most up-to-date and comprehensive review available for the UK.

There were 228 ICUs, 221 combined ICUs with high-dependency units (HDUs) and 263 HDUs in England and Wales in 1998. However, a large number of these critical care services were either single specialty, such as medical or surgical, or served specific groups of patients such as children, those with burns or requiring neurosurgery or cardiac surgery. If these specialist units are excluded, then there were only 128 ICUs, 83 combined ICU/HDUs and 25 HDUs serving adult general patients. The total complement of adult general critical care beds was just over 1400. As result of a government review, £142.4 million were made available for enhancement of critical care services in 2000, and by January 2001 there was a total 1677 ICU beds (79% of which were for adult general use) and 1208 HDU beds (73% for adult general use) (NHS Executive, 2001).

In 1998, the median size of an ICU was 5.3 beds, combined ICU/HDUs had 6 beds and HDUs 4 beds. However, 56% of ICUs, 55% of combined ICU/HDUs and 15% of HDUs reported that additional beds could be opened at short notice by bringing in additional staff. Indirect evidence suggests that there is still a shortfall of critical care beds; an association between discharge at night and higher hospital mortality suggests that there is still pressure on beds as patients are returned to the general ward before they are completely stable (Goldfrad and Rowan, 2000). In an English ICU, just under 30% of patients were discharged with a Therapeutic Intervention Scoring System (TISS) score greater than 20, implying a need for continuing high levels of medical and nursing support (Smith *et al.*, 1999). These patients subsequently had a higher hospital mortality rate than those patients who were more stable when discharged from ICU (21% versus 3.7%).

There was designated senior physician cover in 100% of ICUs, 96% of ICU/HDUs and 21% of HDUs. The median number of daytime weekday consultant sessions (i.e. half-day) was 10 on ICUs, 8 on ICU/HDUs but 0 on HDUs. These critical care units were directed or led by a consultant with designated daytime clinical sessions in 96% ICUs, 80% combined ICU/HDUs and 18% HDUs. These results suggest that management of patients who are moderately ill but potentially unstable (i.e. HDU patients) is not undertaken by senior staff with responsibility for other critically ill patients on the ICU. This implies that while the most severely ill are looked after by appropriately trained senior doctors, less ill patients remain under the care of medical staff whose main interest is not critical illness. However, most adult general units appear to have written guidelines concerning admission (89% ICUs, 82% ICU/HDUs and 94% HDUs) and discharge (80% ICUs, 76% ICU/HDUs and 74% HDUs).

The senior medical staff were supported by dedicated trainee staff in 53% of ICUs, 35% of combined ICU/HDUs and 6% of HDUs. In the UK, the future development of the new specialty depends upon demonstrable competence and capabilities by those practitioners involved in care of patients. This will form the basis of formal training in intensive care medicine which is the responsibility of the Intercollegiate Board for Training in Intensive Care Medicine. The examination set by the Intercollegiate Board, the Diploma of Intensive Care Medicine, is a measure of knowledge-based competency which complements the competency-based training programme and workplace training assessments developed by the Board.

Because of the nature of their illness, critically ill patients and their relatives require considerable nursing input. In the UK, it is generally accepted that critically ill patients require 1:1 nursing care, while for those receiving high-dependency care a lower ratio may be appropriate. The exact nursing establishment for high-dependency care patients will be influenced by the patients' needs and the nursing skill-mix. However, in a large district general hospital supporting all services except hepatology, transplantation, cardiac and neurosurgery, the required nurse to patient ratio on HDU was found to be 2:3 (Garfield et al., 2000). Nursing staff represent the largest component of costs. The median total nursing budgets were £705311 for ICUs, £607056 for combined ICU/HDUs and £251182 for HDUs. However, within these budgets, there appears to be a wide range of nursing skill-mix and expertise that may not necessarily be explained by differences in patient demography.

Critical care in Europe

Geographical differences in the use of, and mortality following, critical care in Europe have been recently described by Thijs (2000) and interested readers should refer to his article. Although it is difficult to give precise figures, results from the EURICUS–1 study suggests there are about 3000 to 4000 ICUs in Western Europe (Reis Miranda et al., 1998). There would appear to be no estimates of the numbers of HDUs in Europe. Three large European studies have been completed (EPIC (Vincent et al., 1995), EURICUS–1 and SAPS II (Le Gall et al., 1993)) and these suggest that ICU mortality is highest in the southern European countries and the UK where ICU mortality generally exceeds 20% (Figure 1.1).

Northern and central European countries have much lower mortalities (i.e. less than 15%). Such differences are difficult to explain; there are recognized differing national death rates but such differences could also be a consequence of inadequate ICU resources. Although there is regional variation within the UK, critical care provision is approximately 3–5 ICU beds per 100000 population. However, by European standards, such provision seems sparse because Germany provides 25, Switzerland 11, the Netherlands 10 and Italy between 4 and 9 per 100000 population (Figure 1.2).

The size of European ICUs varies considerably; 25% of ICUs have more than 10 beds, 57% have between 6 and 10 beds and 18% have less than 6 (Vincent et al., 1997). The UK has a greater proportion of small ICUs with the median size in 1998 being only six. Because of the greater availability of ICU beds in mainland Europe, HDUs may be less common in Europe than the UK. Indeed,

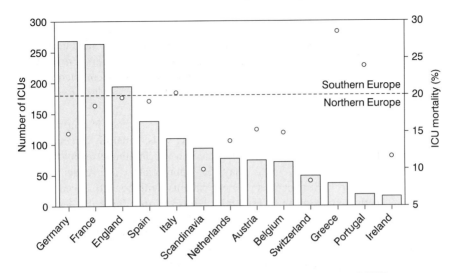

Figure 1.1 The distribution of number of ICUs (solid bars) and ICU mortality (dots) in various European countries with a horizontal line separating the southern European and UK ICUs from northern European ICUs (modified from Thijs, L. G. (2000). Geographical differences in outcome. In *Evaluating Critical Care. Using health services research to improve quality.* (W. J. Sibbald, J. F. Bion, eds) pp 292–308, Springer-Verlag).

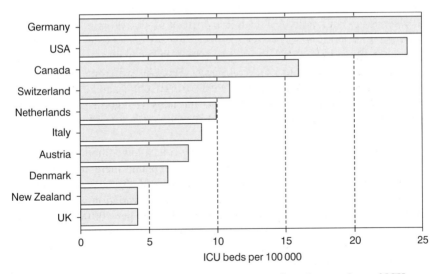

Figure 1.2 The availability of ICU beds expressed as the number of ICU beds per 100 000 general population in North America, New Zealand and Europe (modified from Thijs, L. G. (2000). Geographical differences in outcome. In *Evaluating Critical Care. Using health services research to improve quality.* (W. J. Sibbald, J. F. Bion, eds) pp 292–308, Springer-Verlag).

leading European experts have questioned the value of high-dependency care in the European setting (Vincent and Burchardi, 1999). However, this conclusion may have been influenced by differences in resources and outcomes between countries.

A similar European north-south division exists with respect to distribution of ICU capacity and length of stay (see Chapter 10, Tables 10.1 and 10.2). Other aspects, such as organizational issues, may also be partly responsible. For example, whether the ICU is staffed and patients managed by ICU trained specialists (i.e. the ICU is regarded as 'closed') will influence important outcome measures such as length of stay, mortality and resource use (Carson *et al.*, 1996). With improved training programmes and increasingly widespread recognition of critical care as a specialty, more critical care units are likely to become closed. For example, in a European survey of 200 ICUs almost 90% reported that the ICU staff had responsibility for patient care (Vincent *et al.*, 1997). It has been recognized for some time that coordination and effective communication between critical care professions influences outcome (Knaus *et al.*, 1986). Although all countries would hope to achieve this, it may not have always been developed to the same level.

Meaningful comparisons between European countries are hampered by the lack of directly comparable data. In the UK, independently validated and robust data are collected by critical care units that subscribe to the Intensive Care National Audit and Research Centre's (ICNARC's) case-mix programme. Such a programme greatly facilitates comparative audit between ICUs. European initiatives such as the Patient-centred Acute Care Training (PACT) system have fostered multinational joint enterprises. However, for meaningful national comparisons, robust data, such as that collected by ICNARC, will have to be gathered on a European-wide basis. Until this occurs, explanations concerning differences in outcome will remain largely hypothetical.

Critical care in the USA

Intensive care units in the USA account for only 5–10% of inpatient beds, yet they consume approximately 30% of all inpatient resources, a figure which exceeds 1% of the gross national product (Chalfin *et al.*, 1995). This greater expenditure improves the availability of critical care beds in the USA; the number of beds per 100 000 population in the USA is similar to that of Germany, the European country with the most abundant supply of critical care resources (see Figure 1.2). Consequently a wider spectrum of patients with varying severity of illnesses are admitted to American ICUs. In the UK where intensive care resources are scarce, only the most severely ill patients are admitted to ICU. The distributions of severity of illness as measured by the APACHE III system in large American and English patient cohorts show a marked shift in the distribution of the English patients towards the right. This indicates greater severity of illness in England (Figure 1.3) (Zimmerman *et al.*, 1998; Pappachan *et al.*, 1999).

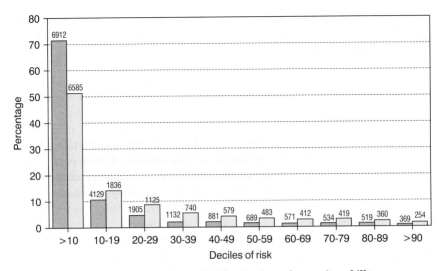

Figure 1.3 A histogram showing the distribution of severity of illness as measured by the APACHE III score in American (dark grey) and English cohorts (light grey). The numbers of patients in each decile of risk is shown on the top of the bars (modified from Zimmerman, J. E., Wagner, D. P., Draper, E. A., Wright, L., Alzola, C., Knaus, W. A. (1998). Evaluation of Acute Physiology And Chronic Health Evaluation III predictions of hospital mortality in an independent database. *Crit. Care Med.*, **26**, 1317–1326 and Pappachan, J.V., Millar, B., Bennett, D., Smith, G.B. (1999). Comparison of outcome from intensive care admission after adjustment for case mix by the APACHE III prognostic system. *Chest*, **115**, 802–810).

In the USA, ICUs may cover the entire spectrum of critical care including both intensive and high-dependency care. Direct comparison between the demographic features of these large databases also reveals significant differences between the continents. Compared to patients in the USA, patients admitted to 17 ICUs in the South of England are more likely to be male, be older than 45 years, have a greater incidence of APACHE III co-morbidities and be more frequently transferred to the ICU from hospital wards or other outlying hospitals. More American patients were admitted directly from the emergency room or another ICU in the hospital. The hospital mortality in England reflected the higher APACHE III scores, being 25.9% versus 17.0% in America.

Critical care facilities in the USA admit a large percentage of 'low risk, monitor only patients'. In an evaluation of a large cohort of 37 688 patients admitted to 285 ICUs in 161 hospitals in the USA, 26 912 patients (71%) had an APACHE III generated risk of hospital death of less than 10% (Zimmerman *et al.*, 1998). Although not directly comparable in terms of risk of hospital death, over 15% of patients in France, Italy, Spain, Portugal, Greece and the UK had APACHE II scores in excess of 20 (Vincent *et al.*, 1995). In Zimmerman's study, most patients (71.5%) were non-operative while almost 80% of postoperative patients (28.5% of all patients) were admitted electively; 39% of patients came from the Accident and Emergency Department. By comparison in Europe, 21% of patients were unscheduled surgical patients and 32% elective surgical admissions (total 53% postoperative patients); the remaining 47% were medical (Le Gall *et al.*, 1993).

These differences in demographic features illustrate the problems of outcome comparison across continents. Accepting that there may be differences in the definitions and methods used to collect the data, the difference in case-mix and patient demography means that crude outcome figures, such as hospital mortality, may not be directly comparable. This is extremely important. While the outcomes (e.g. mortality) chosen to measure any aspect of critical care are likely to be the same worldwide, unless both the characteristics of the patients and the capabilities and capacity of critical care services are carefully controlled, the actual figures may not be comparable. Any reported critical care outcome needs to be interpreted in conjunction with the healthcare system from which the data originated.

Metamorphosis of critical care

The specialty of critical care continues to develop new roles and concepts. One of the most fundamental changes in the UK is the appreciation that critical care is a continuum of illness and that it may be inappropriate to segregate patients according to whether they are located on an ICU, HDU or general ward. It is now recognized that, in the UK, there are moderately ill and potentially unstable patients on the general hospital wards. As these patients may be developing or recovering from critical illness, they may benefit from input from the critical care services while on the general ward.

Unfortunately, the consequences of neglecting sick patients are well recognized. For example, over half the patients admitted to the ICU at Portsmouth, UK, were deemed by two independent assessors to have received suboptimal care on the general wards prior to their admission (McQuillan *et al.*, 1998). The assessors categorized the deficiencies in care as a failure of organization, lack of knowledge, failure to appreciate clinical urgency, lack of supervision and failure to seek advice. Acute physiological disturbance of the cardiorespiratory system, culminating in cardiac arrest, is a frequent prodromal event prior to referral to the intensive care unit. Data from ICNARC shows that just less than 10% of patients presenting to ICUs in England and Wales are admitted following cardiopulmonary resuscitation. There are premonitory signs and symptoms, usually relating to the respiratory or central nervous systems, prior to cardiac arrest (Franklin and Mathew, 1994) and it would seem more appropriate to prevent rather than treat these events.

While there are a number of possible solutions for dealing with this problem, the formation of medical emergency teams has been proposed. These were originally described in Australia (Lee *et al.*, 1995), but more recently, the beneficial effects of such teams have been described in UK practice (Goldhill *et al.*, 1999). The concept of a multidisciplinary team from the critical care services offering advice on management, practical help with procedures, training and education to the staff of the general ward was one of the key recommendations made by the UK Government's most recent review of critical care services (Department of Health, 2000). Because of their expertise in managing critical illness, both nursing and medical professionals in critical care should be able to contribute to the care of all moderately unwell patients throughout the hospital. This concept is the driving force behind the introduction of outreach critical care services and these services are being actively developed. The critical care outreach service is designed to export the expertise of the critical care unit to other areas of the hospital. It is a multidisciplinary approach to identifying patients at risk of developing critical illness so that early intervention or transfer (if appropriate) can be organized. Outreach teams may also follow-up those patients recovering from a period of critical illness. Outreach is intended as a collaboration and partnership between the critical care service and other departments to ensure a continuum of care for patients regardless of location, and should enhance the skills and understanding of all staff in the delivery of critical care (Intensive Care Society, in press). Unfortunately, the outcome and effectiveness of outreach services as organized in the UK is, as yet, unproved and there are no recommendations on how their impact is to be measured.

To complement the care given to patients during their period of acute illness, follow-up support may improve the longer-term outcome from critical illness. Follow-up clinics have tended to concentrate on those patients who were treated on ICU for more than 4 or 5 days and offer rehabilitation to the survivors. While follow-up clinics have only recently been established and are few in number, their results do provide an insight into the problems experienced by patients. During critical illness it is possible to lose 2% of the body's muscle mass per day (Helliwell *et al.*, 1998). Not only does this lead to severe weakness and fatigue but also poor muscle coordination and difficulty swallowing and coughing. Anxiety and depression are common and this may strain relationships with partners and limit social interaction. More severe psychological upset may present as nightmares and delusions. These may be consequences of the initial trauma or the results of the psychological disturbances that developed in ICU. The patient's lack of memory, compounded by a lack of understanding or explanation may aggravate these disturbances. Such non-mortality consequences of critical illness will certainly impinge on other outcomes, such as quality of life.

Future developments in critical care services, such as outreach and follow-up clinics, will expand the variety of outcomes available for measurement. Single outcome measures may be of limited value because each individually fails to capture the entirety of the process of care. As critical care changes from a single therapeutic modality to a complex series of interrelated treatment pathways, clinical outcomes will become more complex and multifaceted and consequently more difficult to define rigorously. Such complexity makes it more difficult to apply them in a uniform and standard manner and allows scope for error in both choice and application.

Outcomes in focus

Critical care outcomes have two important facets. The first is the requirement to measure a suitable outcome and the second is to compare this outcome with an appropriate alternative. Outcomes from critical care can be viewed from at least three perspectives, those of patients, staff and health managers. The patient's perspective, as the consumer and end user of the healthcare system, is of prime importance. Their interest revolves around survival, quality of life and functional ability once they have recovered from critical illness. However, these attributes are the result of the whole hospital episode and intensive care management is only a small part of this process. Quality of life and functional outcome, like long-term survival, is dependent upon the effectiveness of the whole healthcare system including support received in the convalescent period while in the community. Without carefully controlling the effects of support after intensive care, it may be unwise to ascribe changes in long-term outcome measures to ICU management.

Controlling all effects in the post-discharge period will prove difficult. For example, although survival following critical illness is usually measured at hospital discharge, the post-ICU but in-hospital mortality rates can be extremely high. Figures from the UK and elsewhere in Europe suggest that 23–31% of patients may die in hospital but after ICU discharge (Moreno and Agthe, 1999). Once the patients are discharged from ICU, the ICU staff rarely have direct influence over the clinical management during the rest of the hospital stay. Furthermore, we do not know enough about the interaction of the primary pathology and the undesirable complications of intensive care management. For example, victims of serious road traffic accidents may develop post-traumatic stress disorder but ICU management itself can lead to psychosis, anxiety and depression. How much of the patient's psychological change is due to their presenting injury or illness rather than the effects of their management is simply unknown. Whatever the relationship, psychological consequences of the accident or treatment are likely to have serious and adverse effects on the patient's quality of life.

Staff have a duty of care to their patients and to society to ensure that healthcare resources are used appropriately. Staff should ensure that adverse events are minimized. Unfortunately, the incidence of adverse events tends to be higher than anticipated by ICU staff. For example, in a medical ICU in a university hospital 132 (6.6% of 2009) drug administration errors were observed (Tissot *et al.*, 1999). The errors included 41 dose errors, 29 incorrect infusion rates, 24 wrong preparations, 19 physicochemical incompatibilities, 10 incorrect administration techniques, and 9 wrong administration times. Most of the errors were felt to be due to deficiencies in the overall organization of the medication track, patient follow-up and staff training; all of these should be correctable but continuous observation, data collection and audit are necessary for such a quality assurance exercise.

Health managers and politicians focus on outcome measures such as economic analyses and the global performance of the service. Understandably they are not truly interested in outcomes for individual patients. In the UK, modernizing the

Jo Coleman

Information Update Service

Butterworth-Heinemann

FREEPOST SCE 5435

Oxford

Oxon

OX2 8BR

UK

Keep up-to-date with the latest books in your field.

Visit our website and register now for our FREE e-mail update service, or join our mailing list and enter our monthly prize draw to win £100 worth of books. Just complete the form below and return it to us now! (FREEPOST if you are based in the UK)

www.bh.com

Please Complete In Block Capitals

Title of book you have purchased:...

....

Subject area of interest:..

Name:...

Job title:...

Business sector (if relevant):...

Street:...

Town:... County:...

Country:.. Postcode:..

Email:...

Telephone:..

How would you prefer to be contacted: Post ☐   e-mail ☐   Both ☐

Signature:... Date:...

☐ Please arrange for me to be kept informed of other books and information services on this and related subjects (✔ box if not required). This information is being collected on behalf of Reed Elsevier plc group and may be used to supply information about products by companies within the group.

FOR OFFICE USE ONLY

Butterworth-Heinemann,
a division of Reed Educational
& Professional Publishing Limited.
Registered office: 25 Victoria Street,
London SW1H 0EX.
Registered in England 3099304.
VAT number GB: 663 3472 30.

BUTTERWORTH
HEINEMANN

A member of the Reed Elsevier plc group

delivery of critical care is one of the Department of Health's primary objectives. Data concerning activity (augmented care period dataset (NHS Executive, 1996), performance (ICNARC's case-mix program or its equivalent) and costs (cost block dataset (Edbrooke *et al.*, 1999)) should be collected. However, these types of data will provide information about how the system of critical care works rather than measures of the effectiveness of the processes of intensive care, such as organ support.

Thus, when discussing outcome from critical care, the outcome measure chosen depends upon the perspective of the questioner. It is vitally important to be aware of the appropriate use of the outcome measure chosen. For example, outcomes used for research purposes may be different from those used for assessment. Measurements of effectiveness and efficiency may assess performance, while more clinically orientated outcomes will be of interest for research. The outcome measure or tool should be appropriate for its proposed application.

Overcoming the problems

The problems concerning outcomes in critical care can only be resolved using rigorous scientific techniques. Using weak or unscientific methods merely confuses issues and at worst provides false leads and direction. Scientific evaluation involves defining a problem, choosing an intervention (i.e. a clinical, organizational, or managerial change which is thought to influence outcome), choosing an appropriate outcome measure and as far as is possible controlling the confounding influences. It is important to emphasize that under certain circumstances looking at critical care as a single process may be inappropriate. If the aim is to examine the effect of a single therapeutic intervention, such as the effects of steroids (Annane, 2000) or activated Protein C in sepsis (Bernard *et al.*, 2001), then randomized controlled trials are indeed appropriate. However, if the processes or global measures of outcome following critical care are being investigated, single end point randomized controlled trials may not be appropriate. Furthermore, critical care is a series of interdependent therapeutic processes, and looking at each individually may not necessarily give the same result as looking at the whole process.

Experimental design and outcomes

There are several different schemes for classifying study designs but most studies can be divided into observational or interventional (experimental) studies. In observational studies, one or more groups of patients are observed and characteristics about the patients recorded for analysis. Experimental studies involve an intervention or investigated controlled manoeuvre, such as a drug, a procedure or treatment, and focus on the effect of the intervention on the study subjects. Both observational and experimental studies have been used in critical care; however at the moment, observational studies are most frequently used to assess outcomes following critical care.

There are four main types of observational study (Figure 1.4):

1. Case-series – case-series studies describe certain characteristics of a group of patients. The simplest design is one in which the author describes an interesting observation or finding in a small number of patients. Case-series reports generally involve patients over a short period of time and are hypothesis generating for subsequent larger studies. They are important because of their descriptive role in the preparation or precursor for other studies.
2. Case-control – case-control studies start with the presence or absence of an outcome and retrospectively try to detect possible causes or risk factors that may have been suggested in case-series reports or previous studies. Cases in the case-control study are individuals selected on the basis of some disease or outcome while the controls are those patients without the disease or outcome. The history of previous events in both groups of patients is analysed in an attempt to identify a characteristic or risk factor influencing the patients of interest but not the control patients. It is important to emphasize that case-control studies are essentially retrospective.
3. Cohort – the patients in cohort studies are selected by some defining characteristic or characteristics suspected of being a precursor to or risk factor for a disease or outcome. Cohort studies are essentially prospective. Investigators select the subjects at the onset of the study (e.g. ICU admission) and then determine whether the patients have the risk factor (e.g. high APACHE scores) or have been exposed to a risk (e.g. high airway pressures during mechanical ventilation) which might adversely affect their outcome. The patients are followed over a given period of time in order to observe whether these defining characteristics are indeed important in determining outcome. Cohort studies are frequently used for examining non-mortality

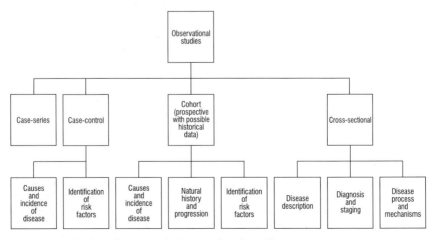

Figure 1.4 A classification of observational studies.

outcomes, such as quality of life or functional outcome following critical care. Historical cohort studies use information collected in the past and saved on records or files. Such studies are still prospective because, although the data on risk factors have already been collected, the study looks forward in time to determine their effect on outcome. The term historical arises because historical information is used (i.e. risk factors were actually evaluated before the onset of the study).

4. Cross-sectional – cross-sectional studies examine data collected on a group of patients during a short period of time rather than over longer periods. Cross-sectional studies are most often used in medicine to describe a disease or to provide information regarding diagnosis or staging of a disease. For example, studies describing the spectrum of acute lung injury or prevalence of certain diseases or pathologies on ICU are cross-sectional studies.

Experimental trials fall into two categories, those with controls and those without (Figure 1.5).

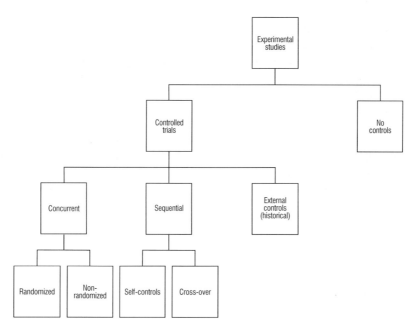

Figure 1.5 A classification of interventional studies.

Controlled trials are studies in which an experimental drug or procedure is compared with another drug or procedure, usually a placebo or the best presently available accepted treatment. Uncontrolled trials are studies in which the investigators' experience with an experimental drug or procedure is described but its treatment effect is not compared to another treatment or outcome. Controlled studies are viewed as having a far greater validity in medicine.

The most robust way to ensure that the subjects and the control patients are similar is to plan interventions for both groups over the same time and in an identical manner. In this way the study achieves concurrent control as opposed to historical control. In order to reduce the chances that the patients or the investigators find what they expect, double-blind trials are designed in which neither the subjects nor investigators know if a subject is in the treatment or control group. Randomized controlled trials provide the strongest evidence for causation and effectiveness; they can be used in intensive care to compare drugs, equipment or treatment modalities. For ethical reasons, randomized controlled trials designed to demonstrate the effectiveness of intensive care management by comparing it to an alternative form of treatment elsewhere in the hospital are probably unworkable.

Providing control in an experimental study can be achieved by using the same group of patients in both experimental and control situations. A cross-over design study uses two groups of patients. One group is assigned to the experimental treatment and the second group is assigned to the placebo or control treatment. After an experimental period, the drug or procedure and placebo are withdrawn from both groups for a 'washout period'. The groups are then given the alternative treatment (i.e. the first group now receives the placebo and the second group the experimental treatment). Unfortunately, because of the rapidly changing physiological state of critically ill patients, cross-over studies are difficult to complete because of a period effect. This describes the situation where some characteristic of the patients has changed during the whole study period so making the two cross-over periods incomparable.

Defining the problem or aim of study

Explicitly defining the problem involves two important tasks; establishing the perspective of the questioner and carefully defining the problem to generate useful results that are of value to the questioner. For example, the outcome measure chosen to answer the simple question 'How effective is your ICU?' will vary. The patient and their relatives may be interested in the risk of mortality. Using severity of illness generated risk of hospital death and the physician's previous experience, a prognosis for that individual patient can be estimated in broad terms. If the same question was directed at the physician in charge of ICU, the response might include a scatter diagram or league table of standardized mortality ratios. In terms of effectiveness, the healthcare provider or decision-maker may be more interested in the cost per ICU survivor in order to compare critical care to other healthcare programmes and so distribute health care resources.

The question also needs to be redefined so that its scope is appreciated prior to the start of the investigation. Once again, the outcome measure chosen to answer the simple question of 'How effective is your ICU?' will vary depending upon the time frame of the study. Is the long-term effectiveness of critical care of interest? If so then the overall effectiveness of critical care will be influenced by the contribution made to the patients' care by the rest of the hospital after ICU discharge. If the short-term effectiveness is under investigation, then as intensive care usually involves stabilizing the most dysfunctional organ system, physicians in critical care may claim that their organ supporting treatments are effective. Most general supportive therapies aim to reverse physiological abnormalities, so buying time for the specific therapy to work. This has been satisfactorily demonstrated with preoperative optimization of high-risk surgical patients. There is now sufficient evidence to suggest that such patients should only be operated on when they have benefited from a period of resuscitation in the critical care unit (Treasure and Bennett, 1999; Wilson *et al.*, 1999). In the short-term, effectiveness can be shown using sequential physiological scoring as it is possible to prevent further deterioration of physiological status of 80% of all critically ill patients over the first 3 days of intensive care admission (Hutchinson *et al.*, 2000) (Figure 1.6).

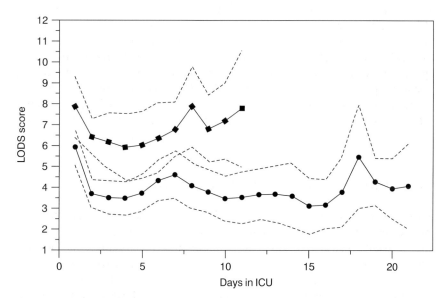

Figure 1.6 The trends in Logistic Organ Dysfunction Score over time for survivors (circles) and non-survivors (squares). The 95% confidence limits of the lines are also shown. Values when less than 10 patients in each group are not shown (modified from Hutchinson, C., Craig, S., Ridley, S. (2000). Sequential organ scoring as a measure of effectiveness of critical care. *Anaesthesia*, **55**, 1149–1154).

This is a short-term outcome measure; it demonstrates the immediate effectiveness of organ support but excludes outcome from the whole process of critical care. However, failure to stabilize a reasonable number of patients may suggest inappropriate or ineffective treatment algorithms or incorrect patient selection.

Choosing an intervention

Interventions in critical care may be broadly classified as clinical, managerial and organizational.

Clinical

Clinical interventions pertain to bedside care of the patient by the multi-disciplinary team. Intensive care management may be divided into general and specific therapies. Specific therapy such as insulin for diabetes, sensitivity guided antibiotic therapy and antidysrhythmics for arrhythmias have all been shown to be effective in randomized controlled trials, albeit outside the ICU. It is the effectiveness of the general supportive measures that remains unclear, primarily because the wide range and combinations of general intensive care management cannot be rigorously controlled so allowing only two alternatives to be properly compared. The treatment pathway chosen for any patient depends upon the sequential interplay of various therapeutic regimens and the patient's response to therapy. If the first pathway proves ineffective, then a second or third is invoked. Restricting the selection of treatment pathways for a randomized controlled trial curtails the options for organ stabilization and so may unbalance the whole treatment regimen. Trying to control the 'chaos' of general intensive care management and standardize it for use in one arm of a randomized controlled trial is likely to be very difficult.

Managerial

Managerial interventions relate to internal administration and running of the critical care unit and there is indirect evidence suggesting that managerial processes in ICUs are important to outcome. In the USA, there appears to be wide variation in ICU mortality and length of admission even when adjusted for patient case-mix. The risk adjusted survival for large diagnostic groups was better at teaching hospitals than other centres and this may have been related to greater physician activity on the ICUs (Zimmerman et al.,1993). However, there is no evidence to support such a distinction in the UK where both teaching hospitals and district general hospitals appear to perform equally well. Changes, such as the introduction of full-time intensive care physicians and the changing from open to closed units resulting in reduced mortality, are examples of positive managerial interventions. However, in all these examples, the end point chosen, mortality, is only partly related to physician activity alone and other factors, such as a change in culture, may also have been important but were simply not captured by the outcome measure chosen.

Organizational

Organizational interventions cover the relationship of the critical care unit to other departments within the hospital and with neighbouring hospitals. Changes in organizational structure of critical care services are usually quantified by observational studies. Such studies tend to reveal associations between outcome and independent variables. It is important to appreciate that such associations may not be causal, especially where there are other possible influences. The recent introduction of high-dependency care has produced indirect evidence of benefit in a number of independent trials. For example, a better match of care required to care provided was achieved after opening a HDU and moving the lower risk, less dependent patients to the new HDU (Fox *et al.*, 1999). While the trauma centre systems works well in the USA, adopting a similar system in the UK where the differences in capabilities of various hospitals is not so great has not produced clear advantages.

Choosing the correct outcome measure

The selected outcome measure must be relevant to the questioner and appropriate to the aspect of critical care under investigation. For example, mortality may be an appropriate outcome measure for the ICU and is clearly highly relevant to the patient; however, mortality may not necessarily be a good outcome measure for high-dependency care. The function of high-dependency care is to observe and monitor moderately and potentially unstable patients, to identify abnormal physiological trends and expeditiously correct these trends before they develop into complications and other morbidities. Thus using mortality as a major outcome measure for high-dependency care may not be correct because HDUs do not provide advanced organ support and mortality rates on such units should be low. Although ICUs and HDUs are part of the critical illness continuum, their functions are different and consequently their outcomes may not necessarily be similar. Complication rates or measures of physiological stability may be more appropriate outcome measures for high-dependency care.

Outcome measures may concentrate on one aspect of outcome; examples of single outcome measures might include mortality, quality of life and functional outcome. However, excellence in one aspect of outcome may be at the expense of another. For example an impressively low standardized mortality ratio might have been achieved by a disproportionately high transfer rate of sick patients to an alternative ICU. A global measure of performance encompassing several measures of outcome would be helpful. Economic costs and length of stay have been offered as a measure of performance but these two aspects still offer a relatively narrow range of outcomes. A possible solution is the radar chart (Moreno, 2000); using standardized definitions and data collection each ICU should be able to plot a variety of outcome measures against recognized performance indicators. Examples might include its occupancy, patient throughput, standardized mortality ratio, percentage of patients stabilized, incidence of adverse events and complications, medical and nursing establishment (Figure 1.7).

The area encompassing the centre of the chart would provide a measure of global ICU performance, accounting for the related factors governing quality, resources and outcome.

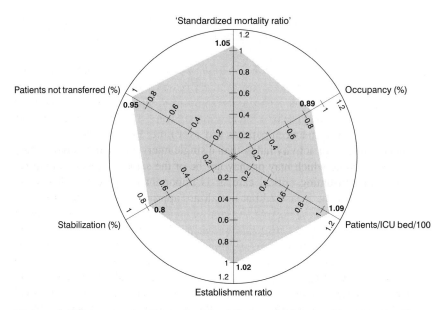

Figure 1.7 An example of a radar chart that could be used to measure the global performance of an ICU. The measures shown need to be transformed so that a larger central shaded area represents better overall performance. Transformations might include representing the standardized mortality ratio (SMR) as '1+(1 − actual SMR)' so that ICUs with low SMRs (i.e. better than average performance) have a larger central area than ICUs with actual SMRs greater than 1. The nursing establishment could be reflected by comparing the actual nurse : bed ratio to a nationally agreed standard for intensive care (e.g. 7.2 whole time equivalents per ICU bed in the UK). The efficiency of the ICU could be captured by the number of patients treated annually per ICU bed (transformed by dividing by 100 to give a figure about one) (Ridley, S. (2001). Critical care outcomes. *Anaesthesia*, **56**, 1–3).

Confounding influences

Confounding influences represent a major hurdle for outcome assessment in critical care. Short-term outcome measures are relevant to the ICU and are usually directly under the critical care staff's control. For example, short-term mortality reflects the ICU and hospital performance, whereas the long-term survival and the consequences of critical illness, such as quality of life, or the psychological problems following critical illness, are dependent upon not just the performance of the ICU but of the whole healthcare system. Clearly the long-term effects of critical illness are of most interest to patients. As the period of follow-up extends, socioecomonic factors also impinge on patients' lives so that it may be impossible to unravel the effects of critical illness from other unrelated factors. A balance between allowing as long as possible for recovery to take place and minimizing the impact of confounding influences is required. Unfortunately, at present there is no evidence to suggest where this balance might lie.

Conclusion

As critical care has developed, its complexity has increased not only in its therapeutic range but also in its reliance on a wide range of hospital personnel. Fortunately for the patient, if they survive, critical illness is only a temporary state and recovery, albeit prolonged, can be anticipated. Therefore outcomes after critical care will vary between patients and over time. Because critical care is a therapeutic process or activity rather than a single intervention, it will have many aspects of outcome which may or may not be of the same interest to all parties delivering or consuming critical care. It is important to appreciate that many outcomes can now be measured but not all are appropriate or relevant to every party. As a result outcome measures may be used inappropriately. An example of inappropriate use may be scatter diagrams or league tables of standardized mortality ratios (SMRs) without a full understanding of how the SMR is generated. It is very important to be aware of the limitations of outcome measures. If applied carelessly or inappropriately, they will hinder, rather than advance our understanding. Practitioners of intensive care have been distracted by doubts concerning their effectiveness. We are fortunate in that we are able to measure numerous aspects of outcome; the subsequent chapters will help us present this information in a way others can understand.

References

Annane, D. (2000). Effects of the combination of hydrocortisone (HC)-fludrocortisone (FC) on mortality in septic shock. *Crit. Care Med.*, **28**, A64.

Audit Commission. (1999). *Critical to Success. The place of efficient and effective critical care services within the acute hospital.* Audit Commission Publications.

Becker, E. L., Lord Butterfield, Harvey, A. M., Heptinstall, R. H., Thomas, L. (1989). *Churchill's Medical Dictionary.* Churchill Livingstone.

Bernard, G. R., Vincent, J. L., Laterre, P-F. *et al.* (2001). Efficacy and safety of recombinant human activated protein C for severe sepsis. *N. Engl. J. Med.*, **344**, 699–709.

Carson, S. S., Stocking, C., Podsadecki, T. *et al.* (1996). Effects of organizational change in the medical intensive care unit of a teaching hospital: a comparison of 'open' and 'closed' formats. *JAMA*, **276**, 322–328.

Chalfin, D. B., Cohen, I. L., Lambrinos, J. (1995). The economics and cost effectiveness of critical care medicine. *Intensive Care Med.*, **21**, 951–961.

Department of Health. (2000). *Comprehensive Critical Care. A review of adult critical care services.* Department of Health.

Edbrooke, D., Hibbert, C., Ridley, S. A., Long, T., Dickie, H. and the National Group on Intensive Care Costing. (1999). A comparative method for costing intensive care. *Anaesthesia*, **54**, 176–180.

Fox, A. J., Owen-Smith, O., Spiers, P. (1999). The immediate impact of opening an adult high dependency unit on intensive care unit occupancy. *Anaesthesia*, **54**, 280–283.

Franklin, C., Mathew, J. (1994) Developing strategies to prevent inhospital cardiac arrest: analyzing responses of physicians and nurses in the hours before the event. *Critical Care Medicine*, **22**, 244–247.

Garfield, M., Jeffrey, R., Ridley, S. (2000). An assessment of the staffing level required for a high-dependency unit. *Anaesthesia*, **55**, 137–143.

Goldfrad, C., Rowan, K. (2000). Consequences of discharges from intensive care at night. *Lancet*, **355**, 1138–1142.

Goldhill, D. R., Worthington, L., Mulcahy, A., Tarling, M., Sumner, A. (1999). The patient-at-risk team: identifying and managing seriously ill ward patients. *Anaesthesia*, **54**, 853–860.

Helliwell, T. R., Wilkinson, A., Griffiths, R. D., McClelland, P., Palmer, T. E. A., Bone, M. J. (1998). Muscle fibre atrophy in patients with multiple organ failure is associated with the loss of myosin filaments and the presence of lysosomal enzymes and ubiquitin. *Neuropathol. Appl. Neurobiol.*, **24**, 507–517.

Hutchinson, C., Craig, S., Ridley, S. (2000). Sequential organ scoring as a measure of effectiveness of critical care. *Anaesthesia*, **55**, 1149–1154.

Intensive Care Society. (in press). *Outreach. An outline for standards of the provision of outreach services.* Intensive Care Society.

Knaus, W. A., Draper, E. A., Wagner, D. P., Zimmerman, J. E. (1986). An evaluation of outcome from intensive care in major medical centers. *Ann. Intern. Med.*, **104**, 410–418.

Le Gall, J. R., Lemeshow, S., Saulnier, F. (1993). A new Simplified Acute Physiology Score (SAPS II) based on a European/North American multicenter study. *JAMA*, **270**, 2957–2963.

Lee, A., Bishop, G., Hillman, K. M., Daffurn, K. (1995). The medical emergency team. *Anaesth. Intensive Care*, **23**, 183–186.

McQuillan, P., Pilkington, S., Allan, A. *et al.* (1998). Confidential inquiry into quality of care before admission to intensive care. *Br. Med. J.*, **316**, 1853–1858.

Moreno, R. (2000). Outcome prediction in intensive care. In *2000 Yearbook of Intensive and Emergency Medicine* (J. L. Vincent, ed.) pp. 825–836, Springer-Verlag.

Moreno, R., Agthe, D. (1999). ICU discharge decision-making: are we able to decrease post-ICU mortality? *Intensive Care Med.*, **25**, 1035–1036.

NHS Executive Committee for Regulating Information Requirements. (1996). *Dataset Change Notice 29/96/P24. Augmented Care Period Data Set.* NHS Executive.

NHS Executive. (2001). *Department of Health Form KH03a.* Department of Health.

Pappachan, J.V., Millar, B., Bennett, D., Smith, G.B. (1999). Comparison of outcome from intensive care admission after adjustment for case mix by the APACHE III prognostic system. *Chest*, **115**, 802–810.

Reis Miranda, D., Ryan, D. W., Schaufeli, W. B., Fidler, V. (1998). *Organisation and Management of Intensive Care.* Springer-Verlag.

Ridley, S. (2001). Critical care outcomes. *Anaesthesia*, **56**, 1–3.

Smith, L., Orts, C. M., O'Neil, I., Batchelor, A. M., Gascoigne, A. D., Baudouin, S. V. (1999). TISS and mortality after discharge from intensive care. *Intensive Care Med.*, **25**, 1061–1065.

Thijs, L. G. (2000). Geographical differences in outcome. In *Evaluating Critical Care. Using health services research to improve quality.* (W. J. Sibbald, J. F. Bion, eds) pp 292–308, Springer-Verlag.

Tissot, E., Cornette, C., Demoly, P., Jacquet, M., Barale, F., Capellier, G. (1999). Medication errors at the administration stage in an intensive care unit. *Intensive Care Med.*, **25**, 353–359.

Treasure, T., Bennett, D. (1999). Reducing the risk of major elective surgery. *Br. Med. J.*, **318**, 1087–1088.

Vincent, J. L., Bihari, D. J., Suter, P. M. *et al.* (1995). The prevalence of nosocomial infection in intensive care units in Europe. Results of the European Prevalence of

Infection in Intensive Care (EPIC) Study. EPIC International Advisory Committee. *JAMA*, **274,** 639–644.

Vincent, J. L., Burchardi, H. (1999). Do we need intermediate care units? *Intensive Care Med.*, **25,** 1345–1349.

Vincent, J. L., Thijs, L. G., Cerny, V. (1997). Critical care in Europe. *Crit. Care Clin.*, **13,** 245–254.

Wilson, J., Woods, I., Fawcett, J. *et al.* (1999). Reducing the risk of major elective surgery: randomised controlled trial of preoperative optimisation of oxygen delivery. *Br. Med. J.*, **318,** 1099–1103.

Zimmerman, J. E., Shortell, S. M., Knaus, W. A. (1993). Value and cost of teaching hospitals: A prospective multicenter, inception cohort study. *Crit. Care Med.*, **21,** 1432–1442.

Zimmerman, J. E., Wagner, D. P., Draper, E. A., Wright, L., Alzola, C., Knaus, W. A. (1998). Evaluation of Acute Physiology And Chronic Health Evaluation III predictions of hospital mortality in an independent database. *Crit. Care Med.*, **26,** 1317–1326.

Patients' and relatives' perspectives

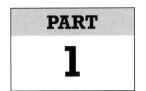

PART

1

Patients' and relatives' perspectives

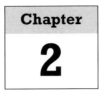

Chapter 2

Mortality as an outcome measure for intensive care

Duncan Young and Saxon Ridley

Introduction

Intensive care is a mixture of diagnostic, therapeutic and operational factors that combine to produce a process of care for the patient. How this process of care affects the patient's chance of recovery, and how to measure its effect, is the essence of outcome research in intensive care. In order to make comparisons between individual intensive care units (ICUs), between ICUs in different countries, or to track changes in the effectiveness of intensive care over time, the whole process is often viewed as a 'black box'. Intensive care research concentrates on the output from the black box, defining suitable outcome measures and relating these to the characteristics of the patients admitted to ICU (the 'input' to the black box or the case-mix). One outcome measure that is commonly used is mortality.

Using the absolute number of deaths within a fixed time period as an outcome measure is of no practical value as the number of patients admitted varies between ICUs and over time. Usually mortality is expressed as a crude mortality rate; the numerator is the number of deaths in a fixed period and the denominator is the number of admissions, or less commonly the number of new patients admitted in the same period (i.e. excluding re-admissions).

Using crude mortality rates as outcome measures in studies to evaluate the process of intensive care has several obvious advantages. Mortality is a binary outcome, and death can be clearly defined and simply recorded. Deaths are recorded by all hospitals as part of their basic data set, and usually the information is available electronically. Death during or following intensive care remains common; in the UK the average mortality within an ICU is about 21% of new admissions. While high mortality rates are distressing, they may allow early detection of the most important influences determining mortality. Mortality rates are also clearly of great importance to patients, relatives and the community at large; they provide a simple and readily understandable measure of the effectiveness of intensive care.

However, for all their convenience, crude mortality rates are a very poor means to assess the performance of intensive care. Large variations in mortality rates will occur depending on when the data are collected. For example in the UK, data from the Intensive Care National Audit and Research Centre (INCARC, 2000b) gives a crude mortality rate in the admitting ICU of 20.9% (deaths in the admitting ICU/new patient admissions). If the mortality calculation includes patients transferred from the admitting ICU to another ICU, the crude mortality rate rises to 21.8%. If the crude mortality rate uses deaths before discharge from the admitting hospital as the numerator, the mortality rises markedly to 29.1%, and if patients who were transferred to other hospitals are also included crude mortality reaches 30.8% (Table 2.1).

Even if the data collection times are standardized, crude mortality rates may still be an imprecise measure of effectiveness of intensive care because they take no account of the variation in the characteristics of the patients entering ICU. This variation is normally termed case-mix. This chapter examines the use and limitations of intensive care and hospital crude mortality rates as outcome measures, and gives some examples of the influence of case-mix. Methods to correct or allow for variations in case-mix are discussed in Chapters 3 and 4.

Table 2.1 Variations in intensive care unit (ICU) mortality depending on data collection time

Rate	Numerator	Denominator	UK rate (%)
Mortality rate in admitting ICU	Deaths before discharge from admitting ICU	All ICU patients admitted during the same period	20.9
Mortality rate for all ICU care	Deaths before discharge from admitting ICU or an ICU to which the patient had been transferred	All ICU patients admitted during the same period	21.8
Mortality rate for all ICU care and subsequent hospital care in the admitting hospital	Deaths before discharge from admitting hospital	All ICU patients admitted during the same period	29.1
Mortality rate for all ICU care and all subsequent hospital care	Deaths before discharge from all hospital care	All ICU patients admitted during the same period	30.8

Mortality within the ICU

If comparisons of effectiveness of care within an ICU over time or between ICUs are to be made, then superficially the ICU mortality would seem the preferred outcome measure, as it is independent of effects of subsequent hospital care. If a clear definition of what constitutes an ICU was available, if discharge policies were similar, if transfers did not occur, if the location where end-of-life care is delivered was standardized, and if expectations of care from families and physicians did not vary, ICU mortality would indeed be a good indicator of ICU effectiveness. However, all these factors will alter the site to which the death is attributed (ICU or hospital) and will markedly affect the ratio of ICU to hospital deaths. Thus comparisons made between ICUs using the ICU mortality rate may simply reflect organizational factors and not quality of care.

Clinical factors influencing mortality in the ICU

Deaths in ICU account for two-thirds of the hospital deaths of patients admitted to ICUs, so factors affecting ICU mortality will necessarily affect hospital mortality. Case-mix is one of the most important factors influencing mortality. The components that define case-mix are the diagnosis, severity of illness, co-morbidity, age and emergency status. ICU mortality is also influenced by the timing and application of treatment and the patient's physiological reserve to respond to that treatment.

Case-mix: underlying disease or diagnosis

The patient's underlying disease clearly has a major impact on their chance of survival. To give two extreme examples, patients admitted to ICU with type 1 respiratory failure (acute hypoxaemic respiratory failure) due to a pulmonary infection following bone marrow transplantation have an expected hospital mortality of about 95% (Rubenfeld and Crawford, 1996; Gruson *et al.*, 1999); the majority of these patients do indeed die on ICU. At the other end of the spectrum, patients admitted following elective aortic aneurysm surgery in the UK have an ICU mortality of 6.6%, while those admitted simply for observation and management of epidural analgesia have an ICU mortality of less than 1% (ICNARC, 2000a). Making comparisons of the effectiveness of care between ICUs or within a unit over time using ICU mortality will be meaningless if the range of presenting conditions is not considered.

However, if a well-defined group of patients with a similar diagnosis can be identified and their severity of illness measured, then ICU mortality does become a useful measure of the effectiveness of the intensive care process if a significant proportion of deaths occur on ICU. Probably the best example of this is an audit of trauma victims ventilated on a single ICU (Watt and Ledingham, 1984). A sudden increase in mortality was noted, although the severity of the injuries (as determined by an Injury Severity Score) remained unchanged. Between 1969 and 1982, mortality in trauma patients had fluctuated between 19% and 29% but suddenly rose to 47% in 1981 to 1982. This increased mortality was confined to patients surviving more than 5 days from injury and was associated with multiple organ dysfunction and infection. The mortality in patients receiving etomidate was 77% while the mortality rate was only 28% in those receiving benzodiaze-pines. Etomidate was subsequently found to inhibit basal cortisol production and abolish the stress response and so probably caused the increased mortality by limiting the patient's response to infection.

Case-mix: severity of illness

Most of the commonly used severity scoring systems (APACHE, SAPS and the MPM models) were developed using hospital mortality as an outcome, and link the severity of illness to a probability of hospital, rather than intensive care, mortality. Hospital mortality is used in these systems as it is less dependent on operational factors (see below), and is clinically and socially more relevant. There are, however, a variety of other severity scoring systems that use ICU, as opposed to hospital, mortality as an outcome measure; these systems demonstrate a clear relationship between severity of illness and ICU mortality. Examples are the PRISM (Pediatric Risk of Mortality) score (Pollack et al., 1988), the SOFA (Sequential Organ Failure Assessment) score (Vincent et al., 1996), the MOD (multiple organ dysfunction) score (Marshall et al., 1995) and ODIN (organ dysfunction/infection) scores (Fagon et al., 1993). Sequential SOFA or MOD scoring also demonstrates the burden of illness of ICU outcome as continuing high SOFA or MOD scores indicate a failure to respond to treatment and are associated with a higher mortality.

The ODIN, SOFA and MOD scoring systems are primarily designed to describe the severity of illness of critically ill patients, rather than predict their hospital mortality. For example, the MOD score was designed as an alternative outcome measure to mortality. As such it is fundamentally different from APACHE II or any of the predictive systems, as it is designed to measure the outcome of the early part of the intensive care process rather than to characterize patients. For this reason, it was optimized to have a wide spread of scores with equal weighting for all organ systems rather than best predictive power. However, to establish criterion validity (how well the new measure performs against a gold standard) it was tested to ensure that increasing organ dysfunction correlated with the best available alternative outcome measure, namely intensive care mortality.

Case-mix: co-morbidity, age and emergency status

As might be expected, increasing age, increasing co-morbidity and admission to the ICU as an emergency as opposed to following elective surgery all increase the probability of death in the ICU (Fagon et al., 1993), much as they increase the probability of hospital mortality in the APACHE, SAPS and MPM models. To date there is no validated means to adjust for these factors when comparing ICU, as opposed to hospital, mortality.

Application and timing of treatment

Application and timing of treatment have been shown to affect ICU mortality. Initially the term 'lead-time' bias was used to describe the beneficial effect on reducing measured physiological derangement by pre-admission resuscitation and organ support. The effect of lead-time bias was to reduce the predicted risk of ICU mortality based on ICU admission severity of illness scoring in critically ill patients who had been ill for some time. It was originally used to explain the higher mortality in patients transferred to larger ICUs after a period of organ support in another unit (Dragsted et al., 1989).

Preoperative optimization for high-risk surgical patients is now recognized as having a beneficial effect in terms of reduced mortality (Boyd et al., 1993; Boyd and Bennett, 1996). Resuscitating patients so that they are in the optimum physiological status prior to surgical insults seems intuitively sensible. However, the reduced subsequent ICU mortality in this patient group, while welcome and encouraging, may skew the overall ICU mortality. The effectiveness of ICU management of other patients may not have improved nor changed and yet the overall ICU mortality will have declined.

Operational factors influencing mortality in the ICU

Even if it were possible to perform robust case-mix adjustment, mortality within the ICU would still be considered a poor outcome measure for determining ICU effectiveness. This is primarily because different operational factors will alter whether the death occurs in or is attributed to the ICU. This may alter the apparent mortality figures even in the presence of equivalent ICU effectiveness. The operational factors most likely to have an effect are admission and discharge policies, bed availability including the availability of high-dependency beds, patient transfers and local treatment protocols including staffing establishment.

Admission and discharge policies

Admission policies can have a major effect on both ICU mortality and hospital mortality. A unit admitting a high proportion of low-risk patients (e.g. patients following elective coronary artery bypass grafting) will have low mortality figures, whereas a unit that admits primarily acute medical admissions will have a higher mortality. These variations in case-mix can to some degree be overcome by quoting condition-specific ICU mortality. However, differences in discharge policies have more subtle effects that will tend to make ICU mortality figures even more unreliable as an outcome measure. One clear example relates to patients who have had treatment withdrawn but are breathing spontaneously. In some ICUs it is viewed as more humane to keep the patient on the ICU and deliver terminal care with the same group of staff who have cared for the patient through their illness. Other units take the view that this care is better delivered in the less technological environment of the general ward. In the first case, the patient's death will be recorded as an ICU death, whereas in the second as a hospital death. Similar scenarios occur with organ donation; if the patient is formally discharged from ICU when they go for organ retrieval in the operating theatre, their death will be counted as part of the hospital rather than the ICU mortality.

Bed availability and designation

The availability and labelling of beds also affects the ICU mortality statistics. Low ICU bed availability alters the distribution of severity of illness in the ICU population, tending to increase the proportion of severely ill patients and hence crude ICU mortality rates. For example, a study was undertaken comparing intensive care in New Zealand and the USA. New Zealand had 1.7% of its hospital beds designated as intensive care beds whereas in the USA, 5.6% of hospital beds were designated as intensive care beds. In New Zealand where ICU beds were more limited, the ICU population was on average more severely ill and contained less elective admissions. As a result, New Zealand units had a higher crude ICU mortality rate (15%) than the USA units (11.7%) (Zimmerman et al., 1988). However, when the hospital mortality was examined it was the same, both corrected and uncorrected for case-mix, suggesting that the additional beds available to the Americans contained patients with a lower mortality risk (or that the additional care did not alter their risk of mortality). The effectiveness of ICU care in both countries was probably the same in spite of the differing ICU mortality rates. A similar pattern was seen when Japanese ICUs (2% of all hospital beds) were compared to USA units (Sirio et al., 1992) (Table 2.2).

There are increasing numbers of high-dependency or intermediate-dependency units being established in the UK. The recorded effects of developing a high-dependency unit (HDU) include an increase in the mean severity of illness on the ICU (Fox et al., 1999), an increase in the total number of patients admitted to the combined ICU/HDU (Dhond et al., 1998), reduced re-admissions (Fox et al., 1999) and a reduction in complications from general surgery (Jones et al., 1999). The effect on the crude ICU mortality rate will critically depend on how the HDU beds are 'badged'. If admissions to HDU are included in the ICU admissions, the overall ICU mortality rate would probably decrease, because of an increased number of admissions with a lower severity of illness. If the HDU beds are not included in the ICU figures the ICU mortality might be expected to increase, as the average severity of illness of the ICU patients will increase. The situation is further complicated by an increasing tendency to have critical care complexes, with flexible use of the beds as either HDU or ICU beds depending on demand and nursing staff availability.

In the UK, ventilated patients are nearly always cared for on the ICU. However, in the USA, increasing cost pressures brought about by managed care and an economically driven healthcare system have led to the establishment of

Table 2.2 The effect of bed availability on intensive care and hospital mortality. Note that limitations on bed availability result in a higher severity of illness as judged by the APACHE II score and fewer elective admissions (data not shown) or 'monitor only' admissions (data not shown), with a resulting high intensive care mortality. The case-mix adjusted predicted hospital mortalities and actual mortalities are not different. This suggests the process of intensive care is as good in Japanese and New Zealand intensive care units as it is in the USA

Country (Year)	Mean APACHE II score	ICU beds as % all hospital beds	Crude ICU mortality (%)	Crude hospital mortality	Predicted hospital mortality
New Zealand (1988)	14.2	1.7	15	18	19.2
Japan (1992)	14.0	2.0	Data not given	16.9	19.2
USA (1988)	10.7	5.6	11.7	19.7	19.2

Data are taken from Zimmerman, J. E., Knaus, W. A., Judson J. A. *et al.* (1988). Patient selection for intensive care: a comparison of New Zealand and United States hospitals. *Crit. Care Med.*, **16**, 318–326 and Sirio, C. A., Tajimi, K., Tase C., *et al.* (1992). An initial comparison of intensive care in Japan and the United States. *Crit. Care Med.*, **20**, 1207–1215.

extended care facilities. These units care for stable patients requiring longer-term high technology care and can accept patients requiring artificial ventilation. They may not be in the same hospital as the ICU. Although they may only accept a limited number of patients, the patients that are cared for in extended care facilities have 50% mortality (Nasraway *et al.*, 2000). If the original ICU mortality rate is calculated excluding these patients the effectiveness of that ICU will be overestimated.

Transfers

Most modern healthcare systems concentrate specialist services in a limited number of centres, to contain costs and maintain a high level of experience among the staff. Many of these specialist services (e.g. cardiac, trauma and neurosurgery, haematology) are relatively frequent users of intensive care services. Some specialist services have a dedicated ICU, but others use the general ICU for support. This distorts the spectrum of severity of illness and diagnosis in the general ICUs in tertiary referral centres. However, in specialist neurosurgical units in the UK, the reverse situation can occur; patients are operated on in the tertiary centre but transferred back to the referring hospital for long-term care and rehabilitation. Clearly the early mortality occurs in the neurosurgical unit but a number of late deaths do occur before ICU discharge in the referring hospital. Overall in the UK, the ICNARC data suggest that a 1% error in mortality rates can be caused by failure to track the patient through the healthcare system to ultimate discharge or death.

Staffing

Comparisons of ICU mortality will be unreliable unless ICUs with similar capabilities are compared. This is particularly relevant with regard to medical staff. Early studies demonstrated the improvement in mortality following the introduction of full-time intensive care specialists (Brown and Sullivan, 1989). Later work has shown how all aspects of ICU performance, including mortality, are improved by changing the organization of the ICU from 'open' (where the referring clinician retains managerial control) to 'closed' (where the critical care specialists assume control of the patient's treatment) (Reynolds et al., 1994).

Family expectations

It is not immediately clear how family expectations might alter ICU outcome. The recognition of futility may lead to a change from full aggressive intensive care to comfort measures only. While some families and religious groups may have difficulty accepting the concept of futile care, in practical terms their reluctance to change the emphasis of care only delays death on the ICU, and does not alter ICU mortality. The reverse situation is where the family or the patient requests a limit on treatment and this may make death more likely. While this might skew ICU mortality statistics, in the UK, this is probably a rare event.

Differences in healthcare systems

When comparisons of the outcome of ICU care are made across different countries, the limitations of ICU mortality as an outcome measure of the intensive care process become even more apparent. In a study of an Indian neurosurgical/neuromedical ICU, Parikh and Karnad (1999) noted an ICU mortality of 36.2%, which is a relatively high figure. This figure may have little to do with the care the patients received in the ICU but rather reflect the population, healthcare and economic systems and culture in which the study was undertaken. The mean age of the patients was 36 years, as opposed to 56 years in ICUs in the UK (Rowan et al., 1993). This is partly due to the general population structure, where only 5% of the Indian population are more than 65 years old against 13 to 16% in the USA and Western Europe respectively. Life expectancy at birth in India is 62 years, against 76 and 78 years in the USA and Western Europe. In addition, the authors suggest that there is a cultural bias towards treating younger patients, both from the physicians and families. Yet in spite of the young patient group who might be expected to survive because of good physiological reserve and infrequent co-morbidity, ICU mortality was high. This is related to the diseases treated; 30% of the patients had infectious diseases (notably malaria and tetanus) that are almost unknown in Europe and the USA and a further 8% had organophosphate poisoning. If the performance of the ICU is to be assessed, such differences in case-mix and the altered age distribution need to be addressed. Even if this was done using hospital mortality as an outcome, none of the present case-mix adjustment methods have been calibrated on an ICU population with a 30% rate of malaria and tetanus, so any differences in standardized mortality ratio (SMR) could easily arise from a failure of the Mortality Prediction Model. Thus the ICU mortality or even hospital mortality figure can only be taken in context, and using it as a single measure to compare ICU performance across healthcare systems may be inappropriate.

ICU mortality as an outcome measure

The main use of ICU mortality as an outcome measure is for audit within an individual ICU. Tracking a unit's mortality over time will allow acute changes and trends to be spotted, hopefully relatively early. This may prompt changes in ICU practice, such as the introduction of a new drug (e.g. etomidate) or a change in bed pressure (e.g. night time discharges). ICU mortality in this form of audit is probably more appropriate when applied to single diagnostic categories rather than across the whole ICU population.

When ICU mortality is used to make comparisons of the effectiveness of care between units, the confounding effects of case-mix, the definition of 'ICU' mortality and operational factors make differences difficult or impossible to interpret.

Hospital mortality

There are large variations in hospital mortality following critical illness. Death within hospital following discharge from intensive care is a distressingly frequent occurrence; figures from the UK and elsewhere in Europe (Moreno and Agthe, 1999) suggest that between 23 and 31% of all hospital deaths in patients admitted to intensive care occur after the patient has left the ICU. The contributing factors have not been closely examined, but presently available data suggest that a combination of clinical and organizational issues may be responsible.

Clinical factors include the type and extent of the pathology precipitating the critical illness. Patients admitted to ICUs with medical problems have higher case-mix adjusted mortality compared with those following surgery. In the UK, the APACHE II probability of hospital death for non-operative admissions is 9% higher than for surgical admissions (23.2 versus 14.1%) (ICNARC, 2000b). This increased risk of hospital mortality also continues following discharge home; the

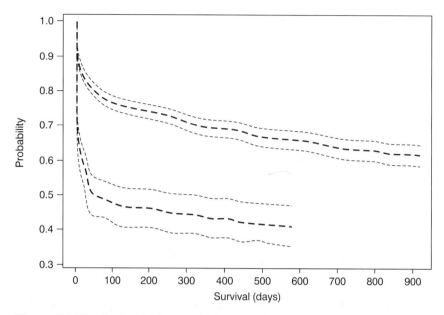

Figure 2.1 The Kaplan-Meier survival curves for medical (solid line, $n =$ 374) and non-medical (dashed line, $n = 1791$) patients; 95% confidence intervals for both curves are shown. The median survival time of medical patients is 40 days (Lam, S., Ridley, S. (1999). Critically ill medical patients, their demographics and outcome. *Anaesthesia*, **54**, 845–852).

median survival time of patients from medical specialties after admission to intensive care was 40 days compared to a median survival time of other patients in excess of 900 days (Figure 2.1) (Lam and Ridley, 1999).

This greater mortality in medical patients probably illustrates the fundamental difference between amelioration and suppression of a medical pathology rather than the excision or correction of surgical pathologies. The effect of pathology can be illustrated by the survival of patients admitted to ICU with cancer. Over a decade ago, Dragsted reported that the survival curve of patients admitted with cancer was consistently worse than other patients at all stages of follow-up (Figure 2.2). At 5 years only 20% of patients admitted to ICU with cancer remained alive compared to 80% of other patients (Dragsted *et al.*, 1990). The physiological reserve of patients and their responsiveness to treatment also affect post-ICU but in-hospital mortality. One of the groups with the highest hospital mortality is elderly patients who only stay for a short time on ICU. Goldhill reported that their in-hospital mortality after ICU discharge was as high as 27% (Goldhill and Sumner, 1998).

The organization and delivery of critical care may affect hospital mortality. If critically ill patients still require a high level of support when they are discharged from an ICU, there is evidence to suggest that they have a higher than average post-ICU hospital mortality. Measuring the patient's dependency using the

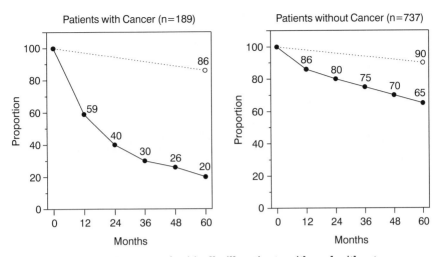

Figure 2.2 Survival curves of critically ill patients with and without cancer (solid lines) compared to an age-matched normal population (dotted lines) (modified from Dragsted, L., Qvist, J., Madsen, M. (1990). Outcome from intensive care IV. A five year study of 1308 patients: long term outcome. *Eur. J Anaesthesiol.*, **7**, 51–61).

Therapeutic Intervention Scoring System (TISS) at discharge, Smith *et al.* (1999) studied 283 ICU survivors of whom 11% subsequently died in hospital. Twenty-one percent of patients discharged with a TISS score of over 20 died, while those discharged with a score of below 10 had a 3.7% mortality. Daly *et al.* (2000) have shown that an increased risk of hospital mortality following intensive care is associated with a higher acute physiology score on the day of discharge (mean 10.1 versus 8.0). Increasing age (mean 65 versus 59 years), the presence of chronic ill health (39 versus 22%) and longer ICU admission (mean 8 versus 3 days) also adversely affected outcome. Early or precipitous discharge is also associated with a higher hospital mortality. Goldfrad and Rowan (2000) reviewed the outcome of patients discharged at night. This study found that night time discharges (defined as discharges between 22:00 to 06:59) had an increased case-mix adjusted risk of hospital death with an odds ratio of 1.33 (95% confidence interval 1.06–1.65). Early or premature discharge implies a continuing high care requirement which, if not provided, leads to higher hospital mortality.

Discharging patients before they are sufficiently stable to be managed on the general ward or discharging them at night may reflect inadequate provision of critical care beds or an imbalance of intensive care to high-dependency care beds. HDUs may improve the quality of care following formal intensive care and so help reduce hospital mortality. Fox *et al.* (1999) and Dhond *et al.* (1998) have separately shown that the development of an HDU reduces the re-admission rate to intensive care. Jones and colleagues (1999) have shown that an HDU reduces the expected complication rate in surgical patients. In a hospital without an HDU the observed to expected ratio for complications was 1.74 compared to 1.09 in patients admitted to an HDU. The commonest complications in patients not receiving high-dependency care were chest infection, arrhythmias and hypotension. While there was no difference in mortality rate between the patient groups, there was a tendency to shorter hospital stay in patients who had been managed on the HDU. Avoiding serious postoperative complications is important as mortality is greater in patients who require a second admission to ICU.

Wallis *et al.* (1997) reviewed the causes of hospital death following discharge from ICU in 1700 patients in a district hospital in the UK over a 5-year period (Table 2.3).

Table 2.3 Causes of death on the ward following ICU discharge

Cause of death	Number	%
Pneumonia (no other major precipitating factor apart from recent critical illness)	43	28.1
Hypoxic brain damage	21	13.7
Structural brain damage (trauma, surgery or cerebrovascular accident prior to ICU admission)	13	8.5
Cerebrovascular accident (occurring during or after critical illness but not the primary event)	12	7.8
Malignancy (direct cause of death)	11	7.2
Myocardial infarction	10	6.5
Renal failure	9	5.9
Multiple organ failure	8	5.2
Sepsis	8	5.2
Thrombo-embolism	5	3.3
Pulmonary aspiration	4	2.6
Hepatic failure	1	0.7
Miscellaneous	4	2.6

Modified from Wallis, C. B., Davies, H. T. O., Shearer, A. J. (1997). Why do patients die on general wards after discharge from intensive care units? *Anaesthesia*, **52**, 9–14.

The main causes of death on the general wards following discharge from ICU were pneumonia, hypoxic or structural brain damage, cerebrovascular accident, malignancy, myocardial infarction, renal or multiple organ failure and sepsis. The management of four of these conditions, namely pneumonia, renal or multiple organ failure and sepsis are certainly within the realms of the critical care services and it is disappointing to see these conditions being responsible for patients' deaths. Frequently the ICU physicians are not involved in decisions concerning the further management of ICU survivors on the general ward and little is known about decision-making processes for general ward patients. Primarily for this reason, it is difficult to attribute the relative proportion of hospital deaths directly to decisions and activity on ICU compared to those occurring in the rest of the hospital stay. In the UK, this may change with the development of intensive care outreach teams (Department of Health, 2000). These teams are similar to the 'Medical Emergency Teams' (Lee *et al.*, 1995) and 'Patient at Risk Teams' (Goldhill *et al.*, 1999) and part of their remit is the continued supervision of patients discharged from the critical care services. An appreciation by the intensive care staff that their responsibility to the patients extends beyond the ICU is probably required; once this occurs then hospital mortality may become a more appropriate outcome measure for critical care.

Hospital mortality is of great interest to the patients and their relatives. Once the patient has left ICU, the relatives' concerns may change from whether or not the patient will survive to how long is the patient going to live and how long will be the recovery. Therefore if the patient dies in hospital after ICU discharge, the relatives may be understandably disappointed that their loved one survived the rigours of intensive care but did not leave hospital. Patients' families may wish to know the chances of their relative returning home to the community and so being able to predict vital status at hospital discharge is an important end point for the consumers of health care.

Alternatives to hospital mortality

Measures of long-term survival may be more useful than either estimates of ICU or hospital mortality. At the moment, long-term survival following intensive care is described in non-standardized calendar periods ranging between 28 days and 5 years. The duration of follow-up period tends to be randomly chosen by the investigator. Long-term survival is a balance between the primary disease that precipitated ICU admission and the incidence of age-related disease, accidents and injury occurring normally in the general population. A more logical length of follow-up may be to the time when mortality can no longer be attributed to either the primary disease precipitating admission or the longer lasting effects of critical illness.

Practicalities of measuring long-term survival

Choice of control group

With appropriate follow-up, it is possible to draw a survival curve for a group of critically ill patients. However, interpretation of the patients' survival requires comparison with an appropriate control group. Two problems need careful consideration. First, which individuals should make up the control group? The ICU patient population is not a representative sample of the general population because ICU patients tend to be chronically ill with pre-existing physiological derangement due to co-morbidity. Comparing their survival with that of an age- and sex-matched normal population may not be appropriate. Even so, this comparison has been most frequently reported because of the relative ease of obtaining death rate data in the national population. Comparing ICU survivors with hospital patients would be a more representative comparison but there may still be real differences due to case-mix. For example, patients with advanced cancer are frequently admitted to hospital but not necessarily to ICU. Ideally ICU survivors should be compared with a group of hospital patients with the same disease who did not develop critical illness and so did not require ICU admission (Figure 2.3). Unfortunately it is difficult to identify this group of patients and even then such a comparison would determine the effect of critical illness rather than the influence of ICU management on survival.

Length of follow-up

Second, the question of how long to follow-up the patients arises. Ideally the ICU survivors should be followed until the gradient of their survival curve parallels

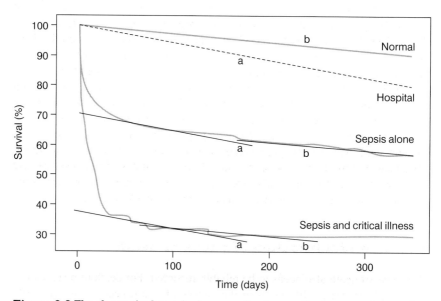

Figure 2.3 The theoretical survival curves for four patient groups (normal individuals, hospital patients, patients suffering from sepsis but not ill enough to warrant ICU admission and critically ill septic patients). Lines marked 'a' or 'b' are parallel with each other, so representing when the survival curves of patients with sepsis parallel the other two possible control groups (Ridley, S. A. (2000) Quality of life and longer term outcomes. In: *Update in Intensive Care and Emergency Medicine 35. Evaluating Critical Care. Using Health Service Research to Improve Quality.* (W. J. Sibbald, J. F. Bion, eds) p. 111, Springer-Verlag).

that of the control group. However, the length of time taken for the gradients of the survival curves to become parallel depends upon the control groups chosen (Figure 2.3). It will take the longest time with an age- and sex-matched normal population and probably the shortest time with hospital patients with the same condition. When the curves of the critically ill patients match those of a comparable population, then the effects of critical illness in combination with the underlying pathological process will have run their course. However, not all the long-term mortality observed in critically ill patients is due to the effects of disease that precipitated their ICU admission. For example, the survival of patients following oesophagogastrectomy is dependent upon their tumour histology while their ICU admission is required for cardiorespiratory observation and monitoring after long and difficult surgery.

Mechanism for notification of death

There are various sources of national or regional population statistics. However, there tends to be a delay in the publication of these figures and, as mentioned above, the patients presenting to ICUs may not be a random selection of the normal population. Theoretically, measurement of mortality should be easy, but the reliability of information concerning survival depends upon a national system that collects these data centrally. For example, the Scandinavian countries have developed an effective system for identifying deaths based upon the individual's unique social security number. In the UK, the Office for National Statistics uses the patients' National Health Service number which is not the same as their hospital number or any other nationally used identifier. If the National Health Service number is not available, then identifying the patients depends upon their addresses and dates of birth. With a mobile population, patients can easily be lost. Contact with their general practitioner may be fruitless if no follow-up details were provided by the patient on moving. Therefore, unless the national system for recording deaths can easily interact with the hospital system, following patients is more difficult because of data collection inadequacies.

Accurate identification of cause of death

The cause of death also needs to be reliably recorded. For death to be genuinely attributable to critical illness, then the causes of death need to be accurately classified. For example, in patients dying of oesophageal cancer following their oesophagogastrectomy who required intensive care admission, there is a clear relationship between the cause of death and critical illness. For other patients, such as those having had an aortic aneurysm repaired but subsequently dying of myocardial infarction due to hypertensive disease, the connection between the pathophysiological insult precipitating ICU admission and the final cause of death is marginal. Under other circumstances, for example accidental trauma, the final cause of death may be completely unrelated to the cause that precipitated

ICU admission. Thus accurate long-term follow-up of critical care survivors not only requires a measurement of the date of death but also the cause of death. Unfortunately, the reliability of death certification, the only information held nationally, is questionable. The disparity between the clinical cause of death and post-mortem findings for patients dying in hospital may be high. Even in the ICU where patients are rigorously investigated and monitored the number of incorrect or missed pathologies may be as high as 33.3% (Gut *et al.*, 1999). The level of accuracy of death certification in the community is unknown and yet this is where the majority of survivors of critical illness will succumb and whence most of the long-term survival data originate.

Statistical analysis

Long-term follow-up of patients requires special statistical techniques because the distribution of survival times is markedly skewed with the highest mortality rate in ICU, a lesser mortality rate in hospital and finally a gradual attrition of patients in the community. Most importantly, special techniques are required because of 'censored' observations. These arise because at the completion of the follow-up period, some patients will still be alive and so their exact survival times are unknown.

Two functions describe the distribution of survival times, the survival function and the hazard function. The survival function is defined as the probability that an individual survives longer than a certain time point, usually denoted by 't' and exemplified by a calendar period (e.g. 55% 5-year survival). The survival curve is a smooth curve of survival probability (S(t)) against time. The hazard function is the probability of death within a time period given that the individual has survived up to the beginning of that time period (known as a 'conditional' probability).

If the patients are all followed-up for the same period of time then analysis is much easier, but the study takes longer to complete because the last patient enrolled in the study period must be followed for the full study period, however long this may be. Under these circumstances, non-parametric summary statistics (e.g. median, interquartile range, and range) and simpler statistical techniques, such as the Wilcoxon rank sum test, can be used to compare survival curves. Unfortunately, in most survival data sets, there are censored observations as patients are lost to follow-up or are alive at the completion of the study. To estimate the survival function of data containing censored observations, the most commonly used technique is the Kaplan-Meier product limit estimator. This procedure involves the continued product of a series of conditional probabilities. For example, the probability of surviving 2 years is the probability of surviving 1 year times the probability of surviving 2 years, having already survived the first year. As the number of patients dying and being withdrawn (i.e. censored) each year determines the probability of survival for that particular year, the censored observations are appropriately accommodated. Kaplan-Meier survival curves are not smooth but have a stepwise change at each alteration in product limit estimator.

Where the data contain censored observations the statistical tests of choice are the following non-parametric tests:

1. Peto/Wilcoxon test. This is a generalization of Wilcoxon's two sample rank sum test. This and the Gehan's Wilcoxon test (another generalization of Wilcoxon's two sample rank sum test) are more powerful than the other tests when the hazard function is constant throughout the study and the data are from a Wiebull distribution.
2. Log-rank or Mantel-Haenszel test compares the number of deaths occurring at each time point with the number that might be expected if the survival curves were similar.
3. Cox-Mantel test is similar to the log-rank test.

All of these tests are illustrated in Lee's textbook on survival data analysis (Lee, 1980). To investigate the causes and significant influences on survival curves, techniques such as Cox's proportional hazard modelling may be used. This involves generating a model in which the dependence of the hazard function on time does not have to be specifically stated. The term 'proportional hazard' arises because for any two individuals in the model the ratio of their hazard remains constant over time. Details of this procedure can be found in Cox and Oates' (1984) short textbook.

Long-term survival

Most of the studies that have followed critically ill patients have matched their survival to that of a normal population, accepting that for the reasons outlined above this may not be the most appropriate control group. Unfortunately, there are conflicting data concerning the length of time required for survival curves to parallel the normal population. Niskanen *et al.* (1996) followed 12 180 Finnish intensive care patients for 5 years. The 5-year survival rate was 66.7% and overall the survival rate paralleled that of the general population at 2 years. However, the time at which this happened varied with diagnostic category. For example, the survival of trauma victims and patients with a cardiovascular diagnosis equalled that of the general population after 3 months (Figure 2.4).

If they survived the initial episode, patients admitted following cardiac arrest had a similar mortality rate as the general population after 1 year. In contrast, there were more deaths than expected throughout the follow-up period among patients with respiratory failure and attempted suicide.

Dragsted *et al.* (1990) followed 1308 patients in Denmark and reported an overall 5-year survival rate of 58%, although once again certain subgroups had much poorer survival (e.g. cancer, medical and older patients). In Sweden, Zaren and Bergstrom (1988) looked at 980 adult patients admitted to ICU and at the end

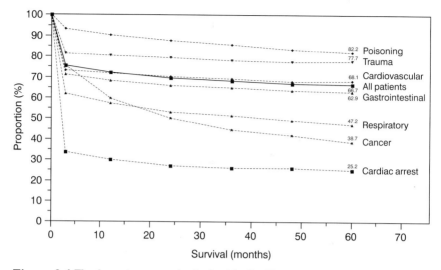

Figure 2.4 The long-term survival of critically ill patients stratified by diagnosis (modified from Niskanen, M., Kari, A., Halonen, P. (1996). Five-year survival after intensive care – comparison of 12 180 patients with the general population. Finnish ICU Study Group. *Crit. Care Med.*, **24**, 1962–1967).

of 1 year 73.6% survived compared to 96% for the normal population. The authors concluded that follow-up was only required for 1 year.

In Scotland, it took 4 years for the survival of 1168 critically ill patients to match that of a normal population, by which time 55% of patients survived (Figure 2.5) (Ridley and Plenderleith, 1994).

Results from East Anglia confirm that, in the UK, the survival of critically ill patients does not match a normal population for at least 2.5 years (Lam and Ridley, 1999). These differences between the length of time taken for a survival curve to match a normal population may have a number of explanations. One of the most pertinent may be the greater severity of illness of patients on ICUs in the UK compared to the rest of Europe. A European study of the organization and management of intensive care in 12 countries found that the mean Simplified Acute Physiology score on UK ICUs was 38.5 compared to an overall mean of 33.6. The hospital mortality was also above average in the UK (31 versus 18%) (Reis Miranda *et al.*, 1998) and so this may partly explain why the survival curve takes longer to become parallel.

Use of long-term survival estimates

Long-term survival data are useful for measuring the natural progression of the disease under present medical and surgical management. Advances in

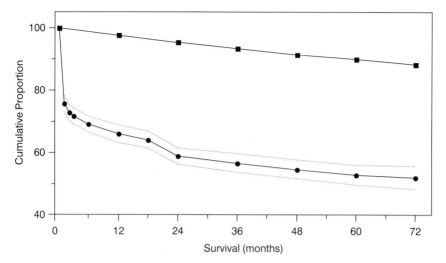

Figure 2.5 The 5-year survival curve of critically ill patients (circles) compared to an age- and sex-matched normal population (squares) (Ridley, S. A., Plenderleith, L. (1994). Survival after intensive care. Comparison with a matched normal population as an indicator of effectiveness. *Anaesthesia*, **49**, 933–935).

medicine and surgery can be assessed by their effect on the survival curves. Long-term survival is also the basis for utility measures such as cost per survivor, the 'time and trade off' methods and the cost per quality adjusted life year. Long-term survival is also useful to allow patients and their relatives a realistic estimate of prognosis. Finally, long-term survival data allow informed debate about triage and admission criteria to critical care.

Conclusion

Mortality is an important outcome measure but it may be a poor reflection of the effectiveness of critical care services. Hospital mortality can be high, especially in the UK and in certain groups of patients. The causes of death after ICU discharge are similar to those seen in ICU; however, the ICU staff are infrequently involved in the management of patients discharged to the general ward. The long-term follow-up of patients is a vital exercise but, at present, the duration of follow-up is not standardized and varies between populations. There are numerous other difficulties relating to identifying and attributing causes of death in survivors of critical illness. Further research is required to quantify the important influences on survival after critical illness.

References

Boyd, O., Grounds, R. M., Bennett, E. D. (1993). A randomized clinical trial of the effect of deliberate perioperative increase of oxygen delivery on mortality in high-risk surgical patients. *JAMA*, **270**, 2699–2707.

Boyd, O., Bennett, E. D. (1996). Enhancement of perioperative tissue perfusion as a therapeutic strategy for major surgery. *New Horiz.*, **4**, 453–465.

Brown, J. J., Sullivan, G. (1989). Effect on ICU mortality of a full time critical care specialist. *Chest*, **96**, 127–129.

Cox, D. R., Oakes, D. (1984). *Analysis of Survival Data*. Chapman and Hall/CRC Press.

Daly, K. J. R., Beale, R. J., Chang, R. W. S. (2000). Ward death following ICU discharge – can it be predicted? Development and validation of a predictive model. *Crit. Care*, **4**, S129.

Department of Health. (2000). *Comprehensive Critical Care. A review of adult critical care services*. Department of Health.

Dhond, G., Ridley, S., Palmer, M. (1998). The impact of a high dependency unit on the workload of an intensive care unit. *Anaesthesia*, **53**, 841–847.

Dragsted, L., Jorgensen, J., Jensen, N. H. *et al.* (1989). Interhospital comparisons of patient outcome from intensive care: importance of lead-time bias. *Crit. Care Med.*, **17**, 418–422.

Dragsted, L., Qvist, J., Madsen, M. (1990). Outcome from intensive care IV. A five year study of 1308 patients: long term outcome. *Eur. J. Anaesthesiol.*, **7**, 51–61.

Fagon, J. Y., Chastre, J., Novara, A., Medioni, P., Gibert, C. (1993). Characterization of intensive care unit patients using a model based on the presence or absence of organ dysfunctions and/or infection: the ODIN model. *Intensive Care Med.*, **19**, 137–144.

Fox, A. J., Owen-Smith, O., Spiers, P. (1999). The immediate impact of opening an adult high dependency unit on intensive care unit occupancy. *Anaesthesia*, **54**, 280–283.

Goldfrad, C., Rowan, K. (2000). Consequences of discharges from intensive care at night. *Lancet*, **355**, 1138–1142.

Goldhill, D. R., Sumner, A. (1998). Outcome of intensive care patients in a group of British intensive care units. *Crit. Care Med.*, **26**, 1337–1345.

Goldhill, D. R., Worthington, L., Mulcahy, A., Tarling, M., Sumner, A. (1999). The patient-at-risk team: identifying and managing seriously ill ward patients. *Anaesthesia*, **54**, 853–860.

Gruson, D., Hilbert G., Portel L. *et al.* (1999). Severe respiratory failure requiring ICU admission in bone marrow transplant recipients. *Eur. Respir. J.*, **13**, 883–887.

Gut, A. L., Ferreira, A. L. A., Montenegro, M. R. (1999). Autopsy: quality assurance in the ICU. *Intensive Care Med.*, **25**, 360–363.

Intensive Care National Audit and Research Centre. (2000a). *Annual Report from the Case Mix Programme Database*. Intensive Care National Audit and Research Centre.

Intensive Care National Audit and Research Centre. (2000b). *Data Analysis from the Case Mix Program Database. Issue 4*. Intensive Care National Audit and Research Centre.

Jones, H. J. S., Coggins, R., Lafuente, J., de Cossart, L. (1999). Value of a surgical high-dependency unit. *Br. J. Surg.*, **86**, 1578–1582.

Lam, S., Ridley, S. (1999). Critically ill medical patients, their demographics and outcome. *Anaesthesia*, **54**, 845–852.

Lee, A., Bishop, G., Hillman, K. M., Daffurn, K. (1995). The medical emergency team. *Anaesth. Intensive Care*, **23**, 183–186.

Lee, E. T. (1980). *Statistical Methods for Survival Data Analysis*, 2nd edn. Lifetime Learning.

Marshall, J. C., Cook, D. J., Christou N. V., Bernard, G. R., Sprung, C. L., Sibbald, W. J. (1995). Multiple Organ Dysfunction Score: a reliable descriptor of a complex clinical outcome. *Crit. Care Med.*, **23**, 1638–1652.

Moreno, R., Agthe, D. (1999). ICU discharge decision-making: are we able to decrease post-ICU mortality? *Intensive Care Med.*, **25**, 1035–1036.

Nasraway, S. A., Button, G. J. *et al.* (2000). Survivors of catastrophic illness: outcome after direct transfer from intensive care to extended care facilities. *Crit. Care Med.*, **28**, 19–25.

Niskanen, M., Kari, A., Halonen, P. (1996). Five-year survival after intensive care – comparison of 12,180 patients with the general population. Finnish ICU Study Group. *Crit. Care Med.*, **24**, 1962–1967.

Parikh, C. R., Karnad., D. R. (1999). Quality, cost, and outcome of intensive care in a public hospital in Bombay, India. *Crit. Care Med.*, **27**, 1754–1759.

Pollack, M. M., Ruttimann, U. E., Getson, P. R. (1988). Pediatric Risk of Mortality (PRISM) score. *Crit. Care Med.*, **16**, 1110–1116.

Reis Miranda, D., Ryan, D. W., Schaufeli, W. B., Fidler, V. (1998). *Organisation and Management of Intensive Care. A Prospective Study in 12 European Countries. Update in Intensive Care and Emergency Medicine.* Springer-Verlag.

Reynolds, H. N., Haupt, M. T., Thill-Baharozian, M. C., Carlson, R. W. (1994). Impact of critical care physician staffing on patients with septic shock in a university hospital medical intensive care unit. *JAMA*, **260**, 3446–3450.

Ridley, S. A., Plenderleith, L. (1994). Survival after intensive care. Comparison with a matched normal population as an indicator of effectiveness. *Anaesthesia*, **49**, 933–935.

Ridley, S. A. (2000). Quality of life and longer term outcomes. In: *Update in Intensive Care and Emergency Medicine 35. Evaluating Critical Care. Using Health Service Research to Improve Quality.* (W. J. Sibbald, J. F. Bion, eds) p. 111, Springer-Verlag.

Rowan, K. M., Kerr, J. H., Major E., McPherson, K., Short, A., Vessey, M. P. (1993). Intensive Care Society's APACHE II study in Britain and Ireland-I: Variations in case mix of adult admissions to general intensive care units and impact on outcome. *Br. Med. J.*, **307**, 972–977.

Rubenfeld, G. D., Crawford, S. W. (1996). Withdrawing life support from mechanically ventilated recipients of bone marrow transplants: a case for evidence-based guidelines. *Ann. Intern. Med.*, **125**, 625–633.

Sirio, C. A., Tajimi, K., Tase, C. *et al.* (1992). An initial comparison of intensive care in Japan and the United States. *Crit. Care Med.*, **20**, 1207–1215.

Smith, L., Orts, C. M., O'Neil, I., Batchelor, A. M., Gascoigne, A. D., Baudouin, S. V. (1999). TISS and mortality after discharge from intensive care. *Intensive Care Med.*, **25**, 1061–1065.

Vincent, J. L., Moreno, R., Matos, R. *et al.* (1996). The SOFA (Sepsis-related Organ Failure Assessment) score to describe organ dysfunction/failure. On behalf of the Working Group on Sepsis-Related Problems of the European Society of Intensive Care Medicine. *Intensive Care Med.*, **22**, 707–710.

Wallis, C. B., Davies, H. T. O., Shearer, A. J. (1997). Why do patients die on general wards after discharge from intensive care units? *Anaesthesia*, **52**, 9–14.

Watt, I., Ledingham, I. M. (1984). Mortality amongst multiple trauma patients admitted to an intensive therapy unit. *Anaesthesia*, **39**, 973–981.

Zaren, B., Bergstrom, R. (1988). Survival of intensive care patients I: prognostic factors from the patients' medical history. *Acta Anaesthesiol. Scand.*, **32,** 93–100.

Zimmerman, J. E., Knaus, W. A., Judson J. A. *et al.* (1988). Patient selection for intensive care: a comparison of New Zealand and United States hospitals. *Crit. Care Med.*, **16,** 318–326.

Chapter 3

Mortality probabilities and case-mix adjustment by prognostic models

Dieter Beck

Scoring systems and prognostic models

Scoring systems have been developed as instruments to standardize the assessment of severity of disease or injury by measuring the impact on functional and anatomical integrity of organ systems or the patient as a whole. Based on these measurements, patients can be stratified into different risk groups that are more or less likely to experience a certain outcome. Risk stratification is essential for describing a patient population and is prerequisite for scientific evaluation of treatment regimens and the comparison of the quality of care between hospitals and healthcare systems. The terms scoring system and prognostic system are often used interchangeably. However, scoring systems are distinct from prognostic models. Scoring systems provide a score for risk stratification and often form the basis for prognostic indices, but they do not convert the score into a probability. By contrast, most of the general intensive care specific prognostic systems are logistic regression models that are designed to predict the probability of hospital death (considered the dependent variable) from one or more explanatory variables. With increasing accountability for the quality and cost of care we deliver, prognostic models will become important instruments for monitoring efficiency and efficacy of intensive care medicine.

Overview: types of scoring systems

Scoring systems that primarily intend to measure severity of disease can be divided into disease- and organ-specific or general models. Organ- and disease-specific systems classify the degree of severity of illness or injury for a particular condition by measuring the level of organ dysfunction or the extent of structural injury. Some scoring methods measure a combination of both physiological and anatomical derangement.

General scoring systems measure the impact of disease or injury on the function of the whole patient. The original APACHE score (Knaus et al., 1981) and the Simplified Acute Physiology Score (SAPS) (Le Gall *et al.*, 1984) were the first physiology based scoring systems for the measurement of disease severity of intensive care patients. By contrast, the Therapeutic Intervention Scoring System (TISS) (Cullen *et al.*, 1976; Keene and Cullen, 1983) was initially developed as a severity of illness index that 'indirectly' measured severity by quantifying the intensity of treatment. Today, it is widely used to assess workload and resource utilization in intensive care (Reis Miranda *et al.*, 1996). A selection of scoring systems used in intensive care is shown in Table 3.1.

The general prognostic models that are mainly used in intensive care today include APACHE II (Knaus *et al.*, 1985), APACHE III (Knaus *et al.*, 1991), SAPS II (Le Gall *et al.*, 1993) and the Mortality Prediction Model (MPM) II (Lemeshow *et al.*, 1993). These systems primarily measure disease severity by patient characteristics and physiology. The Riyadh Intensive Care Program is a mortality prediction algorithm that combines daily APACHE II scores and organ failure coefficients for trend analysis of mortality risks (Chang *et al.*, 1988). As with the general models for adult intensive care patients, the Pediatric Risk of Mortality score (PRISM) was developed for use in paediatric intensive care units (ICUs) (Pollack *et al.*, 1988). A selection of prognostic models used in intensive care is presented in Table 3.2.

General scoring systems and prognostic models in intensive care

Acute Physiology And Chronic Health Evaluation (APACHE)

The original APACHE model was introduced in 1981 (Knaus *et al.*) and represented the prototype of a general physiology based scoring system developed to quantify severity of illness. It consisted of two major components: the acute physiology score (APS) and a pre-admission health evaluation. The method was developed using expert opinion, clinical judgement and evidence from previously published literature. An expert panel of seven physicians selected 34 physiological variables to be included in the score. Weights reflecting the relative importance of each variable on outcome were assigned on a scale from 0 to 4. The sum of the weightings for all variables yields the final APACHE score.

Acute Physiology And Chronic Health Evaluation (APACHE) II

A revision of the original method was introduced in 1985 (Knaus *et al.*). The APACHE II model incorporated three principal components: APS, age, and chronic health evaluation. The number of physiological variables was reduced to twelve, and their relative weights were readjusted, e.g. acute renal failure and the Glasgow coma score were assigned substantially greater weights. In addition, the

Table 3.1 Selection of scoring systems

Scoring system	Acronym	Application	Reference
General			
Therapeutic Intervention Scoring System	TISS	ICU, severity of illness	Cullen et al., 1976
Acute Physiology And Chronic Health Evaluation	APACHE	ICU, severity of illness	Knaus et al., 1981
Simplified Acute Physiology Score	SAPS	ICU, severity of illness	Le Gall et al., 1984
Organ- and disease-specific			
Child's classification	–	Liver disease	Child and Turcotte, 1964
Ranson's criteria	–	Acute pancreatitis	Ranson et al., 1974
Glasgow Coma Scale	GCS	Neurological function	Teasdale and Jennett, 1974
Burn Index	–	Burn injury	Feller et al., 1980
Injury Severity Score	ISS	Trauma	Baker et al., 1974
Trauma score	TS	Trauma	Champion et al., 1981
Trauma and Revised Injury Severity Score	TRISS	Trauma	Boyd et al., 1987

Table 3.2 Selection of prognostic models used in intensive care

Model (country)	Acronym	Year	ICU type	Main measurement	Disease diagnostic coding is required for generating mortality probabilities
Acute Physiology And Chronic Health Evaluation II (USA)	APACHE II	Knaus et al., 1983	General	Severity, physiology based	Yes
Acute Physiology And Chronic Health Evaluation III (USA)	APACHE III	Knaus et al., 1991	General	Severity, physiology based	Yes
Simplified Acute Physiology Score II (Europe and USA)	SAPS II	Le Gall et al., 1993	General	Severity, physiology based	No
Mortality Prediction Model (USA)	MPM	Lemeshow et al., 1993	General	Severity, condition based	No
Riyadh Intensive Care Program (UK)	RICP	Chang et al., 1988	General	Severity, physiology and organ failure	No
Pediatric Risk of Mortality score (USA)	PRISM	Pollack et al., 1988	Paediatric	Severity, physiology based	No

Table 3.3 Acute Physiology And Chronic Health Evaluation (APACHE) II: criteria and definitions for scoring

Acute physiology score points	4	3	2	1	0	1	2	3	4
Rectal temperature (°C)	≥41.0	39.0–40.9		38.5–38.9	36.0–38.4	34.0–35.9	32.0–33.9	30.0–31.9	≤29.9
Mean blood pressure (mmHg)	≥160	130–159	110–129		70–109		50–69		≤49
Heart rate (beats/min)	≥180	140–179	110–139		70–109		55–69	40–54	≤39
Respiratory rate (breaths/min)	≥50	35–49		25–34	12–24	10–11	6–9		≤5
Oxygenation (kPa*)									
$F_iO_2 \geq 0.5$ A-aDO_2	66.5	46.6–66.4	26.6–46.4		<26.6				
$F_iO_2 < 0.5$ P_aO_2					>9.3	8.1–9.3		7.3–8.0	<7.3
Arterial pH	≥7.70	7.60–7.69		7.50–7.59	7.33–7.49		7.25–7.32	7.15–7.24	<7.15
Serum sodium (mmol/l)	≥180	160–179	155–159	150–154	130–149		120–129	111–119	≤110
Serum potassium (mmol/l)	≥7.0	6.0–6.9		5.5–5.9	3.5–5.4	3.0–3.4	2.5–2.9		<2.5
Serum creatinine (µmol/l)	≥300	171–299		121–170	50–120		<50		
Packed cell volume (%)	≥60		50–59.9	46–49.9	30–45.9		20–29.9		<20
White blood cell count ($\times 10^9/l$)	≥40		20–39.9	15–19.9	3–14.9		1–2.9		<1

*If fraction of inspired oxygen F_iO_2 is ≥ 0.5 the alveolar-arterial gradient (A-a DO_2) is assigned points. F_iO_2 is < 0.5 partial pressure of oxygen is used.

Points for creatinine are doubled in the presence of acute renal failure.

Glasgow Coma Scale: score is subtracted from 15 to obtain points. Age < 45 = 0 points, 45–54 = 2, 55–64 = 3, 65–75 = 5, ≥ 75 = 6

Chronic health points (must be present before hospital admission): chronic liver disease with hypertension or previous hepatic failure, encephalopathy or coma; chronic heart failure (New York Heart Association grade 4); chronic respiratory disease with severe exercise limitation, secondary polycythaemia or long-term high dose steroid therapy, leukaemia, acquired immune deficiency syndrome. Five points for emergency surgery or non-surgical patient, 2 points for elective surgical patient.

type of admission (i.e. emergency surgical versus elective surgical or medical) was incorporated in the model (Table 3.3).

The most important modifications were the introduction of a system for diagnostic coding of the primary reason for ICU admission, and the inclusion of a variable for the type of admission (i.e. emergency surgery). The disease classification system consisted of 53 specific disease definitions and five organ system categories. The APACHE II model has probably become the most widely used system in intensive care medicine, but has also been applied to other settings.

Acute Physiology And Chronic Health Evaluation (APACHE) III

A revised version of the APACHE II system was introduced in 1991 (Knaus *et al.*) and had a similar structure to its predecessor; the APACHE III system consisted of a numerical score (range: 0 to 299) reflecting the weights assigned to the variables of three principal data categories: physiological measurements, chronic health status and chronological age. APACHE III uses data from 16 physiological measurements. Five new physiological variables were introduced (i.e. albumin concentration, plasma urea, bilirubin, glucose levels and urine output) and two variables (i.e. potassium concentration and plasma bicarbonate) were omitted. The chronic health component was modified and is now based on seven variables referring to the presence or absence of haematological malignancies, lymphoma, acquired immune deficiency syndrome, metastatic cancer, immune suppression, hepatic failure and liver cirrhosis.

The system for diagnostic coding was also altered. The APACHE III model includes 78 disease definitions to group patients according to the principal reason for ICU admission. The definitions for the type of admission were specified. Patients admitted directly from the operating or recovery room were classified as postoperative (surgical), and are further subdivided according to the urgency of the operation (i.e. elective versus emergency). All other patients are classified as non-operative (medical). In order to assess the impact of therapeutic interventions before ICU admission (lead-time bias), additional information about the patients' treatment location immediately prior to admission was integrated into the APACHE III model. Although the definitions and criteria required for the computation of the APACHE III score were published, the regression coefficients which form the APACHE III equation are not in the public domain and have to be obtained from the developers.

Simplified Acute Physiology Score (SAPS) II

The SAPS was developed in 1984 by independent researchers in an attempt to simplify the original APACHE score (Le Gall *et al.*). Fourteen variables, including chronological age, were selected by regression analysis and were assigned largely the same weights as in the original APACHE score. An updated version (SAPS II) which allowed computation of mortality probabilities was introduced in 1993. The development of the SAPS II prognostic model was based on a cohort of medical and surgical intensive care patients from European and North American hospitals (Le Gall *et al.*, 1993). A set of 37 candidate variables was chosen for clinical reasons by an international team of 'expert' physicians. The final selection and weighting of the variables was achieved by the use of logistic regression techniques. The SAPS II model included 17 variables: twelve physiological measurements, chronological age, type of admission (i.e. unscheduled versus scheduled, surgical versus medical) and three variables relating to pre-existing co-morbidities (i.e. acquired immune deficiency syndrome, metastatic cancer and haematological malignancies). The weights assigned to the 17 variables range from 0 to 26 points. The sum of the weights forms the individual SAPS II score, which can reach a maximum of 158 points. The Glasgow coma score is incorporated as one of the physiological variables. Diagnostic coding of the reason for ICU admission is not required as the developers of SAPS II maintain that diagnostic coding is so difficult in the ICU that it may be unreliable. The variables and criteria for calculating the SAPS II score are summarized in Table 3.4.

Mortality Prediction Models

The Mortality Prediction Models (MPM) are statistically derived prognostic systems and differ in several respects from the empirically derived APACHE and SAPS scores. The MPM models are primarily based on conditions, rather than on physiological data, and contain almost exclusively binary variables that refer to the presence or absence of a certain condition. This reduces the impact of treatment effects on the patients' physiology and hence the extent of measured organ dysfunction as quantified by physiologically based scores.

The development of the initial MPM model was based on the data of a single centre in the USA (Lemeshow *et al.*, 1985, 1988). Applying multiple logistic regression techniques, the developers selected 11 explanatory variables from a pool of 137 background disease- and treatment-related variables at admission and, in addition, 75 variables relating to the first 24 h after admission. The authors described both an admission model (MPM_0) and a model (MPM_{24}) that reflected the first 24 h after ICU admission. In 1993, a major revision of the initial models was presented (Lemeshow *et al.*, 1993). The two models, MPM_0 II and MPM_{24} II together comprising the new MPM II system, were derived from data of critically ill patients from 139 hospitals in 12 different countries. The MPM_{24} II model consists of 13 variables: age, medical and emergency surgical admission, the presence of four co-morbid conditions (i.e. cirrhosis, intracranial mass effect, metastatic cancer, confirmed infection) and five physiological measurements, including coma. The two remaining variables (i.e. mechanical ventilation and vasoactive drugs) refer to therapeutic interventions during the first 24 h of ICU stay. In 1994, the MPM_{24} model was modified to allow prognostication of patients at 48 and 72 h of their ICU stay. The MPM_{48} II and MPM_{72} models use the same variables and regression coefficients as the MPM_{24} model, but the constants of the regression equation were adjusted (Lemeshow *et al.*, 1994).

Table 3.4 Simplified Acute Physiology Score (SAPS) II; criteria and definitions for scoring

Variable	Value	Points	Value	Points	Value	Points	Value	Points	Value	Points	Value	Points
Age (years)	<40	0	40–59	7	60–69	12	70–74	15	75–79	16	≥80	18
Heart rate (beats/min)	<40	11	40–69	2	70–119	0	120–159	4	≥160	7		
Systolic blood pressure (mmHg)	<70	13	70–99	5	100–199	0	≥200	2				
Body temperature (°C)	<39	0	≥39	3								
P_aO_2/F_iO_2 (mmHg)	<100	11	100–199	9	≥200	6						
P_aO_2/F_iO_2 (kPa)	<13.3	11	13.3–26.5	9	≥26.6	6						
Urinary output (l/d)	<0.5	11	0.50–0.99	4	≥1.0	0						
Serum urea level (mmol/l) or	<10	0	10.0–29.9	6	≥30.0	10						
Serum urea nitrogen level (mg/dl)	<28	0	28–33	6	≥84	10						
White blood cell count ($\times 10^9$/l)	<1	12	1.0–19.9	0	≥20.0	3						
Serum potassium (mmol/l)	<3.0	3	3.0–4.9	0	≥5	3						
Serum sodium level (mmol/l)	<125	5	125–144	0	≥145	1						
Serum bicarbonate level (mmol/l)	<15	6	15–19	3	≥20	0						
Serum bilirubin level (μmol/dl)	<68.4	0	68.4–102.5	4	≥102.6	9						
Glasgow Coma Scale	<6	26	6–8	13	9–10	7	11–13	5	14–15	0		
Chronic diseases	Metastatic cancer	9	Haematological malignancy	10	AIDS	17						
Type of admission	Scheduled surgical	0	Medical	6	Unscheduled surgical	8						

Points: points for SAPS II score; F_iO_2: fraction of inspired oxygen; AIDS: acquired immune deficiency syndrome; P_aO_2: points for oxygenation are only assigned in ventilated patients, or if pulmonary artery pressure is monitored; the lowest value of the ratio is used.

Structure of prognostic models

Multiple regression analysis is employed to develop models for prediction of outcome from several explanatory variables. In medicine, regression models relating to patient outcome are termed prognostic models and are used for investigating patient outcome in relation to patient and disease characteristics.

Principles of multiple regression analysis

Multiple regression is a statistical method for estimating the magnitude of the association between exposure and outcome while controlling simultaneously for a number of potential confounding variables. It is an extension of the most basic model describing the relationship between two variables, namely simple linear regression. In simple linear regression, the relationship between the dependent (outcome) variable (Y) and the independent (predictor, explanatory) variable (X) is described by the equation $Y = a + bX$, which when graphically displayed corresponds to a straight line. Linear regression is used to assess the association of one (simple regression) or more (multiple regression) explanatory variables with a continuous outcome variable (e.g. blood pressure).

In medicine, the outcome of interest is often a binary variable, referring to the presence or absence of an event (e.g. disease, death). Logistic regression is a variant of multiple regression, relating binary outcomes to one or more explanatory factors. As with linear regression, the outcome variable (Y) can be expressed as a linear function of the explanatory (predictor) variables ($X_{1+ \ldots +n}$) by the general formula:

$$Y = a + b_1X + b_2X + \ldots + b_nX$$

where a is the constant (also termed the intercept of the regression) and $b_{1+ \ldots +n}$ are the regression coefficients of the respective predictive variables (Hennekens and Buring, 1987).

Basic structure of logistic regression models

Most of the prognostic methods used in intensive care are logistic regression models. The complex underlying mathematical principles are the subject of several textbooks and it is not proposed to discuss this methodology in detail. I shall briefly describe the basic concepts and components of logistic regression models, and the advantages and limitations of their application for prognostic modelling.

In intensive care, the main outcome measure is commonly a binary variable, such as vital status at hospital discharge (i.e. dead versus alive). As mentioned before, logistic regression models are employed when investigating binary patient outcomes in relation to patient and disease characteristics. To estimate the probability of hospital death from binary outcome variables, a 'logistic transformation' of Y needs to be performed. The dependent or outcome variable (Y) in a logistic regression model is defined as the natural logarithm (ln) of the odds of the outcome (also termed the logit). If P denotes the probability of hospital death, then the term $P/(1 - P)$ represents the odds of experiencing the outcome. The log odds or logit is defined as ln $[P/(1 - P)]$ and is a linear function of the predictive variables ($X_{1+ \ldots +n}$). The regression equation can be expressed as follows:

$$Y = \text{logit} = \ln [P/(1 - P)] = a + b_1 X + \ldots + b_n X$$

The probability of hospital death is obtained by transforming the logit according to the following formula:

$$P = e^{\text{logit}}/(1 + e^{\text{logit}}) = 1/(1 + e^{-\text{logit}})$$

By convention, the values for the probability always range between zero and one, but are often expressed as a percentage by simply multiplying by 100. The practical advantage of logistic regression is that, provided the explanatory variables are also binary, the antilogarithms of the regression coefficients are the odds ratios for those variables. Thus, the coefficients can be directly converted into an odds ratio, which is a good estimate of the relative risk associated with a single factor while controlling for the effects of all other variables in the model (Hennekens and Buring, 1987).

Estimation of mortality probabilities using prognostic models

The APACHE II equation gives an example of the structure of a regression model that contains three explanatory variables: (1) APACHE II score; (2) emergency surgery; and (3) diagnosis. The general format of the regression equation is:

$$\text{logit}_{\text{APACHE II}} = \ln [P/(1 - P)]$$
$$= -3.517 + 0.146 \times (\text{APACHE score}) + 0.603 \times (\text{ES}) + [\text{diagnosis}]$$

The constant, or intercept, is -3.517. The coefficient of 0.603 is only relevant for patients who had emergency surgery (ES = 1); for medical or elective surgical patients (ES = 0), this coefficient becomes zero and so the term '$0.603 \times (\text{ES})$' can simply be omitted. The diagnostic weight has to be obtained from a list of 53 specific diagnoses or organ system categories, which are applied if none of the specific diagnoses matches the principal reason for ICU admission.

As an example, take two patients who were admitted to ICU after surgery for gastrointestinal bleeding. Patient A suffered from a major gastrointestinal bleed that required emergency surgery, while Patient B had a less severe bleed and was operated on electively. The 24-h APACHE II scores were 18 and 10, for Patient A and B, respectively. The diagnostic weight for 'GI bleeding, postoperative' (−0.617) is identical for both patients. This results in the following probabilities of hospital mortality:

Patient A:

$$logit_{APACHE\,II} = -3.517 + 0.146 \times \mathbf{18} + \mathbf{0.603} \times \mathbf{1} + [\mathbf{-0.617}] = -0.903$$

Mortality probability: $P = 1/(1 + e^{-logit}) = 1/(1 + e^{0.903}) = 0.288 = 28.8\%$

Patient B:

$$logit_{APACHE\,II} = -3.517 + 0.146 \times \mathbf{10} + 0.603 \times 0 + [\mathbf{-0.617}] = -2.674$$

Mortality probability: $P = 1/(1 + e^{-logit}) = 1/(1 + e^{2.674}) = 0.0654 = 6.5\%$

The relative risk of emergency surgery, expressed by the odds ratio (OR), is calculated as follows:

$$OR = e^{-0.603} = 1.83.$$

Thus, the fact that Patient A had emergency surgery was associated with 1.83-fold increased risk of hospital death adjusted for the effects on outcome of all other variables in the model.

Comparison of mortality probabilities by different models

The SAPS II model is an example of a regression model that includes two explanatory variables: (1) the SAPS II score and (2) a logarithmic transformation of the score, which was introduced to compensate for the skewed distribution in the original dataset (Le Gall *et al.*, 1993). The SAPS II regression equation is expressed as:

$$logit_{SAPS\,II} = \beta_0 + \beta_1 \,(SAPS\,II\,score) + \beta_2 \,[\ln\,(SAPS\,II\,score + 1)]$$
$$= -7.7631 + 0.0737 \,(SAPS\,II\,score) +$$
$$0.9971 \,[\ln\,(SAPS\,II\,score + 1)]$$

where β_0 is the constant or intercept, β_1 and β_2 are the regression coefficients. The criteria used to calculate the SAPS II and APACHE II scores are summarized in Table 3.5.

As an example, if the patient had a total SAPS II score of 49 points. The predicted hospital mortality is:

$$logit_{SAPS\,II} = -7.7631 + 0.0737 \times \mathbf{49} + 0.9971 \,[\ln\,(\mathbf{49} + 1)] = 0.2511$$

Mortality probability: $P = 1/(1 + e^{-logit}) = 1/(1 + e^{-0.2511}) = 0.437 = 43.7\%$

Table 3.5 Comparison of mortality probabilities by APACHE II and SAPS II for a 71-year-old man admitted to ICU from the Accident and Emergency Department. The patient had a diagnosis of abdominal aortic aneurysm and was breathing spontaneously. The fractional inspired oxygen concentration (F_iO_2) was 0.4. For SAPS II: P_aO_2 is only scored in ventilated patients or patients with a pulmonary artery catheter. Type of admission is medical because the patient had no surgical intervention.

Criteria	Value	SAPS II points	APACHE II points
Age	71 years	15	5
Chronic disease	None	0	0
Type of admission	Medical	6	0
Physiology			
Temperature	38.5°C	0	1
Mean blood pressure	60 mmHg	–	2
Systolic blood pressure	85 mmHg	5	–
Heart rate	136 beats/min	4	2
Respiratory rate	28 breaths/min	–	1
Partial arterial oxygen tension P_aO_2	13 kPa	–	0
pH	7.09	–	4
Urine output	0.4 l/d	11	–
Serum sodium	150 mmol/l	1	1
Serum potassium	4.2 mmol/l	0	0
Serum creatinine	145 μmol/l	–	1
Serum bilirubin	81 mmol/l	4	–
Packed cell volume	29%	–	2
White blood cell count	$20 \times 10^9/l$	3	2
Glasgow coma score	14	0	1
Total points		49	22

Using the same physiological and other values, the total APACHE II score for this patient is 22 points; the diagnostic weight for non-operative abdominal aortic aneurysm is 0.731. The patient did not undergo emergency surgery, thus the respective term in the equation becomes zero:

$$\text{logit}_{\text{APACHE II}} = -3.517 + 0.146 \times \textbf{22} + 0.603 \times 0 + [\textbf{0.731}] = 0.426$$

Mortality probability: $P = 1/(1 + e^{-\text{logit}}) = 1/(1 + e^{-0.426}) = 0.460 = 46.0\%$

APACHE II and SAPS II are related models as they have a number of common variables for the calculation of the scores. Therefore, both models can be expected to produce similar, but not necessarily identical, individual mortality predictions. The above example shows that different predictive models can generate different mortality probabilities for the same individual, depending on the variables used. The mortality for the whole population, however, should be similar as described by different models provided they are equally well calibrated (Lemeshow *et al.*, 1995).

Principles of model building and validation

Model building

Multivariable statistical methods are usually employed for model building. The application of these techniques, particularly the selection and categorization of the variables is complex and requires expert guidance. The process of model building includes data collection, definition, categorization and selection of the variables that could be considered for inclusion in the model; it may also involve data transformation and testing for variable interactions. Inaccuracy results from two principal sources, deficiencies in data collection and deficiencies in the standard modelling techniques used to derive the predictive method.

Similar to carefully designed clinical trials, preliminary steps before modelling should include unequivocal variable definition, clear exclusion and inclusion criteria, and the assessment of the reliability of data. Violation of these principles, inadequate sample size and a high frequency of missing data may all contribute to biased or over optimistic predictions of the final regression model (Harrell *et al.*, 1996; Altman and Royston, 2000).

Data reduction and variable selection

For clinical purposes, a predictive method should be based on a small number of explanatory variables that are routinely obtainable and measured reliably. Ideally the variables should not be affected by therapeutic interventions, so that any treatment effect is minimized. Often a large number of possible variables is available. In order to enhance predictive accuracy, the number of variables needs to be reduced or the model should be simplified unless the sample is large. The need to select the important variables from a large pool of 'candidate' variables is the major source for the data-dependency of most prognostic models. This can lead to 'over optimism' regarding the model's predictive performance where the model seems to be better than it actually is.

Different multivariable methods can be applied to derive prognostic models, but all have data-dependent aspects. Multiple regression, using a stepwise selection algorithm (i.e. forward or backward) that is based on multiple sequential hypotheses testing, is the most commonly applied technique for variable selection. In backward multiple regression, for example, all variables considered for inclusion in the model are tested. A P value < 0.05 is often used as the standard inclusion criterion. At each stage, the one variable that makes the least contribution to the variation in outcome is eliminated from further analysis. The stepwise exclusion of 'non-significant factors' continues until all the remaining variables are significant, or until a predetermined limit for the maximum number of variables in the model has been reached. The limitations of this technique are obvious. Altman and Royston (2000) stated that 'this is a fully automated procedure requiring no intellectual input. There is no reason why it should yield the model which is best in a predictive sense'.

An alternative method is best subsets regression. This technique allows a systematic search through different combinations of predictive variables, selecting those subsets that best contribute to the variation in patient outcome. This methodology may have advantages over stepwise variable selection, but has essentially the same limitations. Small sample size aggravates the effects of data-dependent variable selection, increasing the risk of including unimportant variables while, at the same time, omitting important ones (Altman and Royston, 2000). Preselection of potential predictive variables, guided by expert knowledge and clinical judgement, are useful steps for data reduction. Early exclusion (deletion) of candidate variables with little chance of being predictive or measured reliably will result in models with better performance (Harrell and Lee, 1984).

Overfitting

Overfitting is a common problem and results from the inclusion of unimportant variables with no impact on outcome in the model (Harrell *et al.*, 1996). An important aspect is the number of events (e.g. deaths) per variable considered for inclusion in the model. The inclusion of a large number of variables in a regression model may appear to improve prediction in the developmental sample. However, when a data set contains too few outcome events in relation to the number of explanatory variables overfitting of the training (development) data is likely to be present. When applied to an independent sample, the model often has poorer predictive accuracy (Harrell and Lee, 1984; Concato *et al.*, 1995)

In regression analysis, few events per variable may affect the accuracy and precision of regression coefficients for the explanatory variables. Like Type I errors, the null hypothesis that a variable has no impact on outcome may be falsely rejected, or the analysis may lack the power to detect the impact of important variables. It has been suggested that for regression modelling the events per variable should be at least ten times, or even 20 times, the number of explanatory variables included in the model (Harrell and Lee, 1984; Concato *et al.*, 1995).

In logistic regression, the count of the lower number of the binary outcome events (e.g. deaths or survival) is used to calculate the events per variable ratio. Assuming that 10 explanatory variables were examined for their association with 50 deaths in a sample of 1000 patients, then the ratio of events per variable equals 5 (50/10). For continuous outcome variables (e.g. haemoglobin concentration) the events per variable is computed on the entire sample size (1000/10 = 100) (Concato *et al.*, 1995).

Model validation

The performance of statistical models developed for outcome prediction needs to be evaluated. Irrespective of how well a model performs in the developmental sample, a method that is only able to predict outcome in the sample in which it was developed is of no practical worth. The clinical usefulness of a prognostic method is determined primarily by its ability to adapt well to different environments. The wider issue of generalizability – the model's ability to provide accurate predictions in a new series of patients – is not addressed by measuring the apparent accuracy of the model in the developmental sample (Harrell *et al.*, 1996).

The accuracy of predictions commonly decays when prognostic systems are applied to populations that are plausibly related to but different from the developmental cohort. This lack of generalizability is reflected by a model's failure to produce accurate predictions for a similar patient sample from the same centre. Also the model may not be transportable to another location with a new population (Table 3.6).

Table 3.6 Prognostic models: accuracy and generalizability

Terms	Definitions
Accuracy	
Calibration	Degree to which predicted match observed outcomes
Discrimination	Ability to classify correctly patients who do or do not experience the outcome of interest
Generalizability	
Reproducibility	Accuracy of predictions in new sample other than the developmental sample, but from the same institution
Transportability	The accuracy of predictions for patients from a different population, with similar characteristics as the developmental sample, but from a differnt institution

The dissimilarity between patients in different centres or countries is known as case-mix variation. The poor performance of many ICU specific prognostic models applied to new populations has been largely attributed to their failure to adjust appropriately for different case-mix.

Internal and external validation

Validation quantifies the model's ability to measure what it is intended to measure. Internal validation is closely related to the process of model building.

After the model has been developed on the training data (development set), it is then applied to a new sample from the same institution. Internal validation is a prerequisite for the application of a model to other settings, but it does not address the wider issue of transportability. The use of statistical techniques such as shrinkage of the regression coefficients to correct for overfitting may help make the model more transportable (Harrell *et al.*, 1996), but the question as to whether the model provides accurate predictions in a different population can ultimately be answered only by external validation (Wyatt and Altman, 1995). External validation is the most stringent test of validity, and involves the assessment of the model's performance when applied to a new population from a new institution or environment.

Methods for model validation

The principal methods for internal validation of prognostic models are data splitting, cross-validation and bootstrapping. Common to all three methods is the use of validation samples, which are generated from the original dataset using different techniques. The predictive accuracy of the model is then assessed on the validation sample (internal validation) using formal tests of discrimination and calibration. In the case of external validation, the same tests are applied to assess model performance in a new series of patients.

In data splitting, a random portion, for instance, two-thirds of the developmental sample, is chosen for all steps of model development (i.e. data transformation, variable selection, testing for interaction, estimating regression coefficients). The model is then applied to the remaining third (validation sample) for computing calibration statistics and tests of discrimination. Data splitting is simple because all steps involved in model building have to be done only once (Picard and Berk, 1990). Cross-validation repeatedly splits the data and does not rely on a single data split. The size of the development set can be much larger because fewer data are needed for the validation process. Bootstrapping is an alternative method that involves taking a large number of samples for validation with replacement in the original sample. Bootstrapping provides almost unbiased estimates of the predictive accuracy and has the advantage that the entire dataset is used for model development (Efron, 1979; Efron and Tibshirani, 1993).

Quantifying predictive accuracy

Predictive accuracy can be defined as the degree to which predictions match outcomes and consists of two components: calibration (reliability) and discrimination (refinement or spread). Calibration reflects the deviation of individual predicted probabilities from actual outcome, while discrimination is the ability to distinguish between patients who do or do not experience the outcome of interest.

Predictions may therefore be inaccurate in two principal ways. First, the predicted probabilities may be too high or too low (poor calibration) and second, the ranking of the individual risk estimates may be out of order (poor discrimination) (Justice *et al.*, 1999). A third source of inaccuracy may be that the contribution to the overall deviation is exceptionally high for certain subsets of the study population for which the model does not perform well (Miller *et al.*, 1991). One of the reasons why the model's calibration for a new population may deteriorate is simply that the prevalence of outcome events in the new series of patients is much lower or much higher than in the original population.

Testing model performance

Several statistical methods should be employed to assess formally the overall goodness-of-fit of the models. Criteria for evaluating model performance were published by the RAND consensus conference in 1993 (Hadorn *et al.*). It was agreed that measures of calibration and discrimination are complementary.

Using any of the models, a probability of death of 0.3 means that of 100 patients, 30 patients are expected to die. If, in fact, 30 patients die, the predictions are well calibrated. However, this does not allow any inference regarding the individual patients as to who will be among the 30 non-survivors and who will be among the 70 survivors. If the model assigns higher mortality probabilities to individuals who actually survive, while patients with low mortality probabilities die, then the model poorly discriminates between survivors and non-survivors.

Testing discrimination

The testing of model discrimination is based on the concept of sensitivity (true positive rate) and specificity (true negative rate) and is usually assessed by means of 2 by 2 contingency tables, and by receiver operating characteristics (ROC) curves. For prognostic models, the sensitivity is the proportion of patients correctly classified to die, and specificity is the proportion of patients correctly classified to survive. The total correct classification rate is the proportion of all patients, survivors and non-survivors, correctly classified by the model.

Correct classification

Sensitivity, specificity and total correct classification rate can be derived from 2 by 2 contingency tables. Arbitrary cut-off levels are applied to divide the patient sample into two groups, one with individual mortality probabilities below and one with probabilities above the cut-off point. For example, when a cut-off point for mortality probability of 0.5 is used, all individuals with predicted mortalities < 0.5 form one group, and the remaining patients with probabilities ≥ 0.5 constitute the other. By convention, all patients in the group above the cut-off point are classified to die, those in the group below the cut-off point are classified to survive. Clearly, very different patients can be in the same group, and quite similar patients may be allocated to different groups. For instance, patients with probabilities of 0.05 and 0.49 are allocated to the same group and are classified to survive, but individuals with probabilities of 0.49 and 0.51 are assigned to different groups. For clinical reasons, it is not plausible for patients with very different probabilities to experience the same outcome; however, a binary classification implies this (Lemeshow *et al.*, 1995).

Moreover, sensitivity and specificity also depend on the distribution of mortality probabilities. The following hypothetical classification tables illustrate these limitations where a decision threshold of 0.5 is applied to an imaginary sample of 10 000 ICU patients, all of whom have either very low (0.1) or extremely high (0.9) mortality probabilities (Table 3.7a).

Ninety percent of the patients predicted to die, actually died, while 10% of those predicted to live, actually died. The discrimination of the model, as reflected by the total correct classification rate, looks good; it correctly classified death and survival for 90% of the patients.

Table 3.7a Sample A with mortality probabilities of either 0.1 (predicted survivors) or 0.9 (predicted non-survivors) (decision criterion 0.5)

	True dead	*True alive*	*Total*
Predicted dead	2700	300	3000
Predicted alive	700	6300	7000
Total	3400	6600	10000
Sensitivity:	2700/3400 = 79.4%		
Specificity:	6300/6600 = 95.5%		
Total correct classification rate:	(2700 + 6300)/10000 = 90%		

Table 3.7b Sample B with mortality probabilities of either 0.4 (predicted survivors) or 0.6 (predicted non-survivors) (decision criterion 0.5)

	True dead	*True alive*	*Total*
Predicted dead	1800	1200	3000
Predicted alive	2800	4200	7000
Total	4600	5400	10000
Sensitivity:	1800/4600 = 39.1%		
Specificity:	4200/5400 = 77.7%		
Total correct classification rate:	(1800 + 4200)/10000 = 60%		

The calculations are repeated with a second sample of 10 000 patients with a different pattern of mortality probabilities, either 0.4 or 0.6 (Table 3.7b) but the same decision criterion (0.5). By definition, patients with probabilities of 0.4 are predicted to survive, and patients with probabilities of 0.6 are predicted to die. However, this time because of the altered mortality probabilities, 40% actually died, and of those patients predicted to die, only 60% did in fact die. Thus, the sensitivity and total correct classification rate have deteriorated as a result of the distribution of mortality probabilities. These two examples illustrate how the performance of the model is influenced by the estimates of mortality and decision thresholds.

Receiver operating characteristics (ROC) curves

ROC curves are an expression of the relationship between sensitivity (true positive rate) and specificity (true negative rate) of a method, and reflect the model's ability to discriminate correctly between survivors and non-survivors (Hanley and McNeil, 1982). From Table 3.7, it is clear that discrimination cannot be adequately described using a single sensitivity/specificity pair derived from the classification table for a single decision criterion. The ROC curve provides a measure of sensitivity and specificity across the entire spectrum of possible decision criteria, and reflects the proportion of patients who not only died, but who also had higher mortality probabilities than had non-survivors (Ridley, 1998).

ROC curves are constructed by plotting the false positive rate (1 – specificity) against the true positive rate (sensitivity), using values for sensitivity and specificity obtained for 10, or sometimes 20, different thresholds (Figure 3.1).

The curve of a model that discriminates well extends into the left upper corner; the proportion of patients incorrectly classified to die remains low until a high level of sensitivity (i.e. the proportion correctly classified to die) is achieved (Fletcher et al., 1988). Thus, the better the discrimination of the model, the greater is the area under the ROC curve. The curves of models that discriminate less well fall closer to the diagonal line (45 degrees), which indicates discrimination no better than chance (area under the curve = 0.5). An area under the curve of $\geq$ 0.7, is generally regarded as acceptable, values $\geq$ 0.8 and $\geq$ 0.9 indicate good and very good discrimination (Hanley and McNeil, 1982).

Testing calibration or model fit

The model's fit or calibration is commonly tested by Hosmer-Lemeshow goodness-of-fit statistics, and can be graphically displayed using calibration curves.

Hosmer-Lemeshow statistics

Hosmer-Lemeshow C- and H-tests are summary statistics to assess the agreement between the actual and predicted outcomes across the range of estimated risks (Lemeshow and Hosmer, 1982; Hosmer and Lemeshow, 1989). The test basically

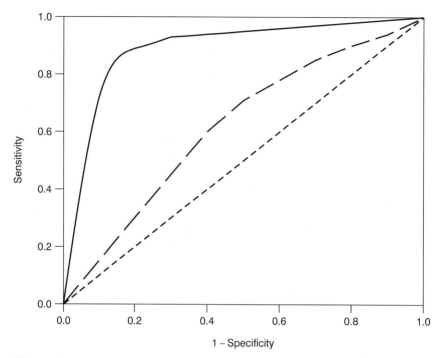

Figure 3.1 Receiver operating characteristics curves. The dotted line (area under the curve = 0.5) indicates that discrimination is no better than chance. The upper curve (solid line) indicates good discrimination (large area under the ROC curve), while the curve that falls closer to the 45 degree line (dashed line) indicates poor discrimination (small area under the ROC curve).

asks whether among 100 patients with predicted mortality probabilities of 0.30, in fact, 30 patients died. Both the C- and H-tests use the same χ^2- like statistic calculated from 2×10 contingency tables with 8 degrees of freedom (df) for the developmental sample and 10 degrees of freedom for the validation sample. The difference between observed and predicted mortality is calculated for each group, and summed across all ranges of observed mortalities. The value of the test statistic increases with increasing differences between expected and observed outcomes providing statistical evidence that the model is not well calibrated (Lemeshow *et al.*, 1995).

The difference between the two tests lies in the criteria applied to group the patients. For the C-test, individual patients are ranked by ascending mortality probabilities and are usually divided into 10 groups with approximately equal numbers of patients (Table 3.8).

For the Lemeshow-Hosmer H-test, 10% risk bands are used to allocate patients to one of ten groups; for example, all patients with predicted risks > 10% and ≤ 20% would be allocated to the second risk band. Patients with predicted risks > 90% would be assigned to the tenth stratum.

Table 3.8 Test of model calibration: Hosmer–Lemeshow C– statistics

Deciles	Patients (n)	Deaths (n)		Survivors (n)	
		Observed	Estimated	Observed	Estimated
0–1.5	1664	22	15.4	1642	1648.6
>1.5–2.9	1665	77	39.5	1588	1625.5
>2.9–5.2	1664	121	67.2	1543	1596.8
>5.2–7.2	1665	166	104.3	1499	1560.7
>7.2–16.7	1665	223	155.0	1442	1510.0
>16.7–26.6	1664	303	233.5	1361	1430.5
>26.6–41.5	1665	534	355.4	1131	1309.6
>41.5–57.5	1664	640	552.8	1024	1111.2
>57.5–66.1	1665	998	885.5	667	779.5
>66.1–100	1665	1335	1373.2	330	291.8
Total	16646	4419	3781.7	12227	12864.3
	$\chi^2 = 287.5$	df = 8,	$P<0.0001$		

Calibration curves

Calibration curves are constructed by plotting the estimated death rates stratified by 5% or 10% intervals of mortality risk (x-axis) against the observed death rates (y-axis). The 45 degree line indicates perfect agreement between observed and predicted outcome. Deviations of the calibration curve above this line indicate that the model underestimated true mortality while curves below the line suggest overestimation of actual mortality (Figure 3.2).

Testing uniformity-of-fit

Poor performance for subsets of the ICU population has been identified as a possible source for the poor fit of logistic regression models. Imperfect characterization of a large subgroup of ICU patients can impair the model's overall goodness-of-fit (Miller *et al.*, 1991). Uniformity-of-fit refers to the model's ability uniformly to adjust across different subgroups of the ICU population. For patients grouped by age, by disease and by location before ICU admission, large variations in the performance of all commonly used models were observed (Rowan *et al.*, 1993a; Moreno *et al.*, 1998b; Pappachan *et al.*, 1999). A simple approach to analysis of model performance for subgroups is to calculate standardized mortality ratios (SMRs) and their respective confidence intervals. Wide confidence intervals or SMRs significantly different from unity may suggest poor uniformity of fit in the population under investigation.

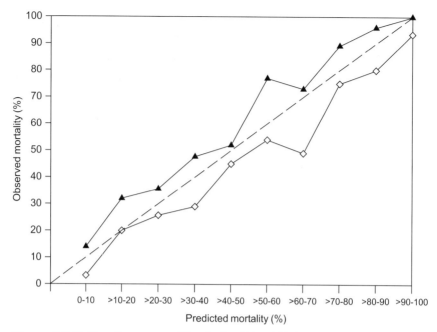

Figure 3.2 Calibration curves. The dashed line (45 degrees) indicates perfect agreement between predicted and observed mortality. Model A (solid triangles) tends to underestimate the actual mortality, the observed mortality is higher than predicted (curve above the diagonal). Model B (open diamonds) overestimates true mortality (curve below the diagonal).

The practical application of prognostic models

All general prognostic models used in intensive care showed good discrimination and calibration for those patients on whom the models were developed and for comparable patient populations from the same institutions used for internal validation. Tests of model discrimination and calibration of the prognostic models on new patients in different hospitals at a later time period (external validation) revealed a different picture. With one exception (Markgraf *et al.*, 2000), all published studies providing detailed information on the assessment of model performance (ROC curves and Hosmer-Lemeshow statistics) show the same pattern: the discrimination is good, but model calibration is imperfect (Teres and Lemeshow, 1998). This pattern is consistent for all commonly used general models, including APACHE III, APACHE II, SAPS II and the MPM II models. The relevant studies that have formally tested model calibration and discrimination on larger samples are summarized in Table 3.9.

In most investigations, external validation was attempted across international borders, raising the additional question as to whether the severity models are exportable. The observed deterioration of predictive accuracy can have several

Table 3.9 External validation of prognostic models with formal testing of discrimination and calibration

Prognostic models	Cohort	ICUs	Year	Time	Countries	Discrimination	Calibration	Reference
APACHE III	1734	10	1990–1991	17	Brazil	0.82	400	Bastos et al., 1996
APACHE III	37 668	285	1993–1996	48	USA	0.89	37	Zimmerman et al., 1998
APACHE III	12 793	17	1993–1995	33	England	0.89	332	Pappachan et al., 1999
SAPS II	1393	99	1994	1	Italy	0.80	71	Apolone et al., 1996
SAPS II	1234	9	1997	6	Austria	0.81	53	Metnitz et al., 1999
APACHE II and APACHE III	1144	1	1993–1996	36	England	0.80 / 0.84	98 / 129	Beck et al., 1997
APACHE II and MPM$_0$	8724	26	1987, 1989	7	Britain and Ireland	0.83 / 0.74	57 / 1737	Rowan et al., 1994
APACHE II and MPM$_0$ and MPM$_{24}$	12 802	137	1991	3	[2]Europe, USA, Canada	0.85 / 0.77 / 0.83	1[1] / 1[1] / 1[1]	Castella et al., 1995
SAPS II and MPM$_0$	10 027	89	1994–1995	4	[3]Europe	0.82 / 0.78	368 / 208	Moreno et al., 1998
SAPS II and APACHE II	982	19	1994–1995	4	Portugal	0.81 / 0.78	28 / 49	Moreno et al., 1997
SAPS II and APACHE II and MPM$_{24}$	1325	3	1994–1995	18	Tunisia	0.84 / 0.82 / 0.88	73 / 25 / 29	Nouira et al., 1998
SAPS II and APACHE II and APACHE III	2661	1	1991–1994	36	Germany	0.85 / 0.83 / 0.85	21 / 12 / 48	Markgraf et al., 2000
SAPS II and APACHE II and APACHE III and MPM$_{24}$	10 393	22	1995–1996	24	Scotland	0.78 / 0.76 / 0.80 / 0.79	142 / 67 / 366 / 101	Livingston et al., 2000b

Year refers to the year(s) of data collection, time refers to the duration of data collection in months; values for discrimination (area under ROC) and calibration (Hosmer-Lemeshow χ^2) are rounded.[1] χ^2 not reported. [2]Ten and [3]thirteen different European countries. In all, but one study, P values <0.001 for χ^2 were reported. Only Markgraf et al. (2000) found a P value >0.1 for the APACHE II model indicating good calibration; for SAPS II and APACHE III, P values were <0.01 and <0.001, indicating poor fit.

causes: differences in case-mix, inaccuracies in disease coding, varying criteria and definitions applied for data collection, differences in the prevalence of outcomes, and the decay of the models over time. Standard models that imperfectly describe a new population can be customized to improve their calibration for the new environment.

Differences in case-mix and model performance

The degree of dissimilarity between the patients in different centres or countries is called case-mix, and adjustment for these differences is essential when comparing outcomes. Disparity between the case-mix of test and reference databases is one of the most important reasons for poor performance of prognostic models when applied to new populations. Prognostic models describe the relation between case-mix and outcome, and if the model includes all important variables and has modelled them appropriately, then the model should perform well in other environments with a different case-mix. If, however, important case-mix factors are not accounted for by the prognostic model, then variation in case-mix can result in quite different model performance in other locations (Altman and Royston, 2000).

Substantial differences in the case-mix of UK patients and the population of the original APACHE II and APACHE III investigations have been reported (Rowan et al., 1993a; Goldhill and Withington, 1996a; Pappachan et al., 1999). The SAPS II and MPM II models also failed to adjust adequately for differences in the case-mix profiles of ICU patients from various European countries (Castella et al., 1995; Apolone et al., 1996; Moreno et al., 1998b). Pappachan reported the results of the largest assessment of the APACHE III model outside the USA and compared the UK with the original data from the USA (Knaus et al., 1991). Patients in England were more likely to be male, older, had greater co-morbidity, and were sicker than the American patients. More British patients were admitted from hospital wards, rather than from the emergency department, and the proportion of emergency surgical admissions was higher. Similar characteristics for British ICU patients were reported by others, using the APACHE II equation (Goldhill and Withington,1996a; Rowan et al.,1993b) for case-mix adjustment.

Measured and unmeasured case-mix factors

Most currently used prognostic models have focused on patient characteristics, deranged physiology and co-morbidities. For example, for the APACHE II model, case-mix is defined in terms of admission diagnosis, surgical status (emergency surgery or not) and severity of disease, expressed by the APACHE II score and its individual components (physiology, age and chronic health). Similiarly, the case-mix factors considered in the SAPS II model are the individual elements that form the SAPS II score. It is increasingly recognized that outcome also depends on a variety of non-clinical factors that are not taken into account, and therefore cannot be adjusted for by the models. Such unmeasured case-mix factors can range from pre- to post-ICU care, and include the organizational and structural framework of care, admission and discharge policies, and the level of discharge facilities available in a particular hospital.

The location of patients before ICU admission is an important case-mix factor, which is not measured by models such as APACHE II, SAPS II and MPM II. By contrast, patient location was introduced as an explanatory variable into the APACHE III system to control for the effects of lead-time bias. Among the main categories for location used by the APACHE III model are operating theatre/ recovery, emergency department, hospital ward and other ICUs. However, this variable accounts for only 1% of the model's explanatory power (Knaus et al., 1991). In the context of prognostic models, lead-time bias refers to the difference in time between hospital and ICU admission. Delayed institution of intensive therapy is assumed to be associated with increased mortality, and patient location serves as an indirect or proxy measure of this delay. A large proportion of patients directly admitted from the emergency department, rather than the hospital wards, is considered as an indicator of timely institution of intensive therapy and improved outcomes. Vice versa, a large number of admissions from the hospital wards tends to reflect delayed intensive therapy and is consequently associated with adverse outcomes.

In fact, several studies demonstrated that patients admitted from hospital wards had significantly higher mortality rates than patients admitted from the emergency department. For the SAPS II and the MPM II models, patient location before ICU admission represents an unmeasured case-mix factor. Moreno (1998a) investigated the performance of both models for European ICU patients. When patients were grouped by location, both models under-estimated actual mortality for admissions from the wards, and overestimated true mortality for patients admitted from the operating theatre and emergency department. The lack of uniform adjustment of the predictive equation for subgroups of patients can indicate variations in case-mix that may produce a distorted image of the performance of ICUs with very high or very low proportions of certain groups of patients.

Quantifying diversity in case-mix

Although analysis of the model's uniformity-of-fit across subgroups of the ICU population can help to identify differences in case-mix, it is difficult to quantify the effects of such differences on the model's overall predictive accuracy for the ICU population as a whole. Murphy-Filkins et al. (1996) analysed the diversity in patient mix on the performance of the MPM_0 admission model. Using computer simulation techniques to vary case-mix, the authors defined a critical percentage for each of the model's variables, above which the model's fit for the population was no longer considered acceptable. A stepwise increase and decrease of the proportions of each of the variables included in the MPM_0 model was performed until a critical limit was reached, at which the model's calibration deteriorated.

This is an important concept because it quantifies the influence of major patient factors on model performance for a particular population. Unlike the APACHE and SAPS systems, the MPM model includes almost exclusively binary variables. For physiology based severity systems, which primarily rely on continuous variables, this concept may not be applicable without modification. A similar approach of critical percentages could possibly be used to quantify the effect of case-mix factors that are not included in the prognostic models.

Diagnostic coding and disease classification

The disease process is a major determinant of hospital mortality. The inclusion of a diagnosis or reason for admission as a predictive variable is a major difference between the APACHE systems and the SAPS II and MPM models. The developers of SAPS II decided not to incorporate admission diagnosis as an explanatory variable because of the complexity of disease definition and the resulting inaccuracies in diagnostic coding. Similarly, detailed diagnostic information is not required for the MPM models. The use of diagnosis as an explanatory variable in a prognostic model requires consistent and reproducible disease definitions, but misclassification is common because of the lack of unequivocal criteria for disease coding.

Wide variations in performance for different diagnostic categories of ICU patients have been reported. This applies to the APACHE, SAPS II and MPM models. The poor uniformity-of-fit across subgroups stratified by disease is partly a reflection of the inaccuracies in diagnostic coding. The validation of APACHE III showed that risk predictions for American patients grouped by disease did not match true mortality for 39% ($n = 14\,690$) of the study sample, and significant differences between the observed and predicted mortalities were observed for 21 of 65 specific admission diagnoses (Zimmerman et al., 1998). The researchers suggested that future efforts should be directed towards improving disease labelling and re-adjustment of the diagnostic weights. In the UK, the APACHE II and III models have been directly compared only once in a single centre study; the results showed poor uniformity-of-fit across subpopulations grouped by diagnostic category for both models, despite an improved APACHE III disease classification system (Beck et al., 1997). Large variations in the performance of the SAPS II and MPM models were also observed in European patients stratified by disease group (Moreno et al., 1998a).

Methods for disease classification

The APACHE system uses a two-tiered system of disease classification. The first component is based on the organ system (e.g. respiratory system) that is mainly affected and the second component relates to the 'specific' disease process. As well as clearly defined diagnoses (e.g. abdominal aortic aneurysm), the APACHE II classification also includes vague conditions, such as 'peripheral vascular surgery'. The APACHE II model contains 53 specific diseases and five organ system categories. APACHE III includes 78 specific conditions, and several organ system groups. If allocation to a specific diagnostic group is not possible, patients are assigned to one of the organ system categories. This can result in heterogeneous patients being grouped in a single system organ.

Potential errors in diagnostic labelling raise the question of what level of diagnostic information is required by predictive models to generate accurate mortality estimates. De Keizer *et al.* (2000) investigated the added value of increasing levels of diagnostic information for the mortality estimates by prognostic models, and showed that more detailed diagnostic information did not provide better mortality estimates. Applying the APACHE II system as the reference model, the authors demonstrated that substitution of the 53 APACHE II diagnostic categories by nine body system categories, and the use of three, instead of two, criteria for the type of admission, resulted in a model with improved discrimination and calibration compared with the reference system.

Regardless of the requirement for prognostic models, detailed diagnostic information is indispensible for the description and characterization of intensive care populations. Attempts have therefore been made to improve the accuracy of disease classification. The Intensive Care National Audit & Research Centre (ICNARC) has developed a five-tiered, hierarchical disease coding system. This method allows the stepwise inclusion of new information. At each level of the hierarchy, a unique code for the relevant information is selected and the final diagnosis is the result of five selections. The same diagnosis can be reached via alternative pathways, using different 'descriptions' of the available diagnostic information. The ICNARC coding method is currently being evaluated and can be expected to facilitate future research on the explanatory value of diagnostic information (ICNARC, 1995). Application of this coding method for a patient who had surgery for a gastric tumour is outlined in Figure 3.3.

Criteria and definitions for data collection

The criteria and definitions for data collection that are required by prognostic models for generating mortality probabilities should be strictly adhered to. Unreliable measurements can have various sources, such as the absence of clear definitions, a large number of missing data (which by convention are then considered normal) and inconsistencies in converting the originally used units of measurement. Some variables, however, are not clearly defined in the original descriptions. Féry-Lemonnier *et al.* (1995) found that the conversion of creatinine values (mg/dl^{-1}) into SI units ($\mu mol/l$) produced upper and lower limits that did not correspond with the original APACHE II description. In addition, in the APACHE II score, the points for serum creatinine are doubled in the presence of acute renal failure, but this condition is not defined in the original publication. The Glasgow Coma Score is another example of a commonly used variable that is prone to misclassification in ICU patients who are sedated and intubated (Livingston *et al.*, 2000a). Rué *et al.* (2000) assessed the MPM_{24} II model and found only moderate interobserver agreement (reliability) for the

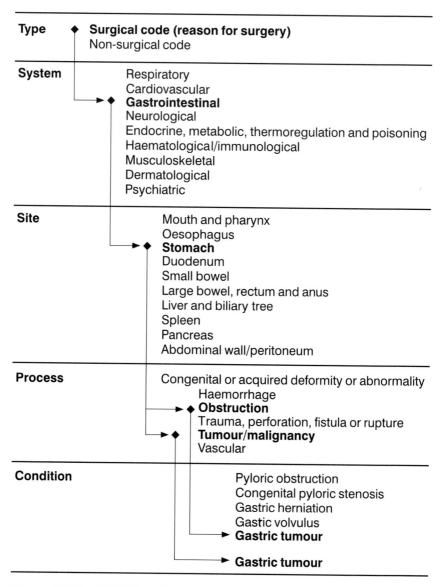

Figure 3.3 The ICNARC coding method: two alternative pathways to determine the final code for the ICU admission diagnosis for a patient after surgery for a gastric tumour. (Modified with permission from De Keizer, N. F., Bonsel, G. J., Goldfrad, C., Rowan, K. M. (2000). The added value that increasing levels of diagnostic information provide in prognostic models to estimate hospital mortality for adult intensive care patients. *Intensive Care Med.*, **26**, 577–584.)

variables 'coma and deep stupor' and 'prothrombin time'. Prothrombin time is often prolonged because of anticoagulant therapy and may reflect treatment effects rather than the underlying pathology.

Goldhill and Withington (1996b) quantified the possible effects of unreliable measurements on the accuracy of APACHE II mortality predictions. Increasing the APACHE II score by 2 or 4 points decreased the standardized mortality ratio (SMR) from its original value of 1.13 to 1.00 and 0.87 respectively. Decreasing the score by the same numbers resulted in an increase of the original SMR to 1.27 and 1.44 respectively. The effects of under- and overscoring are most pronounced for lower risk patients who constitute a large proportion (30–50%) of all ICU admissions. Repeated and systematic assessment of the reliability of the data elements in severity models is necessary to maintain the integrity of prognostic models (Teres and Pekow, 2000).

Prevalence of outcome events

Another reason for the deterioration of the model's fit is that the prevalence of the outcome events in a new series of patients may be higher or lower than in the population in which the model was developed (Miller et al., 1991). This phenomenon was also demonstrated in a computer simulation study; the calibration of the APACHE II model deteriorated significantly with increasing mortality rates (Glance et al., 2000). The original descriptions of the APACHE II and SAPS II models had overall hospital mortality rates of 19.6% and 21.8% respectively. The observed hospital mortality in the external validation of both models in the UK and in Europe was much higher. Italian ICU patients (SAPS II validation) had an overall hospital mortality of 34.1% (Apolone et al., 1996), mortality rates for British ICU patients (APACHE II validation) were 32.1% and 27.0% (Goldhill and Withington, 1996a; Rowan et al., 1993b). The much higher death rates may have contributed to the poor calibration of both models for Italian and British ICU patients.

Decay over time

Severity models probably perform less well over time (Zhu et al., 1996). Diagnostic and therapeutic advances, and the introduction of new treatment strategies may improve outcome for some conditions (e.g. thrombolysis and myocardial infarction), while a changing pattern in medical decision making, such as the earlier withdrawal of active life support (e.g. cardiac arrest) may worsen outcome for other subgroups. However, there is no published evidence that decay over time is a major contributor to the deterioration of a model's predictive accuracy.

The original APACHE III model was developed on data originating from the years 1988 to 1990. External validation of the APACHE III model, based on data collected in the USA between 1993 and 1996 (Zimmerman et al., 1998), does not suggest that performance has decayed over time. For the large group of patients with mortality probabilities between 10% and 40%, the number of observed deaths was consistently higher than predicted. There was closer correspondence between observed and predicted mortality in the higher risk groups (>40%). It seems unlikely that the outcomes for patients with moderate severity of disease should worsen over time while the mortality for the most severely ill remains static (Teres and Lemeshow, 1998). In general, new treatment strategies have had little impact on outcomes for the sickest ICU patients (e.g. sepsis) compared to admission and discharge practices which have undergone drastic changes in the past years.

Model customization

Standard prognostic models that imperfectly characterize the mortality of a specific population can be adjusted by customizing them to obtain more reliable mortality estimates. Models that do not demonstrate good fit for a new population can be customized using techniques that require only minimal adjustments to the original equation. For instance, a change in the prevalence of the outcome events (higher or lower mortality rates) can affect model calibration, which can be adjusted by only changing the intercept of the regression equation (Miller et al., 1991). Other methods include the customization of the coefficients or the logit of the regression equation. Based on the data from the new population, a new logistic regression model is generated using the same variables and weights as does the original method. The structure of the original model remains unaltered, but new estimates for the coefficients are obtained that reflect the characteristics of the population the model was applied to. Customizing the logit involves changes to the structure of the original equation (Zhu et al., 1996). Customization of the original SAPS II and APACHE III models has been successfully employed to improve the models' fit for Italian and Spanish ICU patients (Apolone et al., 1996; Rivera-Fernández et al., 1998).

Therapeutic and technological advances in intensive care may require adaptation of the original models to maintain their predictive accuracy. More importantly, changes in structure, organization and financing of the healthcare systems have profound effects on the provision of care at the hospital and ICU level, and may further degrade the validity of standard severity models. Changing patterns in hospital discharge practice affect the predictive accuracy of models that rely on vital status at hospital discharge as the principal outcome. Earlier discharge of patients from acute care to rehabilitation hospitals, or from tertiary medical centres to the referring hospitals, has become common practice in many countries. Increasing pressure on ICU and hospital beds may result in delayed or refused ICU admission (Smith et al., 1995) and premature ICU discharge (Goldfrad and Rowan, 2000), and will consequently alter the composition of the ICU populations and their mortality.

In these circumstances, customization of the existing models may be useful to maintain their validity over time. No consensus has been reached regarding the intervals at which the customization should be performed (Lemeshow *et al.*, 1995). Despite these limitations, model customization may become an increasingly important means of meeting the demand for robust and useful information on severity of illness, which forms the foundation for evaluating quality, standard and cost of intensive care.

Perspectives

Prognostic models are useful tools for measuring severity of disease and adjusting for differences in case-mix, but they can only measure reliably what they are intended to measure. Case-mix adjustment is the basis for comparative research and evaluation of quality issues and cost of intensive care. Equally important is the detailed description of the diversity in case-mix for ICU populations, since a number of potentially important case-mix factors are not measured by prognostic models.

In many countries, healthcare systems are undergoing rapid transformations which will profoundly affect all levels of medical care provision. With the implementation of new concepts for healthcare financing, based on disease-related groups (DRGs), case-mix adjustment is becoming a major determinant in a process that can be expected to produce the most fundamental changes in the structure of intensive care and hospital medicine for the past 50 years. Standard prognostic models should be (re-)validated and, where appropriate, be adapted by customization to maintain their validity in the face of these dynamic developments. Hospital mortality is the universal outcome measure of almost all prognostic models, but for several reasons may no longer represent an adequate endpoint. The impact of critical illness on functional ability and quality of life is likely to become more important in the future, but the currently used prognostic models lack the ability to estimate these important outcomes.

Conclusion

Scoring systems and prognostic models have been developed as instruments to standardize the assessment of severity of disease. Scoring systems provide a score for risk stratification, but do not convert the score into a probability. Most of the general prognostic systems used in intensive care are logistic regression models that generate mortality probabilities. Prognostic models should ideally be based on a small number of explanatory variables that are routinely available and measured reliably in the clinical setting. The process of developing prognostic methods is complex; in particular, the selection of potentially important variables from a large pool of 'candidate' variables significantly affects the model's ability to produce accurate mortality predictions.

Internal validation is related to the process of model building, and includes testing of model performance in the population on which the model was developed. External validation is a stringent test of the model's generalizability, and involves the assessment of its predictive accuracy in a new series of patients from a different institution. Predictive accuracy consists of two principal components: discrimination and calibration. Internal and external validation should include testing of both components, using receiver operating characteristics curves and Hosmer-Lemeshow statistics. Detailed description of the diversity of the population can help to identify important unmeasured case-mix factors. In addition, the uniformity-of-fit across subgroups of the population should be assessed. All general models used for case-mix adjustment in intensive care showed a similar pattern when applied to new populations: discrimination was good, but calibration was imperfect. Differences in case-mix and inaccuracies in diagnostic coding are probably the main sources for the deterioration of the model's predictive accuracy when applied to new populations. Standard prognostic models that imperfectly describe the mortality experience of a specific population can be customized to obtain more reliable mortality estimates.

Despite the increasingly popular 'assembly-line mentality' and the entrepreneurial beliefs that there are few limits to categorize sick individuals by productivity and economical terms, one should resist the temptation to use prognostic models for purposes for which they were not built. Prognostic systems are, by definition, models. The very nature of a model is that it will always remain an imperfect reflection of reality, and the whole spectrum of reality cannot be reduced to a cluster of numbers. The limitations of prognostic models are inherent to their mathematical structure and to the process of development. Prognostic models are very useful when applied to groups of ICU patients, but the arbitrary nature of converting a binary outcome into a mortality probability precludes the use of these predictions for treatment decisions of individual patients.

References

Altman, D. C., Royston, P. (2000). What do we mean by validating prognostic models? *Stat. Med.,* **19,** 453–473.

Apolone, G., Bertolini, G., D'Amico, R. *et al.* (1996). The performance of SAPS II in a cohort of Italian ICUs: results from GiViTI. *Intensive Care Med.,* **22,** 1368–1378.

Baker, S. P., O'Neil, B., Haddun, W. *et al.* (1974). The Injury Severity Score: a method for describing patients with multiple injuries and evaluating emergency care. *J. Trauma,* **14,** 187–198.

Bastos, P. G., Sun, X., Wagner, D. P. *et al.* (1996). Application of the APACHE III prognostic system in Brazilian intensive care units: a prospective multicenter study. *Intensive Care Med.,* **22,** 564–570.

Beck, D. H., Taylor, B. L., Millar, B., Smith, G. B. (1997). Prediction of outcome from intensive care: a prospective cohort study comparing APACHE II and III in a UK intensive care unit. *Crit. Care Med.,* **25,** 9–15.

Boyd, C. R., Tolson, M. A., Copes, W. S. (1987). Evaluating care: The TRISS method: Trauma score and Injury Severity Score. *J. Trauma,* **27,** 370–378.

Castella, X., Artigas, A., Bion, J., Kari, A. (1995). A comparison of severity of illness scoring systems for intensive care unit patients: Results of a multicenter, multinational study. *Crit. Care Med.*, **23**, 1327–1335.

Champion, H. R., Succo, W. J., Carnazzo, A. J. *et al.* (1981). Trauma score. *Crit. Care Med.*, **9**, 672–676.

Chang, R. W. S., Jacobs, S., Lee, B. (1988). Predicting outcome among intensive care patients using computerised trend analysis of daily APACHE II scores corrected for organ system failure. *Intensive Care Med.*, **14**, 558–566.

Child, C. G., Turcotte, J. C. (1964). Surgery and portal hypertension. In: *The Liver and Portal Hypertension* (C.G. Child, ed.) pp 50–64, Saunders.

Concato, J., Peduzzi, P., Holford, T. R., Feinstein, A. R. (1995). Importance of events per independent variable in proportional hazards analysis I. Background, goals and general strategy. *J. Clin. Epidemiol.*, **48**, 1495–1501.

Cullen, D. J., Civetta, J. M., Briggs, B. A., Ferrara, L. C. (1976). Therapeutic Intervention Scoring System: a method for quantitative comparison of patient care. *Crit. Care Med.*, **2**, 57–60.

De Keizer, N. F., Bonsel, G. J., Goldfrad, C., Rowan, K. M. (2000). The added value that increasing levels of diagnostic information provide in prognostic models to estimate hospital mortality for adult intensive care patients. *Intensive Care Med.*, **26**, 577–584.

Efron, B. (1979). Bootstrap methods: another look at the jackknife. *Ann. Stat.*, **7**, 1–26.

Efron, B., Tibshirani, R. J. (1993). *An Introduction to the Bootstrap*. Chapman and Hall.

Feller, I., Tholen, D., Cornell, L. D. (1980). Improvement in burn care 1965 to 1979. *JAMA*, **244**, 2074–2078.

Féry-Lemonnier, E., Landrais, P., Loirat, P., Kleinknecht, D., Brivet, F. (1995). Evaluation of severity scoring systems in ICUs – translation, conversion and definition ambiguities as a source of inter-observer variability in APACHE II, SAPS and OSF. *Intensive Care Med.*, **21**, 356–360.

Fletcher, R. H., Fletcher, S. W., Wagner, E. H. (1988). *Clinical Epidemiology, the Essentials.* pp 46–51, Williams & Wilkins.

Glance, L. G., Osler, T. M., Papadakos, P. (2000). Effect of mortality rate on the performance of the Acute Physiology and Chronic Health Evaluation II: A simulation study. *Crit. Care Med.*, **28**, 3424–3428.

Goldfrad, C., Rowan, K. (2000). Consequences of discharges from intensive care at night. *Lancet*, **355**, 1138–1142.

Goldhill, D. R., Withington, P. S. (1996a). The effect of casemix adjustment on mortality as predicted by APACHE II. *Intensive Care Med.*, **22**, 415–419.

Goldhill, D.R., Withington, P. S. (1996b). Mortality predicted by APACHE II: The effects of changes in physiological values and post-ICU hospital mortality. *Anaesthesia*, **51**, 719–723.

Hadorn, D. C., Keeler, E. B., Rogers, W. H. *et al.* (1993). Assessing the performance of Mortality Prediction Models. Prepared for the Health Care Financing Administration, US Department of Health and Human Services. Santa Monica, California, RAND/ UCLA/Harvard Center for Health Care Financing Policy Research.

Hanley, J. A., McNeil, B. J. (1982). The meaning and the use of the area under a receiver-operating characteristic (ROC) curve. *Radiology*, **143**, 29–36.

Harrell, F. E., Lee, K. L. (1984). Regression modelling strategies for improved prognostic prediction. *Stat. Med.*, **3**, 143–152.

Harrell, F. E., Lee, K. L., Mark, D. B. (1996). Multivariable prognostic models: issues in developing models, evaluating assumptions and adequacy, and measuring and reducing errors. *Stat. Med.*, **15**, 361–367.

Hennekens, C. H., Buring, J. E. (1987). *Epidemiology in Medicine*. pp 314–321, Little, Brown and Company.

Hosmer, D. W., Lemeshow, S. (1989). *Applied Logistic Regression*. pp 135–149, Wiley and Sons.

Intensive Care National Audit and Research Centre Case Mix Programme. (1995). *Dataset Specification*. Intensive Care National Audit and Research Centre.

Justice, A. C., Covinsky, K. E., Berlin, J. A. (1999). Assessing the generalizability of prognostic information. *Ann. Intern. Med.*, **130**, 515–524.

Keene, A. R., Cullen, D. J. (1983). Therapeutic Intervention Scoring System: update 1983. *Crit. Care Med.,* **11**, 1–5.

Knaus, W. A., Zimmerman, J. E., Wagner, D. P., Draper, E. A., Lawrence, D. E. (1981). APACHE – Acute Physiology and Chronic Health Evaluation: a physiologically based classification system. *Crit. Care Med.,* **9**, 591–597.

Knaus, W. A., Draper, E. A., Wagner, D. P., Zimmerman, J. E. (1985). APACHE II: A severity of disease classification system. *Crit. Care Med.,* **13**, 818–829.

Knaus, W. A., Wagner, D. P., Draper, E. A. *et al.* (1991). The APACHE III prognostic system: risk prediction of hospital mortality for critically ill hospitalised adults. *Chest,* **100**, 1619–1639.

Le Gall, J. R., Loirat, P., Alperovitch, A. *et al.* (1984). A Simplified Acute Physiology Score for ICU patients. *Crit. Care Med.,* **12**, 975–977.

Le Gall, J. R., Lemeshow, S., Saulnier, F. (1993). Development of a new scoring system, the SAPS II, from a European/North American Multicenter Study. *JAMA.,* **270**, 2957–2963.

Lemeshow, S., Hosmer, D. J. (1982). A review of goodness-of-fit statistics for use in the development of logistic regression models. *Am. J. Epidemiol.* **115**, 92–106.

Lemeshow, S., Teres, D., Pastidis, H., Avrunin, J. S., Steingrub, J. S. (1985). A method for predicting survival and mortality of ICU patients using objectively derived weights. *Crit. Care Med.,* **13**, 519–525.

Lemeshow, S., Teres, D., Avrunin, J. S., Gage, R. W. (1988). Refining intensive care unit outcome prediction by using changing probabilities of mortality. *Crit. Care Med.,* **16**, 470–477.

Lemeshow, S., Teres, D., Klar, J., Avrunin, J. S., Gehlbach, S. H., Rapoport, J. (1993). Mortality Probability Models (MPM II) based on an international cohort of intensive care unit patients. *JAMA.,* **270**, 2478–2486.

Lemeshow, S., Klar, J., Teres, D. (1995). Outcome prediction for individual intensive care patients: useful, misused or abused? *Intensive Care Med.,* **21**, 770–776.

Lemeshow, S., Teres, D., Avrunin, J. S. *et al.* (1994). Mortality Probability Models for patients in the intensive care unit for 48 and 72 hours: a prospective, multicenter study. *Crit. Care Med.,* **22**, 1351–1358.

Livingston, B. M., Mackenzie, S. J., MacKirdy, F. N., Howie, J. C. (2000a). Should the pre-sedation Glasgow Coma Score value be used when calculating Acute Physiology and Chronic Health Evaluation scores for sedated patients? *Crit. Care Med.,* **28**, 389–394.

Livingston, B. M., MacKirdy, F. N., Howie, J. C., Jones, R., Norrie, J. D. (2000b). Assessment of the performance of five intensive care scoring models within a large Scottish database. *Crit. Care Med.,* **28**, 1820–1827.

Markgraf, R., Deutschinoff, G., Pientka, L., Scholten, T. (2000). Comparison of Acute Physiology and Chronic Health Evaluation Score II and III and Simplified Acute

Physiology Score II: A prospective cohort study evaluating these models to predict outcome in a German multidisciplinary intensive care unit. *Crit. Care Med.,* **28,** 26–33.

Metnitz, P. G. H., Vesely, H., Valentin, A. *et al.* (1999). Evaluation of an inter-disciplinary data set for national intensive care unit assessment. *Crit. Care Med.,* **27,** 1486–1491.

Miller, M. E., Hui, S. L., Tierney, W. M. (1991). Validation techniques for logistic regression models. *Stat. Med.,* **10,** 1213–1226.

Moreno, R., Morais, P. (1997). Outcome prediction from intensive care: results of a prospective, multicentre Portuguese study. *Intensive Care Med.,* **22,** 177–186.

Moreno, R., Reis Miranda, D., Fidler, V., Van Schilfgaarde, R. (1998a). Evaluation of two outcome prediction models on an independent database. *Crit. Care Med.,* **26,** 50–61.

Moreno, R., Apolone, G., Reis Miranda, D. (1998b). Evaluation of the uniformity of fit of general outcome prediction models. *Intensive Care Med.,* **24,** 40–47.

Moreno, R., Morais, P. (1997). Validation of a simplified Therapeutic Intervention Scoring System on an independent database. *Intensive Care Med.,* **23,** 640–644.

Murphy-Filkins, R. L., Teres, D., Lemeshow, S., Hosmer, D. W. (1996). Effect of changing patient mix on the performance of intensive care unit severity-of-illness models: How to distinguish a general from a specialty intensive care unit. *Crit. Care Med.,* **24,** 1968–1973.

Nouira, S., Belghith, M., Elatrons, S. *et al.* (1998). Predictive value of severity scoring systems: comparison of four models in Tunisian adult intensive care units. *Crit. Care Med.,* **26,** 852–859.

Pappachan, J. V., Millar, B., Bennett, D., Smith, G. B. (1999). Comparison of outcome from intensive care admission after adjustment for case mix by the APACHE III prognostic system. *Chest,* **115,** 802–805.

Picard, R. R., Berk, K. N. (1990). Data splitting. *Am. Stat.,* **44,** 140–147.

Pollack, M. M., Ruttimann, U. E., Gaston, P. R. *et al.* (1988). Accurate predicton of the outcome of Paediatric risk of mortality (PRISM) score. *Crit. Care Med.,* **16,** 1110–1116.

Ranson, J. H. C., Rifkind, K. M., Roses, D. F. *et al.* (1974). Prognostic signs and the role of operative management in acute pancreatitis. *Surg. Gynecol. Obst.,* **139,** 69–81.

Reis Miranda, D., Rijk, A., Schaufeli, W. (1996). Simplified Therapeutic Intervention Scoring System. The TISS–28 items-results from a multicentre study. *Crit. Care Med.,* **24,** 64–73.

Ridley, S. (1998). Severity of illness scoring systems and performance appraisal. *Anaesthesia,* **53,** 1185–1194.

Rivera-Fernandez, R., Vazquez-Mata, G., Bravo, M. *et al.* (1998). The APACHE III prognostic system: customised mortality predictions for Spanish ICU patients. *Intensive Care Med.,* **24,** 574–581.

Rowan, K. M., Kerr, J. H., Major, E., Mc Pherson, K., Short, A., Vessey, M. P. (1993a). Intensive Care Society's APACHE II study in Britain and Ireland-I: Variations in case-mix of adult admissions to general intensive care units and impact on outcome. *Br. Med. J.,* **307,** 972–977.

Rowan, K. M., Kerr, J. H., Major, E., Mc Pherson, K., Short, A., Vessey, M. P. (1993b). Intensive Care Society's APACHE II study in Britain and Ireland-II: Outcome comparisons of intensive care units after adjustment for case mix by the American APACHE II method. *Br. Med. J.,* **307,** 977–981.

Rowan, K. M., Kerr, J. H., Major, E., Mc Pherson, K., Short, A., Vessey, M. P. (1994). Intensive Care Society's Acute Physiology and Chronic Health Evaluation (APACHE

II) study in Britain and Ireland: a prospective, multicenter, cohort study comparing two methods for predicting outcome for adult intensive care patients. *Crit. Care Med., 22,* 1392–1401.

Rué, M., Valero, G., Quintana, S., Artigas, A., Alvarez, M. (2000). Inter-observer variability in the measurement of the Mortality Probability Models (MPM II) in the assessment of severity of illness. *Intensive Care Med., 26,* 286–291.

Smith, G. B., Taylor, B. L., McQuillan, P. J., Nials, E. (1995). Rationing intensive care. Intensive care provision varies widely in Britain. *Br. Med. J., 310,* 1412–1413.

Teasdale, G., Jennett, B. (1974). Assessment of coma and improved consciousness: a practical scale. *Lancet, 2,* 81–83.

Teres, D., Lemeshow, S. (1998). As American as apple pie and APACHE. *Crit. Care Med., 26,* 1297–1298.

Teres, D., Pekow, P. (2000). Assessing data elements in a severity scoring system. *Intensive Care Med., 26,* 263–264.

Wyatt, J. C., Altman, D. C. (1995). Prognostic models: clinically useful or quickly forgotten. *Br. Med. J., 311,* 1539–1541.

Zhu, P. G., Lemeshow, S., Hosmer, D. W., Klar, J., Avrunin, J., Teres, D. (1996). Factors affecting the performance of the models in the Mortality Prediction Model II system and strategies of customisation: A simulation study. *Crit. Care Med., 24,* 57–63.

Zimmerman, J. E., Wagner, D. P., Draper, E. A., Wright, L., Alzola, C., Knaus, W. A. (1998). Evaluation of Acute Physiology and Chronic Health III predictions of hospital mortality in an independent database. *Crit. Care Med., 20,* 1317–1326.

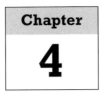

Chapter

4

Case-mix adjustment and prediction of mortality – the problems with interpretation

Owen Boyd

Introduction

The critical care unit is usually a small self-contained area within a larger hospital. Patient numbers are small, but the cost, emotion and time invested in the care of these patients is high. The justification for such expenditure on so few patients with a high mortality rate has been questioned (The King's Fund, 1989). Intensive care practitioners have attempted to collect data, audit results and compare outcomes in order to provide evidence of best practice and the place of intensive care within the health economy.

Crude mortality rates do not allow meaningful comparison between hospitals due to differences in patient demography, referral structure and specialization (Dubois *et al.*, 1987). With regard to intensive care audits, it has therefore been necessary to adjust the interpretation of outcomes based on the case-mix of the intensive care unit (ICU). For example, it clearly would not be appropriate to compare the crude mortality rates of ICUs with predominantly cardiac surgery cases with those treating mostly trauma victims.

One way to adjust for case-mix is to compare diagnostic groups, but in general intensive care practice the number of cases in any diagnostic group may be small so limiting the validity of any comparisons. Some other comparative method is needed. Within ICU practice, outcome of patients is related to their physiological disturbance; indeed the raison d'être of intensive care is to monitor and correct physiological disturbance. A logical step is to develop scoring systems that compare patient outcomes based on groupings of physiological disturbance rather than primary diagnosis.

The most widely used system is the Acute Physiology And Chronic Health Evaluation (APACHE) system, which was originally designed in 1981 (Knaus *et al.*, 1981) but underwent revision in 1985 (Knaus *et al.*, 1985) and again in 1991 (Knaus *et al.*, 1991). The APACHE system is widely used; since 1981, 2005 articles are referenced by the United States National Library of Medicine under the search term 'APACHE'. Most published work concerns APACHE scoring alone or in comparison with other physiological scoring systems. However, it is important to appreciate that wide use of a system does not guarantee validity of the system itself or the results it generates. This chapter will review the uses of scoring systems and case-mix adjustment and the evidence suggesting that these uses are valid and appropriate. The chapter will comment on the abuses and dangers of case-mix adjustment with particular regard to the use of ratios as a method of performance comparison and will look at some of the practicalities limiting the widespread adoption of case-mix adjustment systems.

The use of ratios

Most methods of case-mix adjustment for mortality compare the expected (or predicted) mortality calculated by a scoring system and the observed (or actual) mortality. It is tacitly assumed that if the actual mortality rate is greater than the predicted, then clinical performance is poor; conversely, if the actual mortality rate is less than the predicted, then this is usually regarded as successful clinical performance. To standardize this comparison, it is expressed as a ratio (standardized mortality ratio (SMR)), where a ratio value less than one indicates good performance compared to the original dataset and a value greater than one indicates worse performance. However, there is a fundamental problem when comparing observed and anticipated results, which stems from using comparison data from different datasets. Is it the denominator or the numerator that is different, or have both changed but in differing proportions? The significance of this is demonstrated by a simple example:

> If the ratio of X and Y is R (X/Y = R) and if new values for X and Y are obtained (X_1 and Y_1), the ratio will change to R_1 where $R_1 < R$. If the only presented figures are summary values, R and R_1, it is not possible to calculate whether X (or Y) is greater or smaller than X_1 (or Y_1). Possible options include $X_1 = X$ *and* $Y_1 > Y$, or $X_1 < X$ and $Y_1 = Y$, or that both $X_1 < X$ and $Y_1 < Y$ but the proportional changes from the original values are different.

Expanding this to the example of case-mix adjustment, a change of SMR from 1.0 to 0.7 might be due to:

1. Reduced observed mortality but predicted mortality has remained the same.
2. Increased predicted mortality but observed mortality has not changed.

3. Both observed and predicted mortality reduced but the proportional change in observed mortality is greater so reducing the ratio value.
4. Both observed and predicted mortality have increased but the proportional change in observed mortality is lower.
5. The observed mortality rate falling while the predicted mortality rises.

More information about the observed or predicted mortalities might identify which of the above options is responsible for a change, but the author is not aware of any studies that have presented this important additional data.

Clinical interpretation of SMR results alone is therefore difficult despite the fact that changes in SMR are usually presented as evidence of improved care. These problems are best illustrated by using a hypothetical example in which two patient groups are assumed not to change during two time periods of data collection. Falls in SMR could be due to:

A The reduction in actual mortality rate is real; this is the usually accepted explanation for a fall in SMR. Other explanations such as a difference in the method of recording mortality (e.g. ICU, hospital or 28-day mortality) or changes in ICU discharge policy might be responsible for this reduction.
B There is no change in mortality rate, but the patients treated are sicker and so the predicted risk of mortality has risen.

It is likely that A and B above represent extremes but, in practice, one of the following options is more likely.

C Mortality may have really fallen due to A above. However the 'real' improvement in patient care has been partially hidden due to a decrease in predicted mortality. Because the prediction of mortality is based on the gathering of physiological data, which is itself responsive to treatment, there are many treatments before and during ICU admission that can affect the mortality prediction.
D Mortality rate has actually risen but this worsening of performance is hidden by an even greater rise in predicted mortality.
E A small fall in observed mortality rate has been exaggerated by a small rise in the predicted mortality rate.

Is it right to question the use of case-mix adjustment?

It is widely accepted that mortality rates alone are not reliable enough to compare clinical practice, particularly where case numbers are small and diagnoses are variable and inconsistent (Dubois *et al.*, 1987). It is also accepted that a method of benchmarking ICU practice has become essential in recent years (Angus, 2000), with governmental and non-governmental organizations requiring the collection and processing of data (Audit Commission, 1999; Department of Health, 2000). It is important to question current expectations and practice, especially the relevance of case-mix adjustment when used for comparison purposes. In particular it is important to distinguish whether differences in SMRs should be ascribed to differences in case-mix or poor performance (Apolone, 2000). Apparent differences can be caused by differences in data availability, reliability and collection accuracy, differences from the reference population or sample size (Zimmerman and Wagner, 2000).

Audit is important and costly

Data collection, comparison and analysis is worthwhile to highlight excellence but censure poor practice. Internationally agreed datasets can potentially extend comparison worldwide. However, overall mortality rates are only one dimension of a multidimensional critical care practice (Linde-Zwirble and Angus, 1998). By its nature, mortality concentrates on negative rather than positive attributes of critical care.

Original data sets can be used as a 'control' group for scientific comparison (Lemeshow and Le Gall, 1994). One study examining outcome of critically ill patients treated with intermittent high-volume haemofiltration compared observed mortality with predicted mortality generated from a case-mix adjustment scoring system; the results suggested that intermittent high-volume haemofiltration lowered mortality in ICU patients (Oudemans-van Straaten et al., 1999).

The collection of reliable and robust data is very costly and may distract clinical staff from other aspects of patient care if not adequately resourced. Costs are incurred in training, data collection, checking reliability of data collection and analysis. It must be clear to those involved in data collection, and those financing it, that these costs are worthwhile. It is also imperative that there are no misinterpretations of the data concerning improvements or deficiencies in care, which might result in unsubstantiated censure or adoption of inappropriate practices. The proponents of case-mix adjustment are obliged to ensure that results cannot be misinterpreted, and that not too much reliance is placed on the results.

It is right and necessary to be sceptical and continuously to question methods of case-mix adjustment to eliminate mistakes and offer an alternative explanation if appropriate.

Is there any evidence that SMR reflects quality of care?

The main reason for case-mix adjustment in intensive care is to facilitate outcome comparison while accounting for differing patient populations on different ICUs. It has been suggested that most scoring and case-mix adjustment systems can be used to compare ICU performance and to detect differences in quality of care (Lemeshow and Le Gall, 1994).

Evidence that changes in SMR can identify variations in performance

A number of studies have used changes in SMRs to show supposed changes in performance. Several have examined the effects of reorganization of ICU services on outcome using case-mix adjustment. For example, after reviewing outcome results when new working patterns were introduced, following the appointment of physicians with particular expertise in intensive care medicine, a reduction in SMR was detected. This was attributed to an improvement in care (Blunt and Burchett, 2000). This prompted further calls for full time intensive care physicians on all ICUs (Vincent, 2000). Variations in case-mix adjusted mortality have been used to suggest that right heart catheterization contributes to patient mortality (Connors et al., 1996), prompting far reaching recommendations for right heart catheter use (Dalen and Bone, 1996). While it seems to be generally accepted that case-mix adjusted comparisons of mortality can be used to assess performance variations, is this correct?

The SMR generated by the APACHE scoring system has been compared with hypothesized, independent measures of performance and quality of care (Knaus et al., 1986; Zimmerman et al., 1993a,b). In 1986 Knaus and colleagues (1986) compared the SMRs for the original 13 hospitals that contributed to the APACHE II database with a three-point classification based on their clinical capabilities. There was no clear relationship between the hospital level and the SMR (Boyd and Grounds, 1994); outlying SMRs were generated in both Level I and III hospitals (Knaus et al., 1986). Furthermore, in 1993 when Zimmerman and colleagues (1993a) compared the outcome of patients admitted to 20 ICUs in 18 teaching hospitals with those admitted to 17 non-teaching ICUs, they showed no significant difference in the SMRs of the teaching and non-teaching hospitals. There were, however, significantly lower SMRs in hospitals that were members of the Council of Teaching Hospitals compared to the other hospitals (Zimmerman et al., 1993a).

In a second article, Zimmerman (1993b) performed a much more detailed analysis comparing SMRs from nine of 42 hospitals in the APACHE III database with a quality of care ranking performed by an experienced investigative team. This team of investigators surveyed the ICUs using criteria that had previously been used by Knaus in an attempt to validate the SMR as an objective measure of quality of care (Knaus et al., 1986). As with the previous study there was no relationship between the SMR and the investigators' ranking. These data suggest that, either the assessment team was unable to assess ICU performance, the SMR was not able to quantify performance or neither method could assess performance (Boyd and Grounds, 1994). However, this view has been contested by one of the original authors (Zimmerman et al., 1994).

The authors of the APACHE scoring system draw attention to a number of possible factors that may create errors in estimating the predicted mortality rate, such as unknown patient factors or abnormal case-mixes in particular units. They suggest that these influences may be small but do not provide any data to support their position. In a study from the Mayo Clinic (Marsh *et al.*, 1990), SMRs from ICUs under common management were compared. Given uniformity of policy, staff, and delivery of care, differences in quality would not be expected, and yet surprisingly there were significant differences in the SMRs between the units. The authors of this study suggested that there may have been a failure of the APACHE score to measure factors intrinsic to the disease process in some patients.

Understanding the statistics

The statistical terminology of case-mix adjustment scoring systems and measures of their performance is complicated. Although medical training covers some statistical techniques, particularly those concerned with data description and simple comparisons, most physicians may not understand the relevant statistical techniques used in case-mix adjustment.

The size of a sample reflects the ability of that sample to represent accurately the entire population; this can be expressed as a confidence interval. Usually confidence intervals are quoted at the 95% level, which gives a range or interval of values within which there is 95% chance that the mean of a population will lie. The SMR for each ICU will therefore have a confidence interval and this must be taken into account when considering the variability between ICUs (Randolph *et al.*, 1998). However, following collection of a large amount of ICU data, wide confidence intervals for individual ICUs might rule out meaningful comparisons between them (Sirio *et al.*, 1999). Furthermore, the individual predictions for each patient within the ICU's dataset also has a confidence interval, and this depends on the size of the developmental dataset from which the case-mix adjustment scoring system was devised. This effect may be particularly important if there are variations between the patient group being analysed and the case-mix of the original developmental population.

A number of statistical methods have been used to assess the accuracy of scoring and case-mix adjustment systems. The overall score may show good prediction, for example an SMR of 1.0, but this might hide large over- and underestimates of mortality in certain groups of patients. Receiver operating characteristic (ROC) curves are frequently used to display graphically the accuracy of a prediction model (Figure 4.1) (McNeil and Hanley, 1984), but they have a number of possible errors (Angus, 2000).

The goodness of fit of a model can be described by the Hosmer-Lemeshow C statistic (Lemeshow and Hosmer, 1982), but the limitations of this complex statistic are not widely understood, and it was not reported in the earlier dataset descriptions. Both the ROC curves and the Hosmer-Lemeshow C statistic are described more fully in Chapter 3.

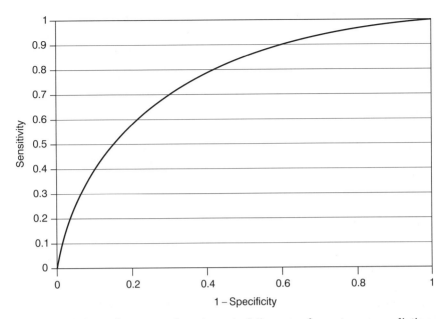

Figure 4.1 A receiver operating characteristic curve for outcome prediction of APACHE II in 1623 patients at the Royal Sussex County Hospital, Brighton. Area under the curve is 0.77 (95% confidence interval 0.74–0.79).

Relevance of single value in clinical terms

The use of a single value to summarize quality of care in an understandable and comparable fashion may be attractive. However, this relies on uniformity of the model's performance across variations in case-mix, treatment changes over time and other factors, such as admission criteria and discharge decision making. Furthermore, there are a number of different case-mix adjustment models that can be used and they do not always produce the same prediction of mortality.

Using formal statistical assessment to compare the performance of the new Simplified Acute Physiology Score (SAPS II) (Lemeshow *et al.*, 1987; Le Gall *et al.*, 1993) and the new admission Mortality Probability Model (MPM II_0) (Teres *et al.*, 1987), Moreno and colleagues (1998a) found very large differences in subgroups of patients where the prediction varied from excellent to almost random. The authors suggested that some of the difficulties of the models accurately to predict mortality could be explained by different patient baseline characteristics (Table 4.1).

They also stressed the importance of evaluating multiple diverse populations to generate the developmental set and of methods to improve the validation set before extrapolations can be made from the validation setting to new independent populations. In a further analysis, the same group (Moreno *et al.*, 1998b) showed that the models themselves may perform badly when applied to new populations outside the original database. For example, the original SAPS and MPM_0 models

Table 4.1 Goodness of fit for SAPS II and MPM II$_0$ based on data from 10 027 patients from a European database

Characteristic	SAPS II			MPM II$_0$		
	ROC	C-statistic	SMR	ROC	C-statistic	SMR
Non-operative						
Cardiovascular	0.833	P<0.001	0.79	0.829	P<0.001	0.71
Respiratory	0.756	P<0.001	1.01	0.692	P<0.001	1.04
Gastrointestinal	0.757	P<0.001	1.31	0.714	P<0.001	1.04
Neurological	0.827	P>0.001	1.09	0.806	P>0.001	0.96
Sepsis	0.776	P<0.001	1.08	0.705	P<0.001	1.14
Trauma	0.855	P>0.001	1.02	0.803	P>0.001	0.88
Metabolic	0.831	P<0.001	0.33	0.792	P<0.001	0.27
Others	0.832	P>0.001	0.89	0.762	P>0.001	0.88
Postoperative						
Cardiovascular	0.839	P>0.001	0.80	0.814	P>0.001	0.86
Respiratory	0.778	P<0.001	0.77	0.758	P>0.001	0.79
Gastrointestinal	0.814	P>0.001	1.01	0.766	P<0.001	1.02
Neurological	0.877	P>0.001	0.82	0.828	P<0.001	0.66
Trauma	0.802	P>0.001	0.79	0.741	P<0.001	0.75
Others	0.771	P<0.001	0.35	0.738	P<0.001	0.34

Adapted from Moreno, R., Apolone, G., Reis Miranda, D. (1998a). Evaluation of the uniformity of fit of general outcome prediction models. *Intensive Care Med.*, **24**, 40–47. Discrimination is analysed by the receiver operating characteristic curve and calibration by the C Statistic (see Glossary for details of interpretation). The data show that calibration is frequently poor for differing diagnostic categories and although discrimination is usually good, there are wide variations in SMRs for different diagnostic groups.

did not accurately predict mortality on an independent large international multicentre ICU patient database (Moreno *et al.*, 1998b). The authors suggest that the results of studies utilizing general outcome prediction models without previous validation in the target population should be interpreted with caution.

Different scoring systems themselves give different predictions for differing populations. Despite having good discrimination, calibration varied between scoring systems in head injury patients (Alvarez *et al.*, 1998) and general ICU patients (Nouira *et al.*, 1998) and were not suitable for patients with renal failure (Fiaccadori *et al.*, 2000). The results of another study led the authors to doubt that one system can be validated in all types of populations for comparisons among different ICUs (Katsaragakis *et al.*, 2000). In a recent German study the original APACHE II scoring system was better calibrated than the newer APACHE III system, possibly as a result of varying case-mix between the two scoring databases (Markgraf *et al.*, 2000). However, contrary to this, it is interesting to note that in an earlier study the newer scoring methods were found to be more accurate than their earlier counterparts (Table 4.2) (Castella *et al.*, 1995).

Variations in case-mix and treatment over time may have contributed to these findings. Other studies continue to emphasize the possible importance of case-mix variations. In a study at the Veterans Affairs Medical Center, the overall mortality was consistent with the predicted mortality; however, the poor fit of the model impaired the validity of the result (Patel and Grant, 1999). The authors suggested that this could be due to erratic quality of care, or differences between the study population and the patient population in the original studies and that the data could not be used to distinguish between these options. In a multicentre

Table 4.2 Comparisons of calibration and discrimination for old and new systems for case-mix adjustment

Case-mix adjustment system	Area under the ROC	C statistic
APACHE		
APACHE II	0.848	–
APACHE III	0.866	–
MPM		
MPM_0	0.766	<0.0001
MPM II_0	0.805	0.0694
MPM_{24}	0.815	<0.0001
MPM II_{24}	0.833	0.1531
SAPS		
SAPS	0.784	–
SAPS II	0.855	–

Adapted from Castella, X., Artigas, A., Bion, J., Kari, A. (1995). A comparison of severity of illness scoring systems for intensive care unit patients: results of a multicenter, multinational study. The European/North American Severity Study Group. *Crit. Care Med.*, **23**, 1327–1335. Interpretations of receiver operating characteristic (ROC) area and the C statistic are given in the Glossary.

study to validate the accuracy of the APACHE II and III systems, the Trauma and Injury Severity Score (TRISS), and a 24-h ICU point system for prediction of mortality in trauma victims (Vassar *et al.*, 1999), none of these systems had an acceptable level of performance when estimating ICU mortality for subsets of patients without head trauma. Another study showed that SAPS lost its discriminative power over time; however, its accuracy of prediction was maintained at an acceptable level in patients who stayed in the ICU no longer than 5 days. The authors postulated that the ICU stay represented a complex variable, which was not predictable, and it was this that influenced the performance of SAPS as data were only collected on the first day (Sicignano *et al.*, 1996).

In an increasingly competitive healthcare market, hospitals with extreme mortality rates have received adverse publicity. This may be unfair. Outcome report cards may be used to compare the quality of healthcare according to use of services, performance of healthcare processes or outcomes across providers, hospitals or other organizations. However, fair analysis of report cards should allow an adequate adjustment of case-mix between providers. In a study of report cards from 1336 patients in a University Hospital, the Veterans Affairs Medical Center and a community hospital, eight different methods were used to adjust for severity of disease. It was found that matching survival prediction depended on the method used for case-mix adjustment with little uniformity being found between the various methods (Poses *et al.*, 2000).

Influences that may change the prediction of mortality

Automated charting

Automated charting of physiological variables is now available with the increasing use of clinical information systems. For scoring systems this may improve accuracy of data collection. By electronically interfacing with the ICU monitor, automated patient data entry into the scoring system is possible. Current prognostic scores can then be made available to the clinician at the bedside (Unertl and Kottler, 1997). Clinical information systems will be more readily available for independent audit of data accuracy, and will reduce the time and cost of data collection. However, the use of clinical information systems may affect data collection such that the patient's score and predicted mortality are altered.

One study in this area has shown that the use of clinical information system charting to acquire the most abnormal physiology values for severity of illness scores and derived prognostic indices results in a higher mortality prediction (Bosman *et al.*, 1998). Predicted mortality increased by 15% for APACHE II compared to manual charting, 25% for SAPS II, and 24% for MPM_0. If these results are substantiated, comparison of patients and/or ICUs based on severity scores may be impossible without standardization of data collection. The authors suggest that the Mortality Prediction Models have to be revalidated and recalibrated when data are collected by a clinical information system. Furthermore, they suggest that every patient record in local, regional, national, or international ICU databases should be marked as being recorded by manual or by clinical information system charting (Bosman *et al.*, 1998). This finding has been confirmed more recently by a study showing that increasing the sampling rate for physiological variables results in higher scores and lower SMRs (Suistomaa *et al.*, 2000). It is interesting to speculate to what the apparent reduction in SMR would be attributed, particularly as the ICUs most likely to implement clinical information systems tend to be larger and may have more full-time staff trained in intensive care medicine.

The availability of bedside laboratory investigations

As well as automated charting, other bedside investigations, such as combined blood gas and biochemical analysis within the ICU might be expected to influence predicted mortality by altering the recorded physiological variables. The importance of small changes in the values collected for physiological data in the APACHE II score has been emphasized by Goldhill and Withington (1996). In a retrospective analysis of 11 348 critically ill patients, increasing scores by two or four points decreased mortality ratios from an original value of 1.13 to 1.00 and 0.89 respectively, while decreasing scores by two or four points to a minimum of zero increased mortality ratios to 1.27 and 1.44 respectively.

There is no published work comparing point of care to laboratory testing for biochemical and haematological variables with regard to the score calculated by ICU severity scoring systems. In theory, two opposite effects may occur. On one hand, predicted mortality might rise as it is probable that abnormal values are more likely to be identified by frequent point of care testing. Contrary to this, it could be argued that more frequent testing allows trends in abnormal values to be quickly identified and more promptly treated, so limiting the ultimate physiological disturbance.

Measuring coma

Many scoring systems include data from the Glasgow Coma Score (Teasdale and Jennett, 1974) to assess the patient's level of consciousness. It has been recognized that the reliability of Glasgow coma scoring is quite variable, largely due to difficulties interpreting the influence of sedative drugs (Angus, 2000). In one study examining interobserver reliability of APACHE scoring, the kappa statistic for APACHE II score components ranged from 0.315 (poor agreement) for the Glasgow Coma Score point allocation to 0.976 (good agreement) for age. Although the mean scores were not significantly different, important discrepancies in some components suggested either inadequate definitions for consistent data collection or inconsistent data collection itself (Chen *et al.*, 1999).

The Scottish Intensive Care Society Audit Group has recently stressed the importance of correct scoring for Glasgow Coma Score (Livingston *et al.*, 2000a). The effect of two different ways of scoring the Glasgow Coma Score on the performance of both APACHE II and APACHE III was assessed using measures of discrimination (the area under the ROC curve) and goodness of fit (calibration curves and the Hosmer-Lemeshow C statistic). The impact of the different scoring techniques produced large numbers of patients whose scores altered. The study concluded that Glasgow Coma Score should be assessed directly whenever possible, but when patients were sedated, using the Glasgow Coma Score recorded before sedation was preferable to the assumption of normality. Differences in scoring techniques for the Glasgow Coma Score might therefore result in wide institutionalized variations in score and predicted mortality for similar groups of patients.

Data collection accuracy

Another cause of interobserver variability is the selection of a diagnosis required in a number of scoring systems. We have previously demonstrated the variation in predicted mortality that arises from different interpretations of diagnosis and scoring for physiological variability in a structured case scenario reviewed by various ICU physicians in the south of England (Millar *et al.*, 1992). Using two fictitious patients we asked intensive care specialists to calculate the scores and predicted mortalities for the data provided. Scores ranged from 2 to 38 for the first 'patient' with predicted mortalities of between 1.0 and 86.2% and from 20 to 40 for the second patient with associated predicted mortalities of 12.8 to 80.7%. Other groups have found similar results when reviewing real data collected from different ICUs (Chen *et al.*, 1999). Although it might be possible to simplify the UK APACHE II model by extending the admission type and substituting the 53 UK APACHE II diagnostic categories with nine body systems without affecting performance (de Keizer *et al.*, 2000), differences in diagnostic categorization might account for present significant variations in predicted mortality and hence SMR.

Accuracy of data collection is prerequisite for useful, reliable and valid results from a scoring system. As well as the effect of small changes in data values discussed above, interobserver variability occurs between ICUs (Chen *et al.*, 1999), but the relevance of this variability in practice has not been investigated. It would be costly and time-consuming to audit data collection accuracy in the day-to-day running of an ICU. Moreover, to standardize data collection and maintain accuracy, retraining of data collection and analysis staff must be ongoing. It is impossible to say whether inaccuracies in data collection are likely to result in an over- or underestimation of predicted mortality. Random inaccuracies might just increase the spread of data while not altering their mean value. However, systematic bias, such as institutionalized inaccuracies concerning the Glasgow Coma Score are more likely to occur in particular patient groups and so might considerably bias the final mean predicted mortality for a particular group.

Variations in appropriateness of clinical targets

Scoring systems were initially designed with ranges of increasingly abnormal values for physiological data. The abnormal values were assigned scores commensurate with the supposed abnormality; such assignment was either done intuitively (Copeland *et al.*, 1991) or by more complex regression statistic models (Knaus *et al.*, 1991). However, changes in practice over time concerning appropriateness of clinical targets may affect the score generated while having an opposite or insignificant effect on actual mortality rates.

Two examples in intensive care practice illustrate this point. First, the use of expensive albumin infusions in critically ill patients has declined sharply

(Patey *et al.*, 1999) since its use has not been shown to improve outcome compared to alternatives (Stockwell *et al.*, 1992) and might even worsen outcome (Cochrane Injuries Group Albumin Reviewers, 1998). The decreased use of albumin exacerbates falls in serum albumin levels which will attract more points for physiological derangement in systems that score serum albumin levels. The increase in score will raise predicted mortality, while the effect on outcome is not clear.

Second, recent studies to determine whether a restrictive or liberal strategy of red cell transfusion in critically ill patients affects outcome, have shown that a restrictive strategy is at least as effective as, and possibly superior to, a liberal transfusion strategy (Hebert *et al.*, 1999). As with albumin levels, this would influence case-mix adjustment systems that use haemoglobin level as part of the predictive physiological data: lower haemoglobin levels would increase the predicted mortality while the restrictive transfusion policy might actually improve outcome (Hebert *et al.*, 1999). From the perspective of interpreting SMRs, a lower transfusion threshold may not alter outcome but would certainly reduce the SMR by increasing the apparent severity of illness of the patients.

Recalibration

Many clinical groups that use case-mix adjustment scoring systems to make comparisons between local ICUs are customizing or recalibrating the models to reflect local practice and results (Rowan *et al.*, 1994; Rivera-Fernandez *et al.*, 1998; Sirio *et al.*, 1999; Metnitz et al., 1999; Livingston et al., 2000b). These groups have decided that it is more important to decide how local hospitals compare with each other than to compare them with different ICUs or other databases. Such recalibration prevents comparisons with data gained from sources outside the recalibration group. Furthermore, a large change in practice might negate the commitment to data collection. For example in the Cleveland quality improvement initiative, the mean SMR fell over the 4 years of the data collection. However, rather than an improvement in care, this fall was probably due to a change in hospital discharge practice whereby patients were discharged earlier to skilled nursing facilities so excluding some patients from the calculation of the SMR (Sirio *et al.*, 1999).

Data manipulation

Data manipulation alters raw data to present the best possible result. It can be applied to case-mix adjustment scoring in numerous ways; any data manoeuvre that increases the prediction of mortality and reduces the measured mortality will reduce the SMR and apparently show an improvement in performance. Without careful external and independent audit, it is difficult to exclude data manipulation. Although the idea of data manipulation is an anathema to the honest clinician, professional standards must be maintained as in the long term an honest presentation of results, even if these results suggest poor performance, will produce better gains in healthcare resources and delivery.

It is particularly difficult to identify data manoeuvres that influence variables that cannot be easily checked by computerized data analysis, such as the diagnostic grouping and the Glasgow coma score. It is also possible to provide 'in house' rules for data collection that maximize the chance of finding the most abnormal value for physiological data and entering it into the appropriate scoring system.

The example of diagnostic weighting is particularly interesting. Frequently a selection of potential diagnoses can be applied to patients admitted to the ICU. The diagnosis specific weighting coefficient is combined with physiological data to calculate a predicted mortality. A legitimate manoeuvre would appear to be to select the diagnosis with the greatest weighting in all cases since combined organ failures tend to have a synergistic rather than additive effect; a computer program could do this automatically and most importantly, independently.

The UK collection of APACHE III data is guided by the Intensive Care National Audit and Research Centre's (ICNARC's) Case Mix Program Dataset Specification (1995). This specification details data collection for patients dying within 8 h of ICU admission and for those dying within 24 h. If the patient dies within 8 h, the data and the patient's death are not added to the results for that ICU. When the patient dies between 8 and 24 h, data are not collected during the patient's terminal phase. It is clear that the most abnormal data are likely to be collected closer to the patient's death, and this would have a strong influence on the predicted mortality.

Changes in measured mortality

At first sight, mortality would appear to benefit from having an absolute definition, and therefore seems to be the perfect endpoint for measurement. However, there are a number of influences that can change the measured mortality for scoring and case-mix adjustment programmes.

The rules for measuring mortality vary between scoring systems and may vary with local customization of such systems. The time of death within the dataset and the methods by which late deaths are excluded from the dataset vary considerably.

ICU scoring and case-mix adjustment programmes will not score patients who die prior to ICU admission. However, variations in admission protocols and facilities within the hospital, such as emergency room resuscitation and recovery facilities and the instantaneous availability of beds on ICU will all influence the number of early deaths on ICU. Such variation may be a function of facilities and procedure rather than quality of care. For example, one hospital may admit unstable patients directly to the ICU for pre-optimization while another hospital may admit these patients to a resuscitation area capable of ventilation and aggressive haemodynamic support outside the formal ICU. Furthermore, cultural differences in the thresholds for withdrawing or limiting invasive and aggressive care may also influence ICU mortality rates. To avoid this problem, rules for the inclusion of deaths occurring after a defined time period of intensive care may be required; one example is the 8 h limit employed in the UK ICNARC dataset (1995).

Inclusion criteria for later deaths are also variable, with some scoring systems including deaths within a defined time period, while others include all hospital deaths. Both of these are susceptible to variations between different hospitals, countries and times. For example, the increased transfer to nursing homes over time in Cleveland may have contributed to falling hospital mortality rates (Sirio *et al.*, 1999) despite no change in overall mortality. Unfortunately, the fall in hospital mortality rate was interpreted as an improvement in care and erroneously led to cessation of the entire Cleveland quality improvement initiative (Burton, 1999).

The link between care and the prediction of mortality

The logical use of case-mix adjustment is for the assessment of quality issues; improvements in care should improve mortality and consequently decrease SMR. This is not necessarily the case. Improved quality of organ support might result in less physiological disturbance and hence lower severity of illness scores. However, the underlying disease process may not have been reversed or affected so that the ultimate outcome of the patient remains unchanged; this would result in an increase in SMR. The relationship between quality of care and SMR is complicated, but is there any evidence that care can affect the prediction of mortality?

Lead-time bias

One of the first recognized effects of care on mortality prediction was that of care given before admission to the ICU on mortality prediction of scores collected after ICU admission. This has been termed 'lead-time bias'. Bion and colleagues (1985) described the effect of patients stabilized prior to transport to a tertiary referral centre showing a marked reduction in the APACHE II score and rise in SMR for the patient group. Other scoring systems also can be affected by lead-time bias. In a study of 76 critically ill patients using APACHE II, APACHE III and SAPS II scoring systems, data were collected either only after ICU admission or both prior to ICU and following admission. The inclusion of data collected in the period prior to ICU admission significantly increased both severity of illness scores and estimated risk of hospital mortality for all three scoring systems. This lead-time bias had most effect in medical patients and on emergency admissions, and least effect in patients admitted from the operating theatre (Tunnell *et al.*, 1998). The level of intensive care management before conventional ICU admission also modifies accuracy of predictive models (Castella *et al.*, 1991).

The effects of therapy

In addition to lead-time bias more subtle effects can occur on the ICU itself. We postulated in a discussion paper that ICU therapy might influence the prediction of mortality and the SMR in unexpected ways (Boyd and Grounds, 1993; Grounds and Boyd, 1997) and, although there was some debate at the time, others have agreed with our contention (Selker, 1993; Shann, 2000).

A number of clinical studies have shown the effects of ICU therapy on scoring prediction and case-mix adjustment. A study of the Injury Severity Score (Baker *et al.*, 1974) failed to differentiate severe injury from mismanagement of injury. The authors found that the Injury Severity Score mixed outcome data with injury severity, incorrectly assigning increased severity to the lesser injuries of mismanaged patients. These findings had important implications for use of the Injury Severity Score in quality of care assessments (Rutledge, 1996). This effect can be exaggerated by scores that use the worst physiological value in the first 12 to 24 h; patients mismanaged in a poorly performing ICU will have higher scores than similar patients managed in a better unit, and the bad unit's high mortality rate may be incorrectly attributed to its sicker patients (Shann *et al.*, 1997).

In other situations where general ICU care is improved, for example by the introduction of full-time intensivists, the lower scores for physiological derangement may be achieved in the better care group (Randolph, 1999; Pronovost *et al.*, 1999; Ghorra *et al.*, 1999). This suggests that full-time medical staff might be able to achieve finer physiological control; however, this is not always the case (Reynolds *et al.*, 1988). The data are confusing because other studies have found more physiological derangement in a 'closed' ICU compared to the same ICU when it was managed as an 'open' ICU (Carson *et al.*, 1996; Hanson *et al.*, 1999). There are a number of explanations such as sicker patients being admitted to the 'closed' ICU, or that the 'closed' ICU collected the worst data because they were looked for more often and better recorded.

Conclusion

The use of scoring systems in intensive care medicine is widespread and is becoming essential benchmarking practice. Scoring systems are used to adjust many diagnoses and severities of illness so that comparisons can be made. It has been suggested that these comparisons will allow identification of good and bad practice, and might be used for comparison of novel therapeutic approaches.

This chapter considered the problems with the interpretation of case-mix adjustment systems and has highlighted the potential misinterpretations. The statistical techniques used for the development and calibration of datasets and scoring systems are complicated and poorly understood by the medical community. Datasets are frequently underpowered for individual ICU decision making. It is possible to change the predicted mortality of the patient group by altering data collection mechanism. Also, it is possible to alter the mortality rate used for calculation of SMR by changing hospital practice and the time-frames for inclusion of patient deaths. Finally, the relationship between quality of care and the prediction of mortality is complex, depending on the timing of care and the influence that good care, or poor care, might have on predicted and actual mortality. It is premature and dangerous to undertake complex comparisons of ICU performance without a full understanding of the problems inherent in case-mix adjustment.

References

Alvarez, M., Nava, J. M., Rue, M., Quintana, S. (1998). Mortality prediction in head trauma patients: performance of Glasgow Coma Score and general severity systems. *Crit. Care Med.*, **26,** 142–148.

Angus, D. C. (2000). Scoring system fatigue and the search for a way forward. *Crit. Care Med.*, **28,** 2145–2146.

Apolone, G. (2000). The state of research on multipurpose severity of illness scoring systems: are we on target? *Intensive Care Med.*, **26,** 1727–1729.

Audit Commission (1999). *Critical to Success. The place of efficient and effective critical care services within the acute hospital.* Audit Commission.

Baker, S. P., O'Neil, B., Haddun, W., Long, W. B. (1974). The Injury Severity Score: a method for describing patients with multiple injuries and evaluating emergency care. *J. Trauma,* **14,** 187–196.

Bion, J. F., Edlin, S. A., Ramsey, G., Ledingham, I. M. (1985). Validation of a prognostic score in critically ill patients undergoing transport. *Br. Med. J.,* **291,** 432–434.

Blunt, M. C., Burchett, K. R. (2000). Out-of-hours consultant cover and case-mix-adjusted mortality in intensive care. *Lancet,* **356,** 735–736.

Bosman, R. J., Oudemane van Straaten, H. M., Zandstra, D. F. (1998). The use of intensive care information systems alters outcome prediction. *Intensive Care Med.,* **24,** 953–958.

Boyd, O., Grounds, R. M. (1993). Physiological scoring systems and audit. *Lancet,* **341,** 1573–1574.

Boyd, O., Grounds, M. (1994). Can standardized mortality ratio be used to compare quality of intensive care unit performance? *Crit. Care Med.,* **22,** 1706–1709.

Burton, T. M. (1999). Examining table: Operation that rated hospitals was success, but the patience died. Cleveland Clinic found faults with CEOs, whose ardor had faded too. Low grades spurred reforms. *Wall Street Journal,* 23 August, p. A1.

Carson, S. S., Stocking, C., Podsadecki, T. *et al.* (1996). Effects of organizational change in the medical intensive care unit of a teaching hospital: a comparison of 'open' and 'closed' formats. *JAMA,* **276,** 322–328.

Castella, X., Artigas, A., Bion, J., Kari, A. (1995). A comparison of severity of illness scoring systems for intensive care unit patients: results of a multicenter, multinational study. The European/North American Severity Study Group. *Crit. Care Med.,* **23,** 1327–1335.

Castella, X., Gilabert, J., Torner, F., Torres, C. (1991). Mortality Prediction Models in intensive care: Acute Physiology And Chronic Health Evaluation II and Mortality Prediction Model compared. *Crit. Care Med.,* **19,** 191–197.

Chen, L. M., Martin, C. M., Morrison, T. L., Sibbald, W. J. (1999). Inter-observer variability in data collection of the APACHE II score in teaching and community hospitals. *Crit. Care Med.,* **27,** 1999–2004.

Cochrane Injuries Group Albumin Reviewers. (1998). Human albumin administration in critically ill patients: systematic review of randomised controlled trials. Cochrane Injuries Group Albumin Reviewers. *Br. Med. J.,* **317,** 235–240.

Connors, A. F., Speroff, T., Dawson, N. V. *et al.* (1996). The effectiveness of right heart catheterization in the initial care of the critically ill. JAMA, **276,** 889–897.

Copeland, G. P., Jones, D., Walters, M. (1991). POSSUM: a scoring system for surgical audit. *Br. J. Surg.,* **78,** 355–360.

Dalen, J. E., Bone, R. C. (1996). Is it time to pull the pulmonary artery catheter ? *JAMA,* **276,** 916–918.

de Keizer, N. F., Bonsel, G. J., Goldfrad, C., Rowan, K. M. (2000). The added value that increasing levels of diagnostic information provide in prognostic models to estimate hospital mortality for adult intensive care patients. *Intensive Care Med.,* **26,** 577–584.

Department of Health. (2000). *Comprehensive Critical Care: A review of adult critical care services.* Department of Health.

Dubois, R. W., Rogers, W. H., Moxley J. H. 3rd, Brook, R. H. (1987). Hospital inpatient mortality; is it a predictor of quality? *N. Eng. J. Med.,* **317,** 1674–1680.

Fiaccadori, E., Maggiore, U., Lombardi, M., Leonardi, S., Rotelli, C., Borghetti, A. H. (2000). Predicting patient outcome from acute renal failure comparing three general severity of illness scoring systems. *Kidney Int.,* **58,** 283–292.

Ghorra, S., Reinert, S. E., Cioffi, W., Simms, H. H. (1999). Analysis of the effect of conversion from open to closed surgical intensive care unit. *Ann. Surg.,* **229,** 163–171.

Goldhill, D. R., Withington, P. S. (1996). Mortality predicted by APACHE II. The effect of changes in physiological values and post-ICU hospital mortality. *Anaesthesia,* **51,** 719–723.

Grounds, R. M., Boyd, O. (1997). Audit using ICU physiology scoring and outcome prediction. *Anaesthesia,* **52,** 916.

Hanson, C. W. 3rd, Deutschman, C. S., Anderson, H. L. 3rd, *et al.* (1999). Effects of an organized critical care service on outcomes and resource utilization: a cohort study. *Crit. Care Med.,* **27,** 270–274.

Hebert, P. C., Wells, G., Blajchman, M. A. *et al.* (1999). A multicenter, randomized, controlled clinical trial of transfusion requirements in critical care. Transfusion Requirements in Critical Care Investigators, Canadian Critical Care Trials Group. *N. Engl. J. Med.,* **340,** 409–417.

Intensive Care National Audit and Research Centre (1995) *ICNARC Case Mix Program Dataset Specification,* Intensive Care National Audit and Research Centre.

Katsaragakis, S., Papadimitropoulos, K., Antonakis, P., Strergiopoulos, S., Konstadoulakis, M. M., Androulakis, G. (2000). Comparison of Acute Physiology and Chronic Health Evaluation II (APACHE II) and Simplified Acute Physiology Score II (SAPS II) scoring systems in a single Greek intensive care unit. *Crit. Care Med.,* **28,** 426–432.

King's Fund. (1989). Intensive Care in the United Kingdom: Report from the King's Fund Panel. *Anaesthesia,* **44,** 428–431.

Knaus, W. A., Draper, E. A., Wagner, D. P., Zimmerman, J. E. (1985). APACHE II: A severity of disease classification system. *Crit. Care Med.*, **13**, 818–829.

Knaus, W. A., Draper, E. A., Wagner, D. P., Zimmerman, J. E. (1986). An evaluation of outcome from intensive care in major medical centers. *Ann. Int. Med.*, **104**, 410–418.

Knaus, W. A., Wagner, D. P., Draper, E. A. *et al.* (1991). The APACHE III prognostic system: risk prediction of hospital mortality for critically ill hospitalized adults. *Chest*, **100**, 1619–1636.

Knaus, W. A., Zimmerman, J. E., Wagner, D. P., Draper, E A., Lawrence, D. E. (1981). APACHE – Acute Physiology And Chronic Health Evaluation: a physiologically based classification system. *Crit. Care Med.*, **9**, 591–597.

Le Gall, J. R., Lemeshow, S., Saulnier, F. (1993). A new Simplified Acute Physiology Score (SAPS II) based on a European/North American multicenter study. *JAMA*, **270**, 2957–2963.

Lemeshow, S., Hosmer, D. W. Jr (1982). A review of goodness of fit statistics for use in the development of logistic regression models. *Am. J. Epidemiol.*, **115**, 92–106.

Lemeshow, S., Le Gall, J. R. (1994). Modeling the severity of illness of ICU patients. A systems update. *JAMA*, **272**, 1049–1055.

Lemeshow, S., Teres, D., Avrunin, J. S., Pastides, H. (1987). A comparison of methods to predict mortality of intensive care unit patients. *Crit. Care Med.*, **15**, 715–722.

Lemeshow, S., Teres, D., Klar, J., Avrunin, J. S., Gehbach, S. H., Rapoport, J. (1993). Mortality Probability Models (MPM II) based on an international cohort of intensive care unit patients. *JAMA*, **270**, 2478–2486.

Lemeshow, S., Teres, D., Pastides, H., Avrunin, J. S., Steingrub, J. S. (1985). A method for predicting survival and mortality of ICU patients using objectively derived weights. *Crit. Care Med.*, **13**, 519–525.

Linde-Zwirble, W. T., Angus, D. C. (1998). Can scoring systems assess ICU performance? *J Intensive Care Med.*, **13**, 155–205.

Livingston, B. M., Mackenzie, S. J., MacKirdy, F. N., Howie, J. C. (2000a). Should the pre-sedation Glasgow Coma Scale value be used when calculating Acute Physiology and Chronic Health Evaluation scores for sedated patients? Scottish Intensive Care Society Audit Group. *Crit. Care Med.*, **28**, 389–394.

Livingston, B. M., MacKirdy, F. N., Howie, J. C., Jones, R., Norrie, J. D. (2000b). Assessment of the performance of five intensive care scoring models within a large Scottish database. *Crit. Care Med.*, **28**, 1820–1827.

Markgraf, R., Deutschinoff, G., Pientka, L., Scholten, T. (2000). Comparison of Acute Physiology And Chronic Health Evaluations II and III and Simplified Acute Physiology Score II: a prospective cohort study evaluating these methods to predict outcome in a German interdisciplinary intensive care unit. *Crit. Care Med.*, **28**, 26–33.

Marsh, H. M., Krishan, I., Naessens, J. M. *et al.* (1990). Assessment of prediction of mortality by using the APACHE III scoring system in intensive-care units. *Mayo Clin. Proc.*, **65**, 1549–1557.

McNeil, B. J., Hanley, J. A. (1984). Statistical approaches to the analysis of receiver operating characteristic (ROC) curves. *Med. Decis. Making*, **4**, 137–150.

Metnitz, P. G., Valentin, A., Vesely, H. *et al.* (1999). Prognostic performance and customization of the SAPS II: results of a multicenter Austrian study. Simplified Acute Physiology Score. *Intensive Care Med.*, **25**, 192–197.

Millar, B., Boyd, O., Henderson, S., Bennett, D. (1992). APACHE II cannot be used to compare performance between intensive care units. *Clin. Sci.*, **82**, 25P.

Moreno, R., Apolone, G., Reis Miranda, D. (1998a). Evaluation of the uniformity of fit of general outcome prediction models. *Intensive Care Med.*, **24**, 40–47.

Moreno, R., Reis Miranda, D., Fidler, V., Van Schilfgaarde, R. (1998b). Evaluation of two outcome prediction models on an independent database. *Crit. Care Med.*, **26**, 50–61.

Nouira, S., Belghith, M., Elatrous, S. *et al.* (1998). Predictive value of severity scoring systems: comparison of four models in Tunisian adult intensive care units. *Crit. Care Med.*, **26**, 852–859.

Oudemans-van Straaten, H. M., Bosman, R. J., van der Spoel, J. I., Zandstra, D. F. (1999). Outcome of critically ill patients treated with intermittent high-volume haemofiltration: a prospective cohort analysis. *Intensive Care Med.*, **25**, 814–821.

Patel, P. A., Grant, B. J. (1999). Application of mortality prediction systems to individual intensive care units. *Intensive Care Med.*, **25**, 977–982.

Patey, R., Wilson, G., Hulse, T. (1999). Albumin controversy continues. Meta-analysis has affected use of albumin. *Br. Med. J.*, **318**, 464.

Poses, R. M., McClish, D. K., Smith, W. R. *et al.* (2000). Results of report cards for patients with congestive heart failure depend on the method used to adjust for severity. *Ann. Intern. Med.*, **133**, 10–20.

Pronovost, P. J., Jenckes, M. W., Dorman, T. *et al.* (1999). Organizational characteristics of intensive care units related to outcomes of abdominal aortic surgery. *JAMA*, **281**, 1310–1317.

Randolph, A. G. (1999). Reorganizing the delivery of intensive care may improve patient outcomes. *JAMA*, **281**, 1330–1331.

Randolph, A. G., Guyatt, G. H., Calvin, J. E., Doig, G., Richardson, W. S. (1998). Understanding articles describing clinical prediction tools. Evidence Based Medicine in Critical Care Group. *Crit. Care Med.*, **26**, 1603–1612.

Reynolds, H. N., Haupt, M. T., Thill-Baharozian, M. C., Carlson, R. W. (1988). Impact of critical care physician staffing on patients with septic shock in a university hospital medical intensive care unit. *JAMA*, **260**, 3446–3450.

Rivera-Fernandez, R., Vazquez-Mata, G., Bravo, M. *et al.* (1998). The APACHE III prognostic system: customized mortality predictions for Spanish ICU patients. *Intensive Care Med.*, **24**, 574–581.

Rowan, K. M., Kerr, J. H., Major, E., McPherson, K., Short, A., Vessey, M. P. (1994). Intensive Care Society's Acute Physiology and Chronic Health Evaluation (APACHE II) study in Britain and Ireland: a prospective, multicenter, cohort study comparing two methods for predicting outcome for adult intensive care patients. *Crit. Care Med.*, **22**, 1392–1401.

Rutledge, R. (1996). The Injury Severity Score is unable to differentiate between poor care and severe injury. *J. Trauma*, **40**, 944–950.

Selker, H. P. (1993). Systems for comparing actual and predicted mortality rates: characteristics to promote cooperation in improving hospital care. *Ann. Intern. Med.*, **118**, 820–822.

Shann, F. (2000). MPM is preferable to APACHE as an intensive care scoring system. *Br. Med. J.*, **320**, 714.

Shann, F., Pearson, G., Slater, A. *et al.* (1997). Paediatric index of mortality (PIM): a Mortality Prediction Model for children in intensive care. *Intensive Care Med.*, **23**, 201–207.

Sicignano, A., Carozzi, C., Giudici, D., Merli, G., Arlati, S., Pulici, M. (1996). The influence of length of stay in the ICU on power of discrimination of a multipurpose severity score (SAPS). *Intensive Care Med.*, **22**, 1048–1051.

Sirio, C. A., Shepardson, L. B., Rotondi, A. J. *et al.* (1999). Community-wide assessment of intensive care outcomes using a physiologically based prognostic measure:

implications for critical care delivery from Cleveland Health Quality Choice. *Chest,* **115**, 793–801.

Stockwell, M. A., Soni, N., Riley, B. (1992). Colloid solutions in the critically ill. A randomised comparison of albumin and polygeline. 1. Outcome and duration of stay in the intensive care unit. *Anaesthesia,* **47**, 3–6.

Suistomaa, M., Kari, A., Ruokonen, E., Takala, J. (2000). Sampling rate causes bias in APACHE II and SAPS II scores. *Intensive Care Med.,* **26**, 1773–1778.

Teasdale, G., Jennett, B. (1974). Assessment of coma and impaired consciousness, a practical scale. *Lancet,* **ii**, 81–84.

Teres, D., Lemeshow, S., Avrunin, J. S., Pastides, H. (1987). Validation of the Mortality Prediction Model for ICU patients. *Crit. Care Med.,* **15**, 208–213.

Tunnell, R. D., Millar, B. W., Smith, G. B. (1998). The effect of lead time bias on severity of illness scoring, mortality prediction and standardised mortality ratio in intensive care – a pilot study. *Anaesthesia,* **53**, 1045–1053.

Unertl, K., Kottler, B. M. (1997). Prognostic scores in intensive care. *Anaesthetist,* **46**, 471–480.

Vassar, M. J., Lewis, F. R. Jr., Chambers, J. A. *et al.* (1999). Prediction of outcome in intensive care unit trauma patients: a multicenter study of Acute Physiology and Chronic Health Evaluation (APACHE), Trauma and Injury Severity Score (TRISS), and a 24-hour intensive care unit (ICU) point system. *J. Trauma,* **47**, 324–329.

Vincent, J. L. (2000). Need for intensivists in intensive-care units. *Lancet,* **356**, 695–696.

Zimmerman, J. E., Knaus, W. A., Wagner, D. P. (1994). Can standardized mortality ratio be used to compare quality of intensive care unit performance? *Crit. Care Med.,* **10**, 1708–1709.

Zimmerman, J. E., Shortell, S. M., Knaus, W. A. *et al.* (1993a). Value and cost of teaching hospitals: a prospective, multicenter, inception cohort study. *Crit. Care Med.,* **21**, 1432–442.

Zimmerman, J. E., Shortell, S. M., Rousseau, D. M. *et al.* (1993b). Improving intensive care: observations based on organizational case studies in nine intensive care units: a prospective, multicenter study. *Crit. Care Med.,* **21**, 1443–1451.

Zimmerman, J. E., Wagner, D. P. (2000). Prognostic systems in intensive care: how do you interpret an observed mortality that is higher than expected? *Crit. Care Med.,* **28**, 258–260.

Chapter 5

Organ dysfunction scores

Jean-Louis Vincent and Daliana Peres-Bota

Introduction

Organ dysfunction is a common event among intensive care patients; indeed almost all critically ill patients will have some degree of organ dysfunction during their hospital stay. Multiple organ failure, the extreme end of the continuum of organ dysfunction, is the leading cause of morbidity and mortality on the intensive care unit (ICU) (Tran *et al.*, 1990; Deitch, 1992; Beal and Cerra, 1994; Moreno *et al.*, 1999). Multiple organ failure has been defined as progressive dysfunction of two or more organ systems following an acute threat to systemic homeostasis (ACCP-SCCM Consensus Conference, 1992), but there is little consensus on which organ systems should be included in this definition, or even on what constitutes 'failure'. Hence, the 'simple' term, multiple organ failure, covers a host of possible combinations and degrees of organ failure or dysfunction. Several systems, the organ dysfunction scores, have thus been developed to describe and quantify the organ dysfunction of individual or groups of ICU patients. In this chapter we will discuss the development, applications and limitations of the organ dysfunction scores most commonly used in adult critically ill patients.

Models for ICU patient description

The organ dysfunction scores allocate specific numerical values to the degree of organ dysfunction in individual ICU patients. By following trends in these values, one can follow the evolution of the organ dysfunction over time. Other methods of describing patient populations have been developed that are non-organ specific and rather describe 'syndromes' of ICU disease; these include the Sepsis Syndrome (Bone *et al.*, 1989a), and the Systemic Inflammatory Response Syndrome (SIRS) (ACCP-SCCM Consensus Conference, 1992). These definitions do not attempt to describe or predict outcome, but were developed to facilitate comparisons between patient groups and to create some uniformity in the assessment of patients for inclusion in clinical trials (Opal, 1998).

'The Sepsis Syndrome' is a term coined by Roger Bone and colleagues (1987, 1989b) in the late 1980s to describe patients with sepsis, and has been used to select patients for entry to several clinical trials of treatments for sepsis. The Sepsis Syndrome is defined as hypothermia (temperature less than 96°F (35.6°C)) or hyperthermia (greater than 101°F (38.3°C)), tachycardia (greater than 90 beat/min), tachypnoea (greater than 20 breaths/min), clinical evidence of an infection site, and at least one end-organ demonstrating inadequate perfusion or dysfunction expressed as poor or altered cerebral function, hypoxaemia (PaO_2 less than 75 mmHg (10 kPa)), elevated plasma lactate, or oliguria (urine output less than 30 ml/h or 0.5 ml/kg body weight/h without corrective therapy). Problems have, however, arisen with the use of this definition, and it is now not widely used; for example, a patient who is clearly septic and fulfills all the criteria but has a temperature of just 38.2°C would not fit the definition and would thus be excluded from trial entry.

SIRS was developed at a North American consensus conference in an attempt to provide standard guidelines to identify patients who were likely to benefit from new anti-sepsis treatments. The SIRS criteria are met when at least two of the following are present:

1. Body temperature greater than 38°C or less than 36°C
2. Heart rate greater than 90 beats/min
3. Tachypnoea (respiratory rate greater than 20 breaths/min or $PaCO_2$ less than 32 mmHg (4.3 kPa))
4. Alterations in white blood cell count (greater than $12 \times 10^9/l$ or less than $4 \times 10^9/l$)

However, these criteria proved to be too sensitive, with the majority of ICU patients, regardless of their disease process, having SIRS at some point during their ICU stay (Rangel-Frausto et al., 1995; Salvo et al., 1995; Bossink et al., 1998). In fact many healthy people could be said to have SIRS when, for example, they run to catch a bus (Vincent, 1997). Studies using SIRS as an entry criterion, will thus include hugely heterogeneous groups of critically ill patients. As such, the SIRS definition is of little practical use and after being 'in vogue' for sometime, many intensivists are no longer using the term.

Mortality versus morbidity

With ever-increasing emphasis on the need to practice effective, but cost-efficient medicine, patient outcomes are being scrutinized across all walks of medicine, including critical care. The ultimate outcome measure for any patient is of course survival (or mortality), and several scoring systems, for example the Acute

Physiology And Chronic Health Evaluation (APACHE) (Knaus *et al.*, 1981), the Simplified Acute Physiology Score (SAPS) (Le Gall *et al.*, 1984) and the Mortality Probability Models (MPM) (Lemeshow *et al.*, 1988) have been developed. All are based on assessment of the patient's severity of illness on admission, which provides a prediction of the likelihood of survival for that patient. However, death is not the only relevant measure of the success or failure of intensive care. Aspects of morbidity during an ICU stay provide crucial information regarding a patient's illness and response to treatment. In addition, while mortality prediction tools provide valuable epidemiological data for clinical trial analysis or comparisons between ICUs, such scores give no detail of what happens to individual patients during their ICU admission. For example, in a clinical trial of placebo versus treatment using mortality as the outcome measure, if the mortality rates of both groups of patients are the same, the treatment would be said to be ineffective, and hence discarded. However, if, in the same trial, measures of morbidity are analysed, the treatment group is shown to have fewer episodes of organ failure, less requirement for mechanical ventilation, shorter hospital stays, etc., this same treatment thus has potentially beneficial effects which were hidden by the initial focus on mortality as the outcome measure. Use of an organ dysfunction score could therefore provide encouraging data and perhaps prevent the loss of a potentially valuable therapeutic agent.

Organ dysfunction scores thus provide valuable data for clinical trial enrolment and evaluation. By providing descriptions of patient populations, they enable quality control comparisons between ICUs and within an ICU over time. With repeated evaluation, they can be used to describe the evolution of organ dysfunction in individual patients, and possibly be used to monitor and guide therapeutic decisions. Importantly, organ dysfunction scores are not developed to assess the probability of mortality, although they do correlate well with outcome (Vincent *et al.*, 1998; Marshall *et al.*, 1995), and these scores should thus be seen as providing complementary information to their close neighbours, the mortality prediction scores, rather than replacing them.

Organ failure scores

Development

The value of a scoring system to classify organ dysfunction was recognized some 30 years ago (Tilney *et al.*, 1973), and other early scores were developed that established cut-off points for organ failure (Fry *et al.*, 1980; Stevens, 1983; Knaus *et al.*, 1985; Goris *et al.*, 1985).

More recently, other systems have been developed to describe organ dysfunction using various techniques, but often based on the work of these earlier studies in critically ill patients (Hebert *et al.*, 1993; Fagon *et al.*, 1993; Marshall *et al.*, 1995; Le Gall *et al.*, 1996; Vincent *et al.*, 1996; Leteurtre *et al.*, 1999). The techniques used in the design of these scores include consensus (Vincent *et al.*,

1996), the Delphi method (Leteurtre *et al.*, 1999) and statistical multiple logistic regression (Le Gall *et al.*, 1996); these methods are discussed in more detail below. Importantly, once created, such scores need to be extensively validated in order to be considered accurate for use in different patient populations; unfortunately this has been achieved for relatively few of the scoring systems. Scores need to show good calibration, discrimination, reproducibility, and transportability across geographic and time boundaries (Justice *et al.*, 1999), so that they can be used by different operators, in different ICUs, in different countries and at different times. This is particularly true for severity indices designed to predict survival. However, organ dysfunction scores are used only to describe organ dysfunction, so how should they be validated? Usually, they have been validated against mortality, even though this is not their primary purpose.

In the development of organ dysfunction scores, several key features of organ dysfunction need to be remembered (Vincent *et al.*, 1996):

1. Organ dysfunction is a process rather than a one-off event. There is a continuum of organ dysfunction from the smallest abnormality to full-blown organ failure. Organ dysfunction scores thus need to be able to measure varying degrees of organ (dys)function.
2. Organ dysfunction is a dynamic process and will alter over time. Organ dysfunction scores thus need to be able to be measured repeatedly.
3. Organ dysfunction scores need to be simple to use. Variables included in the scoring system need to be objective, reliable, and specific for the organ in question, but also routinely available in all ICUs. Ideally the variables should be independent of therapeutic or patient variables to enable comparison between ICUs where treatment protocols may vary.

The choice of organ systems to be included in an organ dysfunction score is debatable, but generally six systems are selected: the respiratory, cardiovascular, coagulation, renal, hepatic and central nervous systems. Other systems sometimes included are the gastrointestinal tract and the immune system. Indeed, with recent interest in the role of the gastrointestinal tract in the development of multiple organ failure (Marshall *et al.*, 1993; Mythen and Webb, 1994), inclusion of this system could be of particular interest. There are, however, limited objective measures of gastrointestinal function. Tolerance to feeding is one possibility, but this is difficult to quantitate objectively. Gastric tonometry may provide a means of monitoring gastrointestinal function, but this technique remains experimental and still controversial; hence this is not widely used.

For each system, various measures of (dys)function can be used (Bertleff and Bruining, 1997) (Table 5.1) and those chosen vary between the different scores (Table 5.2).

The key features of the variables chosen are:

1. Objectivity: for example, the presence of clinical jaundice as a measure of hepatic dysfunction, or confusion as a measure of central nervous system

Table 5.1 Suggested variables used in scoring systems for assessing organ dysfunction

Organ system	Potential variables	Organ system	Potential variables
Pulmonary	Days of mechanical ventilation Respiratory rate Positive end-expiratory pressure (PEEP) Fraction of inspired oxygen (F_iO_2) PaO_2/F_iO_2 $PaCO_2$ Static lung compliance Alveolar arterial oxygen diffusion	Hepatic	Bilirubin concentration Aspartate or alanine aminotransferase concentration Alkaline phosphatase concentration Prothrombin or partial thromboplastin time Glutamate dehydrogenase concentration Lactate dehydrogenase concentration Albumin concentration Clinical jaundice
Cardiovascular	Heart rate Systolic blood pressure Mean arterial pressure Cardiac output or index Pulmonary artery wedge pressure Inotropic support Acidaemia Arrhythmias	Neurological	Glasgow Coma Scale Presence of coma Confusion
Renal	Urine output Serum creatinine concentration Serum urea concentration Blood urea nitrogen (BUN) concentration Creatinine clearance Urinary sodium clearance Need for dialysis	Immunological	White blood cell count Hypersensitivity skin testing
Coagulation	Platelet count Prothrombin time Partial thromboplastin time Presence of disseminated intravascular coagulation (DIC)	Gastrointestinal	Stress ulcer bleeding Acalculous cholecystitis Ileus Amount of nasogastric drainage Malabsorption Gastric intramucosal pH (pHi)

Table 5.2 Comparison between the Multiple Organ Dysfunction Score (MODS), Sepsis-related Organ Failure Assessment (SOFA) and Logistic Organ Dysfunction System (LODS)

	MODS	SOFA	LODS
Developed by	Literature review	Consensus	Multiple logistic regression
Values included in daily score	First morning	Worst daily	Worst daily
Parameter chosen to measure dysfunction:			
Respiratory system	PaO_2/F_iO_2 ratio	PaO_2/F_iO_2 ratio and need for ventilatory support	PaO_2/F_iO_2 ratio and ventilation/CPAP requirements
Cardiovascular system	Pressure-adjusted heart rate (heart rate × [central venous pressure/mean arterial pressure])	Blood pressure and adrenergic support	Heart rate and systolic blood pressure
Renal system	Creatinine concentration	Creatinine concentration or urine output	Creatinine and urea concentrations and urine output
Hepatic system	Bilirubin concentration	Bilirubin concentration	Bilirubin concentration and prothrombin time
Central nervous system	Glasgow Coma Score	Glasgow Coma Score	Glasgow Coma Score
Coagulation system	Platelet count	Platelet count	Platelet count and white blood cell count

dysfunction, are subjective and may lead to different interpretation by different physicians, so rendering the scoring system unreliable.

2. Organ specificity: for example, the prothrombin time can be a measure of dysfunction of both the coagulation and the hepatic systems; metabolic acidosis can indicate cardiovascular failure (lactic acidosis), but may also occur in renal failure and other pathologies.

3. Simplicity: assessment of cardiovascular function in the Multiple Organ Dysfunction Score (MODS) uses the pressure adjusted heart rate, making this a more complex score and thus, possibly, less likely to be used routinely. A small number of variables also makes the scores simpler to use.

4. Availability: the variables selected should be readily available at all institutions if the score is to gain widespread acceptance. A scoring system using tests only available at large university-based ICUs will be of little value to more remote, or less technologically advanced community ICUs, who nevertheless are interested in following the course of organ dysfunction in their patients.

5. Patient independence: selected parameters to be included in a scoring system should also be independent of patient variables, such as gender, age, race, etc.

6. Repeatability: as organ dysfunction is time-dependent, it must be possible to repeat the organ dysfunction score several times, even every day, during an ICU stay. Variables must be chosen which can be easily measured as often as necessary.

7. Therapeutic independence: while it may be ideal for the variable to be independent of therapy, it is not realistic; few variables are truly independent of therapy in the ICU. For example, many of the measures of pulmonary function will be influenced by the ventilatory settings, platelet counts by platelet transfusions, measures of renal function by dialysis, etc.

Utility

Organ dysfunction scores have three main areas of application:

1. Use in clinical trials. In recent years, many potential treatments have been proposed and trialled in patients with sepsis and although all have shown great promise in animal models, few have proved to improve mortality in clinical trials. It is increasingly realized that new trials should include some organ dysfunction scoring system in their protocol, and that the outcome emphasis should not be restricted to mortality and, indeed, trials do now use an organ dysfunction score as part of the outcome assessment (Goncalves et al., 1998; Staubach et al., 1998; Di Filippo et al., 1998; Briegel et al., 1999). Organ dysfunction scores can also be used to account for differences in organ dysfunction at the outset of the study. For instance, differences in mortality rates for the recent study of an anti-TNF antibody (Afelimobab, Knoll AG, Ludwigshafen, Germany) became statistically significant when differences in

SOFA scores were taken into account (unpublished data). Such analysis had been included in the analytic plan, so it should not be considered a *post hoc* analysis. In addition, these scores can be used in patient selection for clinical trials to enable more specific groups of patients to be enrolled.

2. Use in epidemiological studies. Organ dysfunction scores can usefully describe the characteristics of patient populations for epidemiological analysis, comparing different ICUs and the same ICU over time; such evaluations and comparisons may help direct ICU resources most appropriately.

3. Clinical use. Repeated (daily) evaluation of an organ dysfunction score can provide a picture of the evolution of single, and overall, organ dysfunction in individual patients. Such use could provide a means of monitoring and guiding therapy. Evaluation of such results can help improve our understanding of the natural history of the development of organ dysfunction and multiple organ failure and of the interaction between various organ failures. This in turn could help in the development and targeting of new therapies.

Logistic Organ Dysfunction System (LODS) score

The LODS was developed in 1996 using a multiple logistic regression technique on a large database of 13 152 admissions to 137 ICUs in 12 countries (Le Gall *et al.*, 1996). By developing the system using statistical methods, the authors felt that levels of organ dysfunction could be determined objectively, the significance of severity levels for each organ could be easily identified, and the levels of dysfunction could be weighted according to their relative prognostic significance. Unlike the MODS and SOFA, the LODS score is both a global score that summarizes the combined dysfunction across organ systems and a logistic regression equation that can be used to translate the score into a probability of mortality.

Using a development set of 10 547 patients, variables were extracted from the database to define organ dysfunction, based on a combination of 12 variables for six organ systems (neurological, cardiovascular, renal, pulmonary, haematological and hepatic). The worst value in the first 24 h of admission was recorded. Cut-off points were identified to define the ranges of severity for each variable, and multiple logistic regression was used to create the final score. For each system, a score of 0 indicates no dysfunction and a score of 5 represents maximum dysfunction. However, as the LODS score is a weighted system, the relative severity of dysfunction allows for a maximum score of 5 for only the neurological, renal, and cardiovascular systems. For the respiratory and coagulation systems, the maximum score is 3, and for the liver the maximum score is 1. The range of LODS scores is thus from 0 to 22. The LODS score was then validated on 2605 patients in the database, showing good correlation with mortality; a LODS score of 22 being associated with a mortality of 99.7%. The LODS score was designed to be calculated on the first day of admission and has not been validated for repeated use during the ICU stay. It is a more complex system than other organ dysfunction scores.

Multiple Organ Dysfunction Score (MODS)

The MODS was developed initially by John Marshall and colleagues (1995) who performed a literature review of all the studies of multiple organ failure published between 1969 and 1993 to determine which characteristics had been used to define organ failure. Thirty clinical studies involving more than 20 patients were identified. Seven organ systems (respiratory, cardiovascular, renal, hepatic, haematological, gastrointestinal and central nervous system) were included in more than half of these studies and so were selected for analysis in the development of MODS.

The variables identified for each of these organ systems were then evaluated against a set of criteria established by the authors as the ideal descriptor of organ dysfunction for each system. As a result, the PaO_2/FiO_2 ratio was selected for respiratory system assessment; serum creatinine concentration for the renal system; serum bilirubin concentration for the hepatic system; a composite measure, the pressure-adjusted heart rate (heart rate × (central venous pressure divided by mean arterial pressure)) for the cardiovascular system; the platelet count for the haematological system; the Glasgow Coma Score (GCS) for the central nervous system. The gastrointestinal system was eliminated from the score because no reliable, continuous descriptor could be found.

These variables were then assessed for their ability to predict ICU mortality in a population of 692 surgical ICU patients. The first 336 patients were used as the development set to evaluate and calibrate the variables. Calibration involved comparing survivors and non-survivors to ascertain that the mean worst value of each variable was indeed worse in non-survivors, and then the variables were correlated with mortality at differing levels of severity. The variables were graded such that a score of 0 for any variable correlated with an ICU mortality less than 5% while a score of 4 correlated with an ICU mortality greater than, or equal to 50%. Intervals were set so that similar scores for different organ systems correlated with approximately the same ICU mortality. These scores were then tested on the validation set of 356 patients.

A high initial MODS correlated with ICU mortality, while the delta MODS, the increase in the MODS score between admission and the worst MODS recorded during the ICU stay, was even more predictive of outcome. In a group of 368 patients with septic shock, Jacobs and colleagues (1999) showed that maximum and delta MODS mirrored organ dysfunction and could distinguish between survivors and non-survivors, while daily APACHE II and organ failure scores could not. Barie *et al.* (1996) found that in 2295 surgical ICU patients, the MODS score and the APACHE III score were independently predictive of mortality, and suggested that the combined use of the two scores could improve prediction of a prolonged hospital stay.

Sequential Organ Failure Assessment (SOFA)

The SOFA was developed in 1994 during a consensus conference organized by the European Society of Intensive Care and Emergency Medicine (Vincent *et al.*,

1996). The conference included internationally renowned intensivists, predominantly from Europe. The conference participants decided, based on a review of the literature, to limit the number of organ systems included in the score to six (respiratory, cardiovascular, renal, hepatic, central nervous and coagulation systems), to use a score from 0 (normal function) to 4 (most abnormal) for each organ, and to record the worst values on each day. The parameters chosen to represent organ dysfunction in the six organ systems are shown in Table 5.3.

Retrospective analysis of the SOFA score with mortality in a European-North American (ENAS) database of 1643 patients with sepsis, showed an increasing mortality rate with an increasing score. A multicentre, prospective analysis of 1449 patients in 40 ICUs across 16 countries, confirmed the correlation between high SOFA scores for any organ and poor outcome (Vincent et al., 1998). While individual organ scores are important in describing the patient's evolution, the total maximum score is of more use for outcome assessment as it allows the system to assess the cumulative amount of organ dysfunction sustained by the patient during their stay. Multiple organ failure is a dynamic process and different organs will be affected to different degrees at different times; mortality from multiple organ failure is indeed associated with the number of failing organs, the severity to which they are affected and the duration of the failure (Moreno et al., 1999). The total maximum SOFA takes all these facets into account. In the prospective analysis of 1449 patients, a maximum total SOFA score (i.e. the maximum total score reached during the ICU stay) greater than 15 correlated with a mortality rate of 90% (Vincent et al., 1998). Interestingly, in the subgroup of 544 patients who stayed on the ICU for longer than 1 week, the total SOFA score increased in 44% of the non-survivors, but in only 20% of the survivors; 33% of the survivors decreased their SOFA score compared to only 21% of the non-survivors. This stresses the value of repeated calculations of the score, and indeed, sequential analysis, particularly during the first 48 h of ICU stay, provides a good indicator of prognosis (Lopes Ferreira et al., 2001).

The SOFA score has now also been validated in medical cardiovascular ICU patients (Janssens et al., 2000) and in trauma patients (Antonelli et al., 1999). Moreno et al. (1999) showed that both the total maximum SOFA and the change in SOFA correlated with outcome, and concluded that the SOFA score can thus be of use in quantifying the organ dysfunction present on admission, the degree of dysfunction appearing during the ICU stay and the cumulative insult suffered by the patient.

Limitations

Each of the scoring systems discussed above has its own limitations; none is perfect. Some of the problems with these systems are discussed below.

Choice of variables

Ideally, a single variable should be used to assess each organ. A key limitation to the LODS score, apart from its complexity, is the use of multiple variables

Table 5.3 The Sequential Organ Failure Assessment score

SOFA score	0	1	2	3	4
Respiration					
PaO$_2$/F$_i$O$_2$ (mmHg)	>400	≤400	≤300	≤200	≤100
(kPa)	(>53.3)	(≤53.3)	(≤40)	(≤26.6)—with respiratory support—(≤13.3)	
Coagulation					
Platelets, (× 10^3/mm^3)	>150	≤150	≤100	≤50	≤20
Liver					
Bilirubin, (mg/dl)	<1.2	1.2–1.9	2.0–5.9	6.0–11.9	>12.0
(μmol/l)	(<20)	(20–32)	(33–101)	(102–204)	(>204)
Cardiovascular					
Hypotension	No hypotension	MAP <70mmHg	dopamine ≤5 or dobutamine (any dose)*	dopamine >5 or epinephrine ≤0.1 or norepinephrine ≤0.1*	dopamine >15 or epinephrine >0.1 or norepinephrine >0.1*
Central nervous system					
Glasgow Coma Score	15	13–14	10–12	6–9	<6
Renal					
Creatinine, (mg/dl)	<1.2	1.2–1.9	2.0–3.4	3.5–4.9	>5.0
(μmol/l)	(<110)	(110–170)	(171–299)	(300–440)	(>440)
or urine output				or >500 ml/day	or >200 ml/day

Modified from Vincent JL, Moreno R, Takala J, *et al.* (1996). The SOFA (Sepsis-related Organ Failure Assessment) score to describe organ dysfunction/failure. *Intensive Care Med.*, **22**, 707–710. *Adrenergic agents administered for at least 1 hour (doses given are in μg/kg/min) for assessing organ dysfunction. A second important 'ideal' in a variable is that it is treatment independent. In an attempt to fulfill this ideal, John Marshall and colleagues chose to develop a complex variable for cardiovascular assessment in the MODS score. However, while they should be commended for their efforts, we do not think the end result helps the score. First, although not very complicated, the variable still requires a computerized system, and the score is, thus, not immediately available at the bedside. Second, a patient may be about to die and still have acceptable values. For example, two patients, one on noradrenaline 100 μg/min and the other with no vasopressor support, could both have an arterial pressure of 100/60 mmHg, a heart rate of 120/min, and a central venous pressure of 12 mmHg, and yet these two patients are in very different clinical states. One must therefore admit that therapeutic interventions have to be taken into account. Likewise, the PaO_2/FiO_2 ratio is influenced by the positive end-expiratory pressure (PEEP) level, the platelet count by platelet transfusions, etc. In the SOFA score, the use of a treatment-related variable for the cardiovascular system is a potential limitation, although the categories used were kept broad to try to limit any potential problem with different treatment protocols. Nevertheless, the development of a new vasopressor may alter the evaluation process. As an example, introducing vasopressin to raise blood pressure may decrease the cardiovascular SOFA score because the doses of adrenergic agents are decreased, but the patient may not really be improving. As another example, for a SOFA score of 3 or 4 in the respiratory system, some degree of respiratory support is required. However, this was included because while hypoxaemia sometimes improves dramatically with mechanical ventilation or the use of continuous positive airways pressure, the reverse is not true; patients on mechanical ventilation can have a score of 0, 1, or 2 if they have no significant hypoxaemia.

A potential limitation for all the scores is the choice of the Glasgow Coma Score (GCS) as the variable for neurological assessment. Many factors can influence the neurological status in the critically ill, which may not be directly related to the degree of organ dysfunction. For example, the administration of sedative agents may give a spurious GCS. In these conditions, an 'assumed' GCS should be used, i.e. the GCS that the patient would have if not under sedation; admittedly this is not always easy to assess and is open to subjective interpretation.

Evaluation over time

The LODS score was designed to be calculated only during the first 24 h, like the APACHE and the SAPS systems, which were not designed to be repeated over time and have never been well validated for this purpose. As indicated above, multiple organ failure is a process changing over time and should not be considered only on admission. The MODS and SOFA scores can be repeated at regular time intervals and, as mentioned above, an increasing score is associated with a worse prognosis.

Problem of missing values

Missing values can be a problem in score calculation, and there are two ways to deal with this. First, one can consider that the value has remained stable until the next available result; alternatively, one can take the mean of the two values on either side of the missing one. For example if values were recorded as bilirubin 2 mg/dl (33.3 μmol/l), then a missing value, and then a bilirubin of 2.6 mg/dl (43.3 μmol/l). With the first option, the missing value would be counted as 2 mg/dl (33.3 μmol/l), while with the second method, the missing value would be taken as 2.3 mg/dl (38.3 μmol/l). For the SOFA score, we have recommended using the second alternative as the time course of changes in variables is rarely smooth (especially for bilirubin, which is the most commonly missing variable).

Despite their limitations these systems provide essential information regarding organ dysfunction in critically ill patients and are increasingly being included as part of the analysis in clinical trials (Goncalves *et al.*, 1998; Staubach *et al.*, 1998; Di Filippo *et al.*, 1998; Fiore *et al.*, 1998; Briegel *et al.*, 1999; Soufir *et al.*, 1999).

Conclusion

The ability to assess and describe the evolution of organ dysfunction in ICU patients is of great importance for comparisons of patient populations, for clinical trial outcome assessment, and potentially for monitoring individual patients. Various scoring systems have been developed using a variety of methods, and all have their strong points as well as their limitations. Importantly, and in contrast to mortality prediction scores, organ dysfunction scores are able to account for the fact that organ failure is not an all-or-nothing phenomenon but an on-going process varying over time. The scoring systems allocate a score for each organ, enabling the total score to be broken down into its constituents. As such, an accurate picture of the organ function in any patient at any time can be extracted. While not developed to predict mortality, these scores correlate well with outcome, confirming what we already knew, that mortality is associated with the degree of organ dysfunction. Simplicity, reliability and reproducibility of the scores are essential for their widespread acceptance and increasingly we will see such systems employed in daily clinical practice.

References

ACCP-SCCM Consensus Conference. (1992). Definitions of sepsis and multiple organ failure and guidelines for the use of innovative therapies in sepsis. *Crit.Care Med.*, 20, 864–874.

Antonelli, M., Moreno, R., Vincent, J. L. *et al.* (1999). Application of SOFA score to trauma patients. Sequential Organ Failure Assessment. *Intensive Care Med.*, **25**, 389–394.

Barie, P. S., Hydo, L. J., Fischer, E. (1996). Utility of illness severity scoring for prediction of prolonged surgical critical care. *J. Trauma*, **40**, 513–518.

Beal, A. L., Cerra, F. B. (1994). Multiple organ failure in the 1990s. *JAMA*, **271**, 226–233.

Bertleff, M. J. O. E., Bruining, H. A. (1997). How should multiple organ dysfunction syndrome be assessed? A review of the variations in current scoring systems. *Eur. J. Surg.*, **163**, 405–409.

Bone, R. C., Fisher, C. J., Clemmer, T. P. *et al.* (1987). The methylprednisolone severe sepsis study group: A controlled clinical trial of high-dose methylprednisolone in the treatment of severe sepsis and septic shock. *N.Engl. J. Med.*, **317**, 653–658.

Bone, R. C., Fisher, C. J., Clemmer, T. P., Slotman, G. J., Metz, C. A., Balk, R. A. (1989a). Sepsis Syndrome: A valid clinical entity. *Crit. Care Med.*, **17**, 389–393.

Bone, R. C., Slotman, G., Maunder, R., Silverman, H., Hyers, T. M., Kerstein, M. D. (1989b). Randomized double-blind, multicenter study of prostaglandin E1 in patients with the adult respiratory distress syndrome. *Chest*, **96**, 114–119.

Bossink, A. W., Groeneveld, J., Hack, C. E., Thijs, L. G. (1998). Prediction of mortality in febrile medical patients: How useful are systemic inflammatory response syndrome and sepsis criteria? *Chest*, **113**, 1533–1541.

Briegel, J., Forst, H., Haller, M. *et al.* (1999). Stress doses of hydrocortisone reverse hyperdynamic septic shock: a prospective, randomized, double-blind, single-center study. *Crit. Care Med.*, **27**, 723–732.

Deitch, E. A. (1992) Multiple organ failure: Pathophysiology and potential future therapy. *Ann. Surg.*, **216**, 117–134.

Di Filippo, A., De Gaudio, A. R., Novelli, A. *et al.* (1998). Continuous infusion of vancomycin in methicillin-resistant staphylococcus infection. *Chemotherapy*, **44**, 63–68.

Fagon, J. Y., Chastre, J., Novara, A., Medioni, P., Gibert, C. (1993). Characterization of intensive care unit patients using a model based on the presence or absence of organ dysfunctions and/or infection: the ODIN model. *Intensive Care Med.*, **19**, 137–144.

Fiore, G., Donadio, P. P., Gianferrari, P., Santacroce, C., Guermani, A. (1998). CVVH in postoperative care of liver transplantation. *Minerva Anestesiol.*, **64**, 83–87.

Fry, D. E., Pearlstein, L., Fulton, R. L., Hiram, C. P. (1980). Multiple system organ failure: The role of uncontrolled infection. *Arch. Surg.*, **115**, 136–140.

Goncalves, J. A. J., Hydo, L. J., Barie, P. S. (1998). Factors influencing outcome of prolonged norepinephrine therapy for shock in critical surgical illness. *Shock*, **10**, 231–236.

Goris, R. J., te Boekhorst, T. P., Nuytinck, J. K., Gimbrere, J. S. (1985). Multiple-organ failure. Generalized autodestructive inflammation? *Arch. Surg.*, **120**, 1109–1115.

Hebert, P. C., Drummond, A. J., Singer, J., Bernard, G. R., Russell, J. A. (1993). A simple multiple system organ failure scoring system predicts mortality of patients who have Sepsis Syndrome. *Chest*, **104**, 230–235.

Jacobs, S., Zuleika, M., Mphansa, T. (1999). The Multiple Organ Dysfunction Score as a descriptor of patient outcome in septic shock compared with two other scoring systems. *Crit. Care Med.*, **27**, 741–744.

Janssens, U., Graf, C., Graf, J. *et al.* (2000). Evaluation of the SOFA score: A single centre experience of a medical intensive care unit in 303 consecutive patients with predominantly cardiovascular disorders. *Intensive Care Med.*, **26**, 1037–1045.

Justice, A. C., Covinsky, K. E., Berlin, J. A. (1999). Assessing the generalizability of prognostic information. *Ann. Intern. Med.*, **130**, 515–524.

Knaus, W. A., Draper, E. A., Wagner, D. P., Zimmerman, J. E. (1985). Prognosis in acute organ-system failure. *Ann. Surg.*, **202**, 685–693.

Knaus, W. A., Zimmerman, J. E., Wagner, D. P., Draper, E. A., Lawrence, D.E. (1981). APACHE-Acute Physiology And Chronic Health Evaluation: a physiologically based classification system. *Crit. Care Med.*, **9**, 591–597.

Le Gall, J. R., Klar, J., Lemeshow, S. *et al.*, ICU Scoring Group. (1996). The Logistic Organ Dysfunction System: A new way to assess organ dysfunction in the intensive care unit. *JAMA*, **276**, 802–810.

Le Gall, J. R., Loirat, P., Alperovitch, A. *et al.* (1984). A Simplified Acute Physiology Score for ICU patients. *Crit. Care Med.*, **12**, 975–977.

Lemeshow, S., Teres, D., Avrunin, J. S., Gage, R. W. (1988). Refining intensive care unit outcome prediction by using changing probabilities of mortality. *Crit. Care Med.*, **16**, 470–477.

Leteurtre, S., Martinot, A., Duhamel, A. *et al.* (1999). Development of a pediatric Multiple Organ Dysfunction Score: use of two strategies. *Med. Decision Making*, **19**, 399–410.

Lopes Ferreira, F., Peres Bota, D., Bross, A. *et al.* (2001). Serial evaluation of the SOFA score to predict outcome in critically ill patients. *JAMA*, **286**, 1754–1758.

Marshall, J. C., Christou, N. V., Meakins, J. L. (1993). The gastrointestinal tract. The 'undrained abscess' of multiple organ failure. *Ann. Surg.*, **218**, 111–119.

Marshall, J. C., Cook, D. J., Christou, N. V., Bernard, G. R., Sprung, C. L., Sibbald, W. J. (1995). Multiple Organ Dysfunction Score: A reliable descriptor of a complex clinical outcome. *Crit. Care Med.*, **23**, 1638–1652.

Moreno, R., Vincent, J. L., Matos, A. *et al.* (1999). The use of maximum SOFA score to quantify organ dysfunction/failure in intensive care. Results of a prospective, multicentre study. *Intensive Care Med.* **25**, 686–696.

Mythen, M. G., Webb, A. R. (1994). The role of gut mucosal hypoperfusion in the pathogenesis of post-operative organ dysfunction. *Intensive Care Med.*, **20**, 203–209.

Opal, S. M. (1998). The uncertain value of the definition for SIRS. *Chest*, **113**, 1442–1443.

Rangel-Frausto, M. S., Pittet, D., Costigan, M., Hwang, T., Davis, C. S., Wenzel, R. P. (1995). The natural history of the systemic inflammatory response syndrome (SIRS). A prospective study. *JAMA*, **273**, 117–123.

Salvo, I., de Cian, W., Musicco, M. *et al.* The Sepsis Study Group. (1995). The Italian SEPSIS study: Preliminary results on the incidence and evolution of SIRS, sepsis, severe sepsis and septic shock. *Intensive Care Med.*, **21**, S244–S249.

Soufir, L., Timsit, J. F., Mahe, C., Carlet, J., Regnier, B., Chevret, S. (1999). Attributable morbidity and mortality of catheter-related septicemia in critically ill patients: a matched, risk-adjusted, cohort study. *Infect. Control Hosp. Epidemiol.*, **20**, 396–401.

Staubach, K. H., Schroder, J., Stuber, F., Gehrke, K., Traumann, E., Zabel, P. (1998). Effect of pentoxifylline in severe sepsis: Results of a randomized, double-blind, placebo-controlled study. *Arch. Surg.*, **133**, 94–100.

Stevens, L. E. (1983). Gauging the severity of surgical sepsis. *Arch. Surg.*, **118**, 1190–1192.

Tilney, N. L., Bailey, G. L., Morgan, A. P. (1973). Sequential system failure after rupture of abdominal aortic aneurysms: an unsolved problem in postoperative care. *Ann. Surg.*, **178**, 117–122.

Tran, D. D., Groeneveld, A. B. J., Vander Meulen, J. *et al.* (1990). Age, chronic disease, sepsis, organ system failure, and mortality in a medical intensive care unit. *Crit. Care Med.*, **18,** 474–479.

Vincent, J. L. (1997). Dear Sirs, I'm sorry to say that I don't like you. *Crit. Care Med.*, **25,** 372–374.

Vincent, J. L., de Mendonça, A., Cantraine, F. *et al.* (1998) Use of the SOFA score to assess the incidence of organ dysfunction/failure in intensive care units: Results of a multicenter, prospective study. *Crit. Care Med.*, **26,** 1793–1800.

Vincent J. L., Moreno, R., Takala, J. *et al.* (1996). The SOFA (Sepsis-related Organ Failure Assessment) score to describe organ dysfunction/failure. *Intensive Care Med.*, **22,** 707–710.

Chapter 6

Non-mortality outcome measures

Saxon Ridley

Introduction

Non-mortality outcome measures are vitally important to the surviving patients as they encompass most of the basic aspects of life. Non-mortality outcome measures can be broadly divided in those that measure functional status and those that measure quality of life (the latter being more fully discussed in Chapter 7). While the patient is critically ill on the intensive care unit (ICU), the most frequently asked question is whether or not the patient is going to survive. However, having left the ICU, the patients and their relatives become more interested in how the patient is going to survive. With the shortcomings of mortality as a measure of effectiveness being appreciated, non-mortality measures will take greater prominence as the primary outcome of healthcare systems. The long-term consequences of critical illness itself are beginning to be recognized and these will be measured by non-mortality outcome measures.

Definitions and classification

Most non-mortality outcome measures can be divided into those that measure quality of life or functional status. Quality of life can be defined as a concept encompassing a broad range of physical and psychological characteristics and limitations that describe an individual's ability to function and derive satisfaction from doing so. It is most important to stress that quality of life includes an element of satisfaction. Health related quality of life is the level of well-being and satisfaction associated with an individual's life and how this is affected by disease, accident and treatments. On the other hand, functional outcome is an assessment of the patient's physical and mental capability. It is not the same as quality of life because functional outcome does not include a measure of satisfaction or well-being. Furthermore, functional outcome is not necessarily related to quality of life in that the same degree of physical incapacity may impinge on patients' quality of life quite differently. Functional outcome can be objectively assessed by a third party, something that is not possible with the uniquely subjective health related quality of life. Functional outcome is frequently and incorrectly used interchangeably with quality of life; although the two may measure similar aspects of life, they are not the same and should not be considered as such.

Problems with non-mortality outcome measures

The problems relating to non-mortality outcome measures concern the performance and application of these measures.

Performance

Critical care is a relatively modern specialty and so the consequences, both physical and mental, of life-threatening critical illness are also new. Attempts to quantify these consequences need special tools or measurement devices. Generally such measurement tools have been designed for use in other areas of medicine or on different populations of patients. Non-mortality outcome measures have been frequently used in chronic diseases such as diabetes, hypertension, rheumatoid arthritis and parkinsonism. The performance of these tools may not be as good in a new population, such as critical illness survivors, when compared with the patient group for whom the tool was designed. Performance essentially quantifies how consistently and accurately the measurement tool measures what it purports to measure and is summarized in the psychometric properties of the measurement device. There are many aspects to psychometric testing but from the perspective of outcome assessment, the most important are:

1. Validity, which assesses how well the measurement tool actually measures what it claims to measure.
2. Reliability, which attempts to quantify the amount of true error versus measurement error (i.e. quantify the signal to noise ratio).

Validity

Validity is an assessment of whether the measurement tool actually measures what it is meant to measure. There are several aspects to validity and the most important relating to outcome measurement are:

1. Concurrent validity where the tool under investigation is compared to the results of a concurrently administered tool. The agreement between the two sets of results can then be quantified and as such reflects concurrent validity.
2. Criterion validity assesses the performance of the new measure as assessed against a previously established standard method. Unfortunately, in critical care there is really no recognized method nor tool that could be regarded as standard.
3. Construct validity is where the ability of the tool to detect clinically established or theoretical constructs is tested. For example, a tool measuring functional outcome might be expected to show a poorer outcome in amputees.
4. Content validity is an assessment of whether the tool measures the entire range of possible outcomes. Content validity tests whether there are basement or ceiling effects. These occur when patients' outcomes are grouped at the highest or lowest parts of the response range. Basement or ceiling effects tend to occur where the distribution of results is highly skewed.

Nearly all outcome assessment tools were developed for use outside critical care. As with any tool, outcome measures may not work well if applied to a different patient population. Before investigating the changes following critical illness, the researcher would be well advised to measure the psychometric properties of the outcome tool as some of the variation in the results might be due to systematic bias produced by the measurement tool itself.

Reliability

Reliability refers to inter- (between) and intra- (within) observer agreement in the use of any outcome measure and represents the agreement, uniformity and standardization in data collection. In general, the greater the subjectivity involved in application of the outcome measure the poorer the reliability of the system. For example, estimating physical performance as 'poor', 'good' or 'excellent' will be less reliable than quantifying the distance walked in metres before fatigue.

The intra-observer reliability estimates the error, usually random, in any measured score. A measured score may be considered a sum of the true value plus an error measurement (Table 6.1). Similarly the variability (i.e. variance) within a group of scores is a sum of the variance of the true scores plus the variance of the error. Reliability quantifies the ratio of the true score variance over the variance of the observed score and so is an estimate of the amount of variable error in a score or scale. Reliability ranges between 0 and 1, having a value of 0 when the measurement involves nothing but error and reaching 1 when there is no variable error in the measurement at all. A reliability coefficient of greater than 0.7, suggesting that no more than 30% of the score is due to error, has been used as a statistical standard (Brazier *et al.*, 1992).

Estimates of score and error variances, and hence intra-observer reliability, can be measured by a variety of techniques which include test/re-test (measuring

Table 6.1 The relationship between the measured score, true score, error and reliability

---

As:

   Measured score = True score + Error

Then:

   $(\sigma_{\text{Measured score}})^2 = (\sigma_{\text{True score}})^2 + (\sigma_{\text{Error}})^2$ where $(\sigma)^2$ is the variance

Consequently:

   Reliability $= (\sigma_{\text{True score}})^2/(\sigma_{\text{Measured score}})^2$

---

fluctuations in performance from one session to another), parallel test (where two measuring systems are administered at the same time), split half tests (where the results of the test are divided and the correlation between them measured) and the Kuder-Richardson or Hoyt methods based on analysis of variance of items within a test (e.g. variations in measurement of physical performance compared to variations in the physical role of the Short Form 36) (Helmstader, 1964).

Measuring reliability is important because it divides the error into true variation related to the outcome of interest and variation due to the measurement technique. The total variation influences the confidence we can have in any results or significant changes reported.

Application

Application of the outcome measure can introduce new sources of error. The three possible sources are:

1. Whether the outcome measure is to be delivered by telephone, by post, or by structured interview.
2. If outcome is to be assessed by a third party (surrogate answers), some measure of the inter-observer agreement is required.
3. Timing of the measurement because once the patient returns home, other socioeconomic factors, which are totally unrelated to critical illness, start to influence non-mortality outcome.

Delivery

Questionnaires concerning outcome have been specially designed to be delivered to the patient either by post, over the telephone or by structured interviews. The choice of application is usually determined by resources, in both time and finance, available to the researcher. Interviews can allow extensive questioning and areas of confusion to be addressed but they are time consuming to perform. Postal questionnaires rarely have response rates above 60% and it is difficult to draw conclusions about the patients who have not replied. Their failure to respond may be related to a poor outcome rather than an incorrect postal address.

Surrogate answers

Survivors of critical illness may not be able to cooperate to answer a questionnaire. Under these circumstances a third party or surrogate will have to interpret the questions and answer on behalf of the patient. This may be unreliable because of the personal attributes of many of the non-mortality outcome measures used after critical illness. Only very close relatives or partners who care for the patients are really qualified to act as proxy respondents, and even then surrogate answers are more reliable in the physical rather than the psychosocial domains (McCusker and Stoddard, 1984; Rothman *et al.*, 1991; Rogers *et al.*, 1997). Medical and nursing staff should not offer their own assessment of a patient's quality of life as these have been shown to be erroneous (Uhlmann *et al.*, 1998). Different statistical methods are required for measuring inter-observer reliability. Inter-observer reliability can be measured by the intra-class correlation coefficients for continuous variables or the kappa statistic in its various forms (i.e. weighted or unweighted) for categorical or grouped data (Altman, 1991).

Timing

The results obtained will depend upon case-mix, patient selection and the confounding influences of socioeconomic changes that affect the whole population. For example, Figure 6.1 represents the theoretical recovery of pre-morbid quality of life in the survivors of critical illness.

The line representing recovery following cardiac surgery exceeds pre-morbid levels because surgery had a therapeutic effect and the patient's life is improved. The other two lines represent two patients recovering following emergency aortic aneurysm repair. One patient made a good recovery in terms of quality of life but the other suffered a stroke 2 months after ICU discharge. This resulted in a dense hemiparesis, and despite some recovery, significantly impaired long-term quality of life. Quality of life after the stroke will be poor but unless precise details about the timing of the stroke are elicited, this poor recovery of quality of life will be ascribed to the aneurysm repair and associated critical illness.

The rate of recovery of the individual components such as quality of life and functional outcome following critical illness is unknown. It is unlikely that the rates of physical recovery and improvements in quality of life are identical and follow the same time course. There will be a balance between allowing as full a recovery of quality of life as possible and avoiding other socioeconomic influences which impinge upon quality of life but may only be indirectly associated with critical illness. Major life events such as marriage, divorce, unemployment may make the interpretation of changes in quality of life in relation to intensive care much more difficult (and hence dangerous). Not enough is known about the recovery of quality of life to make recommendations concerning appropriate measurement points. Many of the non-mortality outcome measures have been designed for, or applied to, patients with chronic diseases such as hypertension and arthritis. Theoretically, clinical changes in such

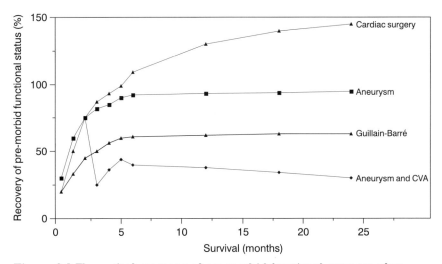

Figure 6.1 Theoretical recovery of pre-morbid functional outcome after cardiac surgery, emergency aneurysm repair and recovery from Guillain-Barré syndrome. The recovery after cardiac surgery should be excellent because the surgery is designed to relieve symptoms and improve exercise tolerance. Recovery of muscle power after Guillain-Barré syndrome may not be complete and this will impinge upon the physical aspects of functional outcome. Following aortic aneurysm repair, the patients should return to a normal functional outcome so long as they do not suffer another serious complication such as a stroke (CVA) (reproduced from Ridley, S. A. (2000). Quality of life and longer term outcomes. In: *Update in intensive care and emergency medicine 35. Evaluating Critical Care* (W. J. Sibbald, J. F. Bion, eds), p. 114, Springer-Verlag).

conditions should be gradual rather than the faster recovery usually expected after critical illness. The responsiveness of tools designed for more chronic and stable conditions may not be adequate for critical care. Finally, any changes need to be compared to a suitable baseline and there is little evidence to suggest that ICU patients have the same distribution of pre-morbid physical and psychosocial attributes as the general population.

Non-mortality outcome measures

A number of non-mortality outcome measures have been used following intensive care and these may be broadly categorized into six classes. These outcome measures, the frequency with which they have been used and their psychometric properties are more fully presented in a systematic review undertaken by the Intensive Care National Audit and Research Centre (Hayes *et al.*, 2000).

Physical impairment and disability

As mechanical ventilation is a key therapeutic modality on ICU, measures of physical impairment have concentrated on the respiratory system. Assessment of respiratory function has included:

1. Respiratory volumes (e.g. total lung capacity, forced vital capacity)
2. Gas flow (e.g. forced expiratory volume in 1 second)
3. Pulmonary diffusing capacity (usually for carbon monoxide)
4. Assessment of the upper airway (usually by endoscopy or radiology looking for tracheal stenosis).

Measurement of these outcomes requires formal pulmonary function tests and hence active cooperation by the patient. Pulmonary function testing is well validated outside critical care but the psychometric properties of these tests have not been rigorously assessed in the survivors of acute illness. However, as the long-term pathophysiological consequences of acute respiratory distress syndrome or other forms of acute lung injury may be similar to other chronic diseases, checking the psychometric properties in critical care survivors may not be as important as for other outcome categories (see later). Most studies in the survivors of critical illness have reported an impairment or departure from normality. However, measures assessing function may not correlate with quality of life or general well-being (van der Molen *et al.*, 1997). These respiratory outcome measures have rather limited application in outcome analysis except for those patients admitted with or who developed acute lung injury and other causes of severe respiratory impairment while on ICU.

Functional status

Functional status measures may be broadly classified as general or disease-specific measures. For example, the New York Heart Association classification (Criteria Committee of the New York Heart Association, 1964) is a disease-specific classification that was originally designed for patients with congestive cardiac failure. The classification grades physical activities from I to IV (Table 6.2).

The New York Heart Association classification has been used in critically ill patients who have undergone cardiac or thoracic surgery (Kumar *et al.*, 1995; Trouillet *et al.*, 1996) but concerns about its use have been raised (Goldman *et al.*, 1982) because of apparent high inter-observer variation. Understandably, the New York Heart Association classification appears not to have been used in the adult general intensive care population. Another disease-specific measure of functional status is the Walk test for chronic heart and lung disease (Guyatt *et al.*, 1985). This involves the patient completing a straight 33 metre course as many times as possible within the allotted 6 minutes. The measurement properties of disease-specific measures in critical care survivors are either unknown or limited. These tools are clearly of use in the specific population for whom they were

Table 6.2 The New York Heart Association classification for patients with cardiac failure

Class	Clinical symptoms
I	No functional limitation
II	Slight functional limitation. Fatigue, palpitations, dyspnoea or angina on ordinary physical activity, but asymptomatic at rest
III	Marked functional limitation. Symptoms on less than ordinary activity, but asymptomatic at rest
IV	Inability to perform any physical activity, with or without symptoms at rest

designed but it is difficult to see how their application in the survivors of general critical care can be justified.

Generic measures of functional status look at broader aspects of physical capability and usually examine the Activities of Daily Living. One well-known example is Katz's Activities of Daily Living, which grades performance from A to G on six daily functions (bathing, dressing, going to the toilet, moving, continence and feeding) (Katz et al., 1963, 1970). Katz's Activities of Daily Living were originally developed from results obtained from elderly patients with fractured necks of femur and were later used to assess treatment in rheumatoid arthritis and stroke. Table 6.3 describes the range of the daily activities and from the table it is clear that patients need to be severely limited before they score a higher grade.

The application of the Activities of Daily Living as a primary outcome measure to critical care survivors may be flawed because of the possible basement or ceiling effects and its developmental population being mainly elderly but not ICU survivors.

Even so the Activities of Daily Living have been used in a number of studies examining patients' functional outcomes following critical illness. In elderly patients, functional outcome appears to return to pre-morbid levels after 6 months to a year (Chelluri et al., 1993) and there was no difference in recovery of function status between the over and under 65 year olds (Rockwood et al., 1993). In a general adult ICU population of 1746, the SUPPORT (Study to Understand Prognoses and Preferences for Outcomes and Risks of Treatment) study reported a tripling in incidence (to 34%) of severe functional limitations at 2 months; unfortunately this particular study did not follow the patients for longer so it is not known how many improved or deteriorated further (Wu et al., 1995). Following neurosurgical intensive care, recovery of functional status at a mean follow-up time of 2.2 years (range 1–3 years) as measured by Activities of Daily Living was poor. Only 23% of 122 survivors scored above the threshold value for moderate to minimal disability (Cho et al., 1997).

Table 6.3 Definitions of limitations in the Activities of Daily Living; the summary grade A to G depends upon the number and specific type of limitation

Activity	Possible range
Bathing	1 Receives no assistance (getting in and out of the bath on own) 2 Receives assistance in bathing only one part of the body (e.g. back or leg) 3 Receives assistance in bathing more than one part of the body
Dressing	1 Dresses completely without assistance 2 Dresses completely except for tying shoes 3 Receives assistance in getting clothes or in getting dressed, or stays partly or completely undressed
Toiletting	1 Goes to the toilet, cleans self and arranges clothes without assistance 2 Receives assistance going to the toilet, cleaning self and arranging clothes or uses bedpan at night 3 Does not physically go to the bathroom or toilet
Moving	1 Moves in and out of bed or chair without help 2 Moves in and out of bed or chair with assistance 3 Does not get out of bed
Continence	1 Completely continent 2 Occasional 'accidents' 3 Supervision required or catheter is used or is incontinent
Feeding	1 No assistance 2 Feeds self but requires help cutting meat or buttering bread 3 Receives help feeding or is fed by tubes or intravenous fluids

Modified and shortened for illustrative purposes from Katz, S., Downs, T. D., Cash, H. R., Grotz, R. C. (1970). Progress in development of the index of ADL. *Gerontologist*, **10**, 20–30.

The Karnofsky Index is another general functional outcome measure that has been applied to the survivors of critical illness. The Karnofsky Index was developed as a measure of overall health in lung cancer patients treated with nitrogen mustards (Karnofsky *et al.*, 1948). The scores range from 0 (dead) to 100 (normal) (Table 6.4).

The scaling takes account of the presence of symptoms, the ability to work, physical activity and self-care. However, its reliability has been questioned because of a basic problem with the scale in that elements (e.g. symptoms, activities or self-care) do not appear on all scale points so that variable interpretations are possible for a given patient status. Along with Katz's Activities of Daily Living, the Karnofsky Index has been investigated for validity and responsiveness over time in only a small number of studies involving critical care survivors.

Unfortunately, most outcome measures examining functional status were developed for use in fields other than critical care. If the study patient population is different from the developmental group, then the psychometric properties of the outcome measure may change, rendering the results more difficult to interpret. However, functional status measurement is very important because, not

Table 6.4 The Karnofsky Index

Descriptive criteria	Scale
Normal, and no complaints	100
Able to carry on normal activities; minor signs or symptoms of disease	90
Normal activity with effort	80
Cares for self. Unable to carry on normal activity or do active work	70
Requires occasional assistance but able to care for most needs	60
Requires considerable assistance and frequent medical care	50
Disabled; requires special care and assistance	40
Severely disabled; hospitalization indicated although death not imminent	30
Very sick. Hospitalization necessary. Active supportive treatment necessary	20
Moribund	10
Dead	10

Modified and shortened for illustrative purposes from Karnofsky, D. A., Abelmann, W. H., Craver, L. F., Burchenal, J. F. (1948). The use of the nitrogen mustards in the palliative treatment of carcinoma. *Cancer*, **I**, 634–656.

only does it usefully quantify physical capacity, in elderly patients it is an important predictor of mortality following discharge from ICU. Inouye *et al.* (1998) modified the Activities of Daily Living to concentrate on instrumental activities (e.g. using the telephone, shopping, using transport, cooking, housekeeping, taking medicine and handling finances) and found that functional status measures were strong predictors of 90-day and 2-year mortality. Functional status is one of the most important outcome measures of critical care because it will determine the level of independence enjoyed by the patient. Although several measures have been used, none was developed specifically for use in critical care survivors and the number of studies measuring functional status is rather limited. More work in this important area is required.

Mental function

As with functional status, mental function outcome measures may be divided into generic and disease-specific measures. Four generic measures have been applied to critical care survivors; these are the Profile of Mood State (POMS) (McNair *et al.*, 1992), Hospital Anxiety and Depression Scale (HADS) (Zigmond and Snaith, 1983), Centre for Epidemiology – Depression Scale (Radoff *et al.*, 1977) and Beck Depression Inventory (Beck *et al.*, 1961). The first two have been used most frequently in the UK and assess anxiety as well as depression.

The POMS scale was developed to assess mood in psychiatric outpatients. The scale assesses mood by ranking 65 adjectives, as opposed to symptoms, on a five-point scale that ranges from zero for 'not at all' to four for 'extremely', based on how the patients felt throughout the previous week. A total score can be calculated as can six subscale scores for mood or affect. The six subscales cover tension – anxiety, depression – dejection, anger – hostility, vigour – activity, fatigue – inertia and confusion – bewilderment (Table 6.5).

The higher the score the greater the disturbance experienced with the exception of the vigour – activity scale. The POMS scale has been reported in five papers concerning critically ill patients. Jones *et al.* (1994) reported the validity of the POMS scale when they compared the POMS scale to Patrick's Perceived Quality of Life Questionnaire. Correlation coefficients (r^2 values) of just under 0.5 were

Table 6.5 Profile of Mood State (POMS) score. The patients are offered a list of adjectives and asked to score how they were feeling in the past week using the following scale: 0 = Not at all; 1 = A little; 2 = Moderately; 3 = Quite a bit; 4 = Extremely. Adjectives used in first three descriptive scales

Tension – anxiety scale	Depression – dejection scale	Anger – hostility scale
Tense	Unhappy	Angry
Shaky	Sorry	Peeved
On edge	Sad	Grouchy
Panicky	Blue	Spiteful
Relaxed	Hopeless	Annoyed
Uneasy	Unworthy	Resentful
Restless	Discouraged	Bitter
Nervous	Lonely	Ready to fight
Anxious	Miserable	Rebellious
	Gloomy	Deceived
	Desperate	Furious
	Helpless	Bad-tempered
	Worthless	
	Terrified	
	Guilty	

found in two measures (fatigue – inertia and tension – anxiety). Jones reported that, at 2 and 6 months, approximately half the patients were suffering from some degree of anxiety, although the spectrum of POMS scores was wide. At 6 months following discharge the POMS tension – anxiety scores were correlated with the anger – hostilities ($r^2 = 0.44$) and fatigue – inertia ($r^2 = 0.45$) scores. Depression – dejection scores were associated with confusion – bewilderment ($r^2 = 0.64$). This pattern of scores or cluster of symptoms suggests that anxiety and depression following intensive care should be a recognized problem.

The HADS score was developed in non-psychiatric patients to measure mood disorders and depression; it contains 14 items assessing depression and anxiety, and scores the responses on a four point scale. This scale is widely used in hospital settings as a screening instrument for anxiety disorders and depressive illnesses. It does not contain questions pertaining to somatic complaints, making it is less likely to be confounded by the direct effects of physical, as opposed to psychological, conditions (Table 6.6).

Both of the subscales (one for depression and one for anxiety) have threshold scores (>8) above which a clinical disorder is likely. Scores from the two subscales may be combined to produce a HADS full-scale score. A total score of over 12 is indicative of a clinical disorder.

Table 6.6 The items of the Hospital Anxiety and Depression Scale grouped according to whether they are measuring anxiety or depression.
Respondents are offered a choice of options (e.g. 'Most of the time', 'A lot of the time', 'From time to time, occasionally' and 'Not at all') which are scored on a four point scale (from zero to three inclusive).

	Question or Comment
Anxiety	I feel tense or 'wound up'
	I get a sort of frightened feeling as if something awful is about to happen
	Worrying thoughts go through my mind
	I can sit at ease and feel relaxed
	I get a sort of frightened feeling like 'butterflies' in the stomach
	I feel restless as if I have to be on the move
	I get sudden feelings of panic
Depression	I still enjoy the things I used to enjoy
	I can laugh and see the funny side of things
	I feel cheerful
	I feel as if I am slowed down
	I have lost interest in my appearance
	I look forward with enjoyment to things
	I can enjoy a good book or radio or TV programme

The psychometric properties of the HADS score have been infrequently measured in critically ill patients. Dixon *et al.* (1997) used the HADS score (and Nottingham Health Profile) to investigate whether there was any association between quality of life and mental outcome after intensive care and satisfaction with intensive care services; no association was found.

The single disease-specific measure that has been used in critical care survivors is the Impact of Events Scale (IES) (Horowitz *et al.*, 1979). The scale has been used outside critical care for measuring post-traumatic stress in individuals following disasters such as oil-rig sinking and fires (Ersland *et al.*, 1989; Hytten and Hasle, 1989). The IES consists of 15 symptom-items that respondents rate according to the frequency of occurrence in the last 7 days, on a scale marked 0 (Not at all), 1 (Fairly), 3 (Sometimes) and 5 (Often). It has two subscales; the first pertains to re-experiencing the trauma (e.g. nightmares) and contains seven items while the second refers to avoiding situations and thoughts that are associated with the trauma (eight items) (Table 6.7).

Scores on the IES subscales for intrusions and avoidance have been stratified as < 9 mild or absent symptoms, 9 to 19 medium level of symptoms and > 20

Table 6.7 The 15 items of the Impact of Events Scale. The patients are asked to score ('Not at all', 'Rarely', 'Sometimes', 'Often') how true each of the comments were for them in the past week

---

Intrusion items

    I had waves of strong feelings about it
    Other things kept making me think about it
    I thought about it when I did not mean to
    Pictures about it popped into my mind
    Any reminder brought back feelings about it
    I had trouble falling asleep or staying asleep because pictures or thoughts about it that came into my mind
    I had dreams about it

Avoidance items

    I was aware that I still had a lot of feelings about it, but I did not deal with them
    I avoided letting myself get upset when I thought about it or was reminded about it
    I tried to remove it from memory
    I tried not to talk about it
    My feelings about it were kind of numb
    I felt as if it had not happened or was not real
    I stayed away from reminders of it
    I tried not to think about it

Modified and shortened for illustrative purposes from Horowitz, M., Wilner, N., Alvarez, W. (1979). Impact of Events Scale: A measure of subjective distress. *Psychosom. Med.*, **41**, 209–218.

high levels of symptoms (maximum possible score 75). Scores above 30 on the IES indicate severe psychological trauma symptoms and individuals scoring in this range are likely to meet diagnostic criteria for post-traumatic stress disorder (Robbins and Hunt, 1996). Briere and Elliott (1998) have shown that scores on the IES are skewed; individuals who are not psychologically traumatized score close to zero while those who have suffered a wide range of traumatic experiences had higher scores (Table 6.8).

Table 6.8 The summary statistics illustrating the differences in distribution of the scores on the Impact of Events Scale's two subscales between traumatized and non-traumatized members of the public

	Mean (standard deviation)	Median	Mode
No trauma history (n = 138)			
Total score	8.1 (12.3)	1.0	0.0
Intrusion	3.9 (6.2)	1.0	0.0
Avoidance	4.2 (6.8)	0.0	0.0
Trauma history (n = 360)			
Total score	16.7 (17.9)	11.0	0.0
Intrusion	7.0 (9.2)	5.0	0.0
Avoidance	8.5 (9.6)	5.0	0.0

Modified from Briere, J., Elliott, D. M. (1998). Clinical utility of the Impact of Events Scale: Psychometrics in the general population. *Assessment* **5**, 171–180.

Patients recovering from severe non-central nervous system traumatic injury had a mean score of 30.6 at 3 months after injury (Richmond *et al.*, 1998). High scores on the intrusion subscale (20 and over) is an independent risk factor for severe disability at 3 months (predicted risk 2.9, 95% confidence limits: 1.1–7.7) (Richmond *et al.*, 1998).

Neuropsychological function

The classical roles of neuropsychology are to enrol the psychologist's help in the early identification of the nature and location of lesions disrupting brain function and to extend understanding about psychological processes themselves. Neuropsychological testing examines higher central nervous system function. The tests are generally complex and use a battery of tests assessing neuropsychological function. Testing usually requires face-to-face interviews, specialist equipment and an appropriately trained tester. They measure attention, perception, cognitive flexibility, information processing and visual memory. These tests have been used for patients with head injury, but are probably rather limited for the general

ICU patient because of their complex application. Examples of tests that have been used after critical illness include Trailmaking Tests A and B (Reitan, 1958), Wisconsin Card Sorting test (Heaton, 1981) and Benton's test for visual retention (Benton, 1984).

The Wisconsin Card Sorting test has been used to demonstrate rigidity and cerebral impairment in patients who have suffered frontal lobe damage. This rigidity may be expressed in several ways:

i.   inability to shift from one concept to the next
ii. perseveration of stereotype behaviour
iii. sensitivity to the effect of set.

The Wisconsin Card Sorting test involves reordering a series of cards and can be used to look for problems in patients with frontal lobe damage as they are likely to have difficulties with conceptual shifts. Benton's test for visual retention involves copying designs from memory and predominantly tests the right hemisphere. The patients are shown one of fifteen designs and are asked to identify a chosen design from a selection of four. Trailmaking Tests A and B were not designed for use on their own but they are short and are good at identifying patients with brain damage. The trailmaking tests involve timed task completion.

Overall neuropsychological function measures brain impairment and as such may be of limited value in the assessment of adult survivors of general critical illness. The psychometric performance of these tools in this group of patients is largely unknown.

Measures of recovery

The extent of recovery may be measured in a multi-item scale such as the Glasgow Outcome Scale which has four grades of recovery (good, moderate disability, severe disability and vegetative state) (Jennett and Bond, 1975). The scale was originally intended to assess recovery 6 months after head injury. However, it was expanded and used to show that mental handicap (usually personality changes) contributed more significantly to overall social disability than did neurological (i.e. physical) deficits (Jennett et al., 1981). The Glasgow Outcome Scale is primarily designed for use after neurosurgical intensive care and so its performance in the adult general population of critically ill patients is unknown. Simple single item scales such as returning to work or independent living have been used but their simplicity limits their usefulness as there are many grades of employment and varying levels of support available to maintain independence.

Quality of life

Measures of quality of life have been widely used outside critical care. Such measures may be general or disease specific. In the critical care setting, quality of life has been most frequently measured using tools such as the Sickness Impact Profile (Bergner *et al.*, 1981), Nottingham Health Profile (Hunt *et al.*, 1985) and the Short Form 36 (Ware *et al.*, 1993). Gill and Feinstein (1994) randomly selected 75 articles reporting quality of life and found that 136 of 159 instruments used had been used only once. When assessing critical care, investigators frequently fail to report the psychometric properties of the instrument they use and rarely report the steps they have taken to ensure adequacy of the sample size. Investigators should be encouraged to select the tools that are specifically designed for the area of outcome in which they are interested (physical impairment, functional status, mental or neuropsychological function, recovery or quality of life). Quality of life is comprehensively discussed in the following chapter.

Non-mortality consequences of critical illness

Although the outcome measures listed above have been used in critical care survivors, they may not be sufficiently comprehensive to detect actually what troubles the patients. While follow-up clinics have only recently been established and are few in number, their results provide an insight into the problems experienced by patients. During critical illness it is possible to lose 2% of the body's muscle mass per day. Not only does this lead to severe weakness and fatigue but also poor muscle coordination and difficulty swallowing and coughing. Anxiety and depression are common and this may strain relationships with partners and limit social interaction. More severe psychological upset may present as nightmares and delusions. These may be consequences of the initial trauma or the results of the psychological disturbances that developed in ICU. The patient's lack of memory, compounded by a lack of understanding or explanation, may aggravate these disturbances. Such non-mortality consequences of critical illness will certainly impinge on quality of life. Therefore, it may be more fruitful initially to look at specific outcomes perceived as problems by the patient rather than attempt to interpret the results of global non-mortality outcome measures.

Conclusion

Unfortunately, there are still many problems and inadequacies with our understanding and appreciation of outcomes following critical care. Until follow-up of patients is standardized in terms of duration, it will be difficult to explore fully the influences that affect survival. Many non-mortality outcome measures have been used but their application to critical care survivors may not have been appropriate. Follow-up clinics have identified the types of long-term problems experienced by the patients and it may be more appropriate to quantify rigorously these problems prior to investigating global changes in quality of life or functional status.

References

Altman, D. G. (1991). *Practical Statistics for Medical Research.* Chapman and Hall.

Beck, A. T., Ward, C. H., Mendelson, M. *et al.* (1961). An inventory for measuring depression. *Arch.Gen. Psychiatr.*, **4**, 561–571.

Benton, A. L. (1984). *Revised Visual Retention Test: Clinical and Experimental Application.* Psychological Corporation.

Bergner, M., Bobbitt, R. A., Carter, W. B., Gilson, B. S. (1981). The Sickness Impact Profile: development and final revision of a health status measure. *Med. Care*, **19**, 787–805.

Brazier, J. E., Harper, R., Jones, M. N. B. (1992). Validating the SF–36 health survey questionnaire: new outcome measure for primary care. *Br. Med. J.*, **305**, 160–164.

Briere, J., Elliott, D. M. (1998). Clinical utility of the Impact of Events Scale: Psychometrics in the general population. *Assessment*, **5**, 171–180.

Chelluri, L., Pinsky, M. R., Donahoe, M. P., Grenvik, A. (1993). Long-term outcome of critically ill elderly patients requiring intensive care. *JAMA*, **269**, 3119–3123.

Cho, D.-Y., Wang, Y.-C. (1997). Comparison of the APACHE III, APACHE II, and Glasgow Coma Scale in acute head injury for prediction of mortality and functional outcome. *Intensive Care Med.*, **23**, 77–84.

Criteria Committee of the New York Heart Association (1964). *Nomenclature and Criteria for Diagnosis of Disease of the Heart and Blood Vessels.* Little Brown.

Dixon, J. J., Manara, A. R., Willatts, S. M. (1997). Patient and relative satisfaction with intensive care. Importance of duration and quality of life. *Clin. Intensive Care*, **8**, 63–68.

Ersland, S., Weisaeth, L., Sund, A. (1989). The stress upon rescuers involved in an oil rig disaster. 'Alexander L. Kielland' 1980. *Acta Psychiatr. Scand.*, **80**, S38–49.

Gill, T. M., Feinstein, A. R. (1994). A critical appraisal of the quality of quality-of-life measurements. *JAMA*, **272**, 619–626.

Goldman, L., Cook, E. F., Mitchell, N. *et al.* (1982). Pitfalls in the serial assessment of cardiac function states: How a reduction of 'ordinary' activity may reduce the apparent degree of cardiac compromise and give a misleading impression of improvement. *J. Chron. Dis.*, **35**, 763–771.

Guyatt, G. H., Sullivan, M. J., Thompson, P. J. *et al.* (1985). The 6-minute walk: a new measure of exercise capacity in patients with chronic heart failure. *Can. Med. Assoc. J.*, **132**, 919–923.

Hayes, J. A., Black, N. A., Jenkinson, C. *et al.* (2000). Outcome measures for adult critical care: a systematic review. *Health Technol. Assess.*, **4**, 1–111.

Heaton, R. K. (1981). *Wisconsin Card Sorting Test Manual.* Psychological Assessment Resources.

Helmstader, G. C. (1964). *Principles of Psychological Measurement.* Appleton-Century-Crofts.

Horowitz, M., Wilner, N., Alvarez, W. (1979). Impact of Events Scale: A measure of subjective distress. *Psychosom. Med.*, **41**, 209–218.

Hunt, S. M., McEwen, J., McKenna, S. P. (1985). Measuring health status: a new tool for clinicians and epidemiologists. *J. R. Coll. Gen. Pract.*, **35**, 185–188.

Hytten, K., Hasle, A. (1989). Fire fighters: a study of stress and coping. *Acta Psychiatr. Scand.*, **80**, S50–55.

Inouye, S. K., Peduzzi, P. N., Robison, J. T., Hughes, J. S., Horwitz, R. I., Concato, J. (1998). Importance of functional measures in predicting mortality among older hospitalized patients. *JAMA*, **279**, 1187–1193.

Jennett, B., Bond, M. (1975). Assessment of outcome after severe brain damage. *Lancet*, **1**, 480–484.

Jennett, B., Snoek, J., Bond, M. R., Brooks, N. (1981). Disability after severe head injury: observations on the use of the Glasgow Outcome Scale. *J. Neurol. Neurosurg. Psychiatr.*, **44**, 285–293.

Jones, C., Griffiths, R. D., MacMillan, R. R., Palmer, T. E. A. (1994). Psychological problems occurring after intensive care. *Br. J. Intensive Care*, **4**, 46–53.

Karnofsky, D. A., Abelman, W. H., Craver, L. F., Burchenal, J. H. (1948). The use of nitrogen mustards in the palliative treatment of carcinoma. *Cancer*, **I**, 634–656.

Katz, S., Downs, T. D., Cash, H. R., Grotz, R. C. (1970). Progress in development of the index of ADL. *Gerontologist*, **10**, 20–30.

Katz, S., Ford, A. B., Moskowitz, R. W., Jackson, B. A., Jaffe, M. W. (1963). Studies of illness in the aged. The index of ADL: A standardized measure of biological and psychosocial function. *JAMA*, **185**, 914–919.

Kumar, P., Zehr, K. J., Chang, A., Cameron, D. E., Baumgartner, W. A. (1995). Quality of life in octogenarians after open heart surgery. *Chest*, **108**, 919–926.

McCusker, J., Stoddard, A. M. (1984). Use of a surrogate for the Sickness Impact Profile. *Med. Care*, **22**, 789–795.

McNair, D. M., Lorr, M., Droppleman, L. F. (1992). *EdITS Manual for the Profile of Mood States*. Educational and Industrial Testing Service.

Radoff, L. S. (1977). The CES-D scale: a self report depression scale for research in the general population. *Appl. Psychol. Measurement*, **1**, 385–401.

Reitan, R. M. (1958) *Trail-making Manual for Administration, Scoring and Interpretation*. Indiana University Medical Center.

Richmond, T. S., Kauder, D., Schwab, C. W. (1998). A prospective study of predictors of disability at 3 months after non-central nervous system trauma. *J. Trauma*, **44**, 635–643.

Robbins, I., Hunt, N. (1996). Validation of the IES as a measure of the long-term impact of war trauma. *Br. J. Health Psychol.*, **1**, 87–89.

Rockwood, K., Noseworthy, T. W., Gibney, R. T. *et al.* (1993). One-year outcome of elderly and young patients admitted to intensive care units. *Crit. Care. Med.*, **21**, 687–691.

Rogers, J., Ridley, S., Chrispin, P., Scotton, H., Lloyd, D. (1997). Reliability of the next of kin's estimate of critically ill patients' quality of life. *Anaesthesia*, **52**, 1137–1143.

Rothman, M. L., Hedrick, S. C., Bulcroft, K. A., Hickman, D. H., Rubenstein, L. Z. (1991). The validity of proxy-generated scores as measures of patient health status. *Med. Care*, **26**, 115–124.

Trouillet, J. L., Scheimberg, A., Vuagnat, A., Fagon, J. Y., Chastre, J., Gibert, C. (1996). Long-term outcome and quality of life of patients requiring multidisciplinary intensive care unit admission after cardiac operations. *J. Thorac. Cardiovasc. Surg.*, **112**, 926–934.

Uhlmann, R. F., Pearlman, R. A., Cain, K. C. (1988). Physicians' and spouses' predictions of elderly patients' resuscitation preferences. *J. Gerontol.*, **43**, M115–121 (Abst).

van der Molen, T., Postma, D. S., Schreurs, A. J., Bosveld, H. E., Sears, M. R., Meyboom de Jong, B. (1997). Discriminative aspects of two generic and two asthma specific instruments: relation with symptoms, bronchodilator use and lung function in patients with mild asthma. *Qual. Life Res.*, **6**, 353–361.

Ware, M. K., Snow, K. K., Kosinski, M., Gandek, B. (1993). *SF–36 Health survey: Manual and interpretation guide*. The Health Institute, New England Medical Center.

Wu, A. W., Damiano, A. M., Lynn, J. *et al*. (1995). Predicting future functional status for seriously ill hospitalized adults. The SUPPORT prognostic model. *Ann. Intern. Med.*, **122,** 342–350.

Zigmond, A. S., Snaith, R. P. (1983). The Hospital Anxiety and Depression Scale. *Acta Psychiatr. Scand.*, **67,** 361–370.

Chapter 7

Quality of life after critical care

D. Jim Kutsogiannis and Tom Noseworthy

Measurement of health-related quality of life

Measuring health and outcomes of therapies and interventions is central to understanding the value of healthcare; critical care is no exception. From a broader perspective, measurement is fundamental to analysing differences in health and predicting the need for care (Clancy and Eisenberg, 1998; McDowell and Newell, 1996). Health and well-being are multidimensional. Their dimensions encompass real-life consequences for individuals, how they perceive and are able to live with such consequences. Accordingly, measurement of health and well-being embraces health-related quality of life (HRQL) which includes values, preferences and perceptions related to health, as well as functionality and symptoms of ill health (Juniper *et al.*, 1996; Feeny *et al.*, 1996; Guyatt *et al.*, 1993). In this context, it is important to differentiate between health status and HRQL. Health status is primarily concerned with the measurement of physical, functional, emotional, and mental well-being, whereas quality of life incorporates specific values and preferences of patients, including elements such as work, friendships and family life (Table 7.1) (Bergner, 1985; Gill and Feinstein, 1994).

Understanding HRQL relies on proper measurement. However, the ability to define and measure HRQL with some degree of certainty poses difficulties not encountered in measuring physiological processes, such as blood pressure.

Fundamental to understanding the tools for and limitations of HRQL measurement is an appreciation of development and validation of specific questionnaires. An overview of basic psychometric theory related to HRQL measurement is provided in Chapter 6 and a more detailed discussion of this topic may be found elsewhere (Carmenes and Zeller, 1981; Streiner and Norman, 1989; Nunnally and Berstein, 1994). Instruments used to measure HRQL are composed of individual *items* or questions to which a specific *scale* (continuous

Table 7.1 The conventional dimensions of health status

---

1 The genetic foundation or inherited characteristics that form the basic structure on which all other aspects of health status must build.
2 The biochemical, physiological or anatomical condition, which includes disease, disability, or handicap, whether obvious or not.
3 The functional condition, which includes performance of all the usual activities of life, such as working, walking, and thinking.
4 The mental condition, which includes self-perception of mood and emotion.
5 The health potential of the individual, which includes longevity, functional potential, and the prognosis of disease and disability.

Bergner, M. (1985). Measurement of health status. *Med. Care*, **23**, 696–704.

or categorical) is attached. Items are often grouped into categories called *domains or dimensions,* which attempt to measure specific attributes such as physical or social function. The entire group of domains collectively comprises the measurement *instrument*. Depending on the type of HRQL instrument, the final measurement may be expressed as a *profile* of domain scores or as an *aggregate* score. Both profile and aggregate scores have been used in populations of critically ill patients. Profiles have been used as measures in the Short Form–36 (SF–36) (Ware, 1993) and the Nottingham Health Profile (Hunt *et al.*, 1981) which contain 8 and 13 subscales respectively. Aggregate scores have been used in the Sickness Impact Profile (Bergner *et al.*, 1981) and Spitzer's Quality of Life Index (Spitzer *et al.*, 1981).

Ultimately, the measurement of HRQL involves both a theoretical framework to describe the determinants of HRQL, as well as an empirical framework with which to operationalize the theory into observable responses, as a questionnaire or scale. As discussed in Chapter 6, the two properties used to evaluate the extent to which a given instrument reflects the proposed theory are reliability and validity. Reliability relates to the consistency of repeated measurements and is formally defined as the variance of the true score divided by the variance of the observed score (where the observed score equals the sum of the true score and random error). Measures of reliability include the test-retest, alternative-form, split-halves, and the internal consistency methods. The most commonly used measures in the intensive care literature include the test-retest and the internal consistency methods (Carmenes and Zeller, 1981). The test-retest method involves administering the instrument to the same population on two different occasions; the reliability is measured as the correlation between the two sets of scores. This method is limited because there is always uncertainty as to whether low reliability results from an unreliable instrument or real changes in individuals' responses. The internal consistency method usually employs *Cronbach's alpha* and requires only single administration of the instrument. Calculating Cronbach's alpha involves tabulating all items within the instrument, determining the correlations between all of the items and the mean inter-item correlation; calculation of the coefficient alpha is then based on the mean inter-item correlation values. Cronbach's alpha increases as the average correlation among items increases or as the number of items increases.

Validation of an instrument may take many forms and is more difficult to achieve; it is perhaps best thought of as a process of hypothesis testing. In essence, the successful 'validation' of an instrument in a given population implies that one may make meaningful inferences about a specific population based on their scores on the instrument. In general, validation has been defined as whether or not an instrument measures what it is purported to measure. Validity is subdivided into content, criterion and construct validity (Streiner and Norman, 1989; Nunnally and Bernstein, 1994) (Table 7.2).

Criterion validity may be further subdivided into concurrent or predictive validity and construct validity is subdivided into discriminant and convergent validity. Content validity requires a theoretical conceptual framework that the instrument must capture. These concepts must be adequately sampled and

Table 7.2 Definitions of validity and its subdivisions

Content validity
The theoretical or conceptual framework upon which a specific instrument is founded.

Criterion validity
The statistical (empirical) correlation between a specific instrument and other physical or health measure known as a criterion measure.

Concurrent criterion validity
The specific instrument and criterion measure are administered or determined simultaneously and statistical correlations are determined between the instrument and criterion measure.

Predictive criterion validity
The criterion measure is administered or determined after the administration of the specific instrument and the predictive performance of the instrument assessed.

Construct validity
The ability of a specific instrument to measure what it purports to measure. Construct validity is established over time by confirming both theoretical and empirical hypotheses in different populations.

Convergent construct validity
The magnitude of the correlation between the specific theoretical constructs of the instrument and other measures of the same construct.

Discriminant construct validity
The magnitude of the lack of correlation between specific theoretical constructs of the instrument and measures which are theoretically dissimilar.

represented in the instrument in order to obtain proper inferences from its use. Unfortunately, there is no statistical test that measures the adequacy of content validity. Criterion validity is the correlation of the instrument with some other physical or health measure (known as a criterion measure). Criterion validity is purely a statistical assessment with no absolute requirement for basis within a theoretical framework. Criterion validity may be concurrent, whereby the instrument and criterion measure are administered simultaneously; or predictive, where the criterion measure is administered some time after the instrument is administered and the predictive performance of the instrument assessed. Construct validity is the most difficult form of validity to achieve in HRQL measurement. Hypothesized attitudes and behaviours (known as constructs), which are thought to determine HRQL, require testing over time so that an accurate description of HRQL can be made and tested against predictions of a subject's HRQL. Consequently, construct validity cannot be established by one study but requires several studies each testing new hypotheses with the specific instrument. This process involves learning about the construct, formulating new hypotheses and subsequently testing them. Both theoretical and empirical aspects are required in this validation process. Convergent validity describes how closely the theoretical constructs are related to other measures of the same construct. Discriminant validity measures the lack of correlation between the instrument and measures which are theoretically dissimilar.

Finally, it is important to note that the validity of an instrument is dependent on its reliability. Mathematically, the greatest validity an instrument can achieve is the square root of its reliability coefficient (Streiner and Norman, 1989). Consequently, reliability limits an instrument's validity. Furthermore, the construct or criterion validity of an instrument may be poor because (Cronbach and Meehl, 1955):

1. the instrument is good, but the theoretical framework used to generate the instrument is wrong
2. the theoretical framework is correct, but the instrument is not sensitive enough to discriminate between populations
3. the instrument lacks construct validity, or
4. both the theoretical framework is wrong and the instrument lacks construct validity.

Health-related quality of life following intensive care unit discharge

Most literature pertaining to HRQL following critical illness was published over the past decade, with only a few longitudinal evaluations of HRQL. Studies have employed both generic and disease-specific instruments encompassing a heterogeneous group of domains. Generic HRQL instruments attempt to capture a broad range of domains across a spectrum of patient populations. They enable comparisons of the relative impact of therapies and health programmes across populations. However, generic instruments are generally not as responsive to changes over time in specific illnesses when compared to disease-specific instruments. For example, the Medical Outcomes Study Short Form, a generic measure, was used to assess health outcomes in hospitalized patients; however, low baseline Medical Outcomes Study Short Form scores prevented detection of further declines in HRQL in the follow-up period. This has been described as a *basement* or *floor* effect (Bindman *et al.*, 1990). In contrast, disease-specific instruments focus on diseases, individuals, or symptoms and complaints and are generally better able to detect subtle changes in HRQL over time. While they provide tangible and relevant information, they may not provide comprehensive information and are less generalizable across different patient populations.

Whether generic or disease-specific instruments are used largely depends on the study goals and availability of required data. Clearly, more can be accomplished by using a combination of generic and disease-specific measures, although the cost and effort is greater. While research and understanding of HRQL associated with critical care may be in its infancy, it is better measured and understood in other medical conditions (Feeny and Torrance, 1989; Guyatt *et al.*, 1991; Hillers *et al.*, 1994; Osoba, 1995).

In determining the aspects of life to be included in instruments measuring HRQL, a system of classification by health-related domains has been widely adopted. At least five specific domains have been categorized and include pain and impairment, functional status and mobility, social role, satisfaction and perceptions, and death. All measures of HRQL should include one or more of these domains. Varying degrees of detail will be needed for general and specific measures.

Recently, investigators have moved beyond simple Mortality Prediction Models and have included the assessment of morbidity, disability, and quality of life following critical care. The growing importance of HRQL as a relevant outcome measure, in addition to mortality, has been recognized and recommended by a consensus conference of the European Society of Intensive Care Medicine (Suter *et al.*, 1994), as well as by prominent reviewers (Brooks *et al.*, 1995). Despite this, the lack of a universal standard for HRQL measurement after critical care has been emphasized. In a systematic review of 1073 articles relevant to the practice of adult intensive care, only 1.7% included quality of life measures (Heyland *et al.*, 1998a). Of the few studies that included some measurement of quality of life after intensive care unit (ICU) discharge, comparisons between studies were limited because of the wide variety of instruments used.

HRQL instruments have examined critically ill patients or subgroups based on age, case-mix, or length of ICU stay. Literature measuring HRQL can be divided into four general types:

1. qualitative or methodological reviews and recommendations about the existing literature (Suter *et al.*, 1994; Brooks *et al.*, 1995; Heyland *et al.*, 1998a)
2. descriptions of HRQL (Daffurn *et al.*, 1994; Sawdon *et al.*, 1995)

3. evaluations of either validated or non-validated original instruments developed specifically for assessing quality of life after ICU admission (Patrick *et al.*, 1988; Rivera Fernandez *et al.*, 1991, 1996; Vazquez Mata *et al.*, 1992; Rustom and Daly, 1993; Munn *et al.*, 1995; Capuzzo *et al.*, 1996, 2000a,b; Brooks *et al.*, 1997)

4. reports using one or more previously validated instruments developed to measure both generic domains and disease-specific quality of life, but not necessarily specific to critical care (Ridley and Wallace, 1990; Hulsebos *et al.*, 1991; Ridley *et al.*, 1994, 1997; Konopad *et al.*, 1995; Tian and Reis Miranda, 1995; Chrispin *et al.*, 1997; Rogers *et al.*, 1997; Hurel *et al.*, 1997; Ortiz *et al.*, 1998; Perrins *et al.*, 1998; Short *et al.*, 1999; Heyland *et al.*, 2000; Pettila *et al.*, 2000; Garcia Lizana *et al.*, 2000).

Ten studies using newly developed instruments for assessing quality of life after critical care have been published within the past 13 years, and eight of these provided some estimate of the instruments' validities. The instruments constructed specifically for the general ICU population are outlined in Table 7.3.

Table 7.3 Instruments measuring HRQL specifically for populations of general adult critically ill patients

---

Measures of reliability and validity published:
    Perceived Quality of Life scale (PQOL)
    Quality of life–Italian (QOL-IT)
    Quality of life–Spanish (QOL-SP)

Measures of reliability and validity not published or limited:
    Health questionnaire – Munn *et al.* (1995)
    Health questionnaire – Brooks *et al.* (1997)
    Health questionnaire – Rustom and Daly (1993)

Seventeen studies used either a previously validated instrument for measuring generic and/or disease-specific domains of HRQL or modified previously validated tools (Table 7.4).

These instruments were not initially developed for studying critically ill patients.

The domains studied include physical and physiological measures, Activities of Daily Living, degree of dependence, employment, emotional status, social functioning and self-Perceived Quality of Life. Typically the physical and physiological domains include mobility, weakness, measures of oral communication, ability to think and remember, ability to drive a vehicle, regular medication usage, re-admission to hospital, disturbance of sleep, pain perception and intensity and sphincter control. The Activities of Daily Living domain include bathing, dressing and preparing meals. Dependence covers place of residence (e.g. nursing home) and degree of physical dependence. Items within the

Table 7.4 Validated instruments for measuring generic or disease-specific health related quality of life

---

Generic Instruments
   EuroQol (Brooks, 1996)
   Sickness Impact Profile (SIP)
   Short Form (SF–36)
   General Health Questionnaire 28-item version (Goldberg and Hillier, 1979)
   Nottingham Health Profile
   Spitzer's Quality of Life Index

Disease specific instruments
   Rosser's Disability Categories (Kind *et al.*, 1982)
   Katz's Activities of Daily Living
   Rosenberg Self-esteem Scale (Rosenberg, 1965)
   The Impact of Events Scale (Horowtiz and Wilner, 1979)
   The Psychological General Well-being Schedule (Dupuy, 1984)
   Karnofsky Scale (Grieco and Long, 1984)

---

employment domain include the capacity to work and satisfaction with current income. Emotional status encompasses a broad array of measures including happiness, energy, strength of relationships with family and friends, self-respect, respect by others, meaning and purpose of life, anxiety and depression, sexual relationships, personal appearance, spiritual satisfaction, somatic symptoms, sense of self-worth, control over life and elements embodying stress following traumatic life events. Contribution to the community, leisure activities, social appearance, social relationships and isolation, hobbies and holidays are characteristics of the social domain. Finally, general questions pertaining to overall self-perceived quality of life may be included as a separate domain.

HRQL instruments developed specifically for ICU populations

Of the instruments developed specifically to measure HRQL of ICU populations, reliability or validity measures have been published for the Perceived Quality of Life scale (PQOL) (Patrick *et al.*, 1988), the Quality of Life-Italian (QOL-IT) (Capuzzo *et al.*, 1996), and the Quality of Life-Spanish (QOL-SP) (Rivera Fernandez *et al.*, 1991) measures.

The PQOL is an 11-item measure of need and satisfaction (Table 7.5). This instrument has proven internal consistency and reliability (Cronbach's alpha coefficient = 0.88 out of a maximum of 1.00). However, the criterion validity of its various social characteristics may be limited (R^2 = 0.18 to 0.50). Its concurrent validity is also poor when compared to other generic measures

Table 7.5 Perceived Quality of Life questions

		(a)	(b)

How satisfied are you with the following aspects of your life?
Please score on a scale of 0 to 100 (0 = not satisfied at all, 100 = completely satisfied).
(a) Before your admission to ICU (b) At present

	(a)	(b)
1 The state of your health	score____	score____
2 Your ability to think and remember	score____	score____
3 How happy you are	score____	score____
4 How much you see your family and friends	score____	score____
5 The help you get from your family and friends	score____	score____
6 Your contribution to the community	score____	score____
7 Your activities outside	score____	score____
8 How your income meets your needs	score____	score____
9 How you are respected by others	score____	score____
10 The meaning and purpose of your life	score____	score____
11 With working/not working/retirement	score____	score____

From Thiagarajan, J., Taylor, P., Hogbin, E., Ridley, S. (1994). Quality of life after multiple trauma requiring intensive care. *Anaesthesia*, **49**, 211–218.

(sickness impact score ($R^2 = -0.49$); the Psychological General Well-being Schedule ($R^2 = 0.54$)).

In the original description of the PQOL scale, the mean score (out of a total of 100 points for maximum satisfaction) at a median of 19 months following ICU discharge was 75. This compared favourably to a mean score of 79 in a group of healthy, elderly patients living in the community. The PQOL scale has also been incorporated into a larger instrument by other investigators who have demonstrated, not surprisingly, that patients who are admitted with a good pre-admission quality of life suffer a significant decrease in quality of life, whereas those with a lower pre-admission quality of life do not experience a significant change (Perrins *et al.*, 1988).

The QOL-IT is an instrument with six domains which initially encompassed residence, physical activity, social life, Perceived Quality of Life, oral communication and functional limitation; the residence domain has been excluded in the most recent revision (Capuzzo *et al.*, 2000a, b) (Table 7.6).

Of 152 respondents to the original instrument, 6 months after discharge from critical care, physical activity decreased in 31%, social function in 32% and functional capacity increased in 30%. The reliability and validity of the revised five-domain instrument has been subsequently studied. In a sample of 36 patients, the inter-observer reliability, and the agreement between patients' and families' retrospective responses was excellent with weighted kappa values of 0.99 and 0.78 respectively (Capuzzo *et al.*, 2000a). Contrary to findings of other studies (McCusker and Stoddard, 1984; Rothman *et al.*, 1991), the closeness of relationship, gender or living arrangements did not influence the strength of

Table 7.6 Italian quality of life questionnaire. There are five items and a range of scores from 0 (perfect quality of life) to 20 (worst quality of life)

Questions	Score
Physical activity:	
Do you perform these physical activities?	
Working out of home	0
Going up one floor without trouble	1
Carrying a full shopping bag	2
Going for a walk	3
Doing the housework	4
Washing and dressing yourself	5
Confined to a chair and bed	6
Social life:	
Do you perform these activities?	
Leisure activities (i.e. sport, hobbies)	0
Contacting friends	1
Reading newspapers	2
Watching the television	3
Contacting only relatives	4
Perceived Quality of Life:	
How do you feel about your quality of life?	
Best	0
Good	1
Fair	2
Poor	3
Worst	4
Oral communication (interviewer):	
How is the speech?	
Normal	0
Understandable, close to the patient	1
Understandable, but dialogue not maintained	2
Incoherent speech	3
Functional limitation (interviewer):	
Is there functional limitation, considering age?	
No	0
Mild limitation	1
Severe limitation	2
Totally dependent	3

Capuzzo, M., Grasselli, C., Carrer, S., Gritti, G., Alvisi, R. (2000b). Validation of two quality of life questionnaires suitable for intensive care patients. *Intensive Care Med.*, **26**, 1296–1303.

agreement. A subsequent study aimed at demonstrating the construct and criterion validity of the QOL-IT showed a significant correlation between the QOL-IT and an independent measure of functional limitation and chronic disease in the same Italian population of critically ill patients (Capuzzo et al., 2000b).

The QOL-SP has sound psychometric properties focusing mainly on functional status by including questions pertaining to capacity to work, physical dependence, movement and exercise, oral communication, requirement for regular medications, and sphincter control (Table 7.7).

After its initial development, a study of 606 patients demonstrated worse HRQL up to 12 months after ICU discharge, with the exception of those patients with the worst initial QOL-SP score, whose HRQL improved at 12 months (Vazquez Mata et al., 1992). The dependence of follow-up HRQL on pre-ICU admission HRQL is further supported by a study using the PQOL scale (Perrins et al., 1998). Only the initial QOL-SP score and age, but not APACHE II score, were predictive of the levels of HRQL at 12 months. Arguably, the most likely explanation for the poor criterion validity between the QOL-SP and APACHE II scores is that the theoretical framework suggesting an association between the two is false; however, it is important to appreciate that possible limitations in the QOL-SP's construct validity cannot be excluded. The QOL-SP has been subsequently expanded into a 15-item validated instrument developed specifi-cally for critical care by the Spanish 'Project for the Epidemiological Analysis of Critical Care Patients' (Rivera Fernandez et al., 1996). The revised 15-item instrument had three domains (basic physiological measures, normal daily activities, and emotional state). This proved to have good internal consistency (Cronbach's alpha coefficient = 0.85), and reproducibility ($R^2 > 0.90$) within and between various populations. The QOL-SP has content validity in support of its theoretical framework, as evidenced by the extraction of three distinct a priori domains in factor analysis techniques. Further evidence for the reliability and validity of the QOL-SP has come from studies of Italian ICU patients (Capuzzo et al., 2000a,b). Inter-observer reliability and agreement between patients' and relatives' retrospective responses were excellent with weighted kappa values of 0.99 and 0.82 respectively. Moreover, the construct validity of the QOL-SP instrument has been strengthened by demonstrating significant correlations between the QOL-SP and an independent measure of functional limitation and chronic disease in the same population.

Three studies have utilized ICU-specific instruments with no or limited estimates of reliability and validity. The first used an instrument consisting of eight items, with an emphasis on HRQL as opposed to functional status. Of 504 survivors of critical care surveyed 3 months after hospital discharge, 47% reported their health as good to very good, fair in 42% and poor or very poor in 11% (Munn et al., 1995). Patients' activity levels were unchanged in 59%, lower in 33% and higher in 8% of respondents. In another study using the ICU-specific health-related quality of life questionnaire containing 13 scales and four single-item questions, 238 patients were studied 16 months after ICU discharge and compared with a random community sample (Brooks et al., 1997). Critically ill patients described more physical symptoms, greater depression and dependence

Table 7.7 Some of the questions about the normal daily activities from the second version of the Spanish quality of life questionnaire. The other domains are four questions about physiological activities and three questions about emotional state. The scores for this questionnaire range from 0 to 29 where a score of 0 is normal and an increasing score corresponds to worsening quality of life

---

Tolerance of major effort

Can the following activities be carried out?

Walking 5 kilometres	Yes/No
Running 1 kilometre	Yes/No
Going up four floors without shopping	Yes/No
Practising a sport requiring a high level of physical effort such as football, tennis, swimming, or similar	Yes/No

0 – Can carry out at least one of these activities
1 – Can carry out none of these activities

Walking

Is there difficulty with walking?

0 – No
1 – Yes, walks with help (crutch or people)
2 – Yes, does not walk, and uses wheelchair
3 – Yes, is permanently bedridden and depends on others

Mobility

Is there difficulty in making normal journeys?

0 – No, can make all the normal journeys
1 – Yes, only moves about the immediate locality
2 – Yes, only moves about the house
3 – Yes remains in his/her room

Dressing

Does the patient have difficulty in getting dressed?

0 – No
1 – Yes, needs some help
2 – Yes, and is totally dependent on others

Work activities or activities appropriate to age

Are there difficulties with the patient's work?

0 – No
1 – Yes. He/she has difficulties, but works as before
2 – Yes. Works only part-time or has changed to a job requiring minimum effort
3 – Does not work because of his/her condition

For patients retired due to age, the question is: are there difficulties with the patient's activities as a retired person?

0 – No, continues with regular scheduled activities
1 – Yes, continues with regular scheduled activities but with difficulty
2 – Yes, activities are no longer regular, and are only sporadic, or have been changed for alternatives requiring less activity
3 – Yes, and has completely abandoned them

From Rivera Fernandez, R., Sanchez Cruz, J. J., Vazquez Mata, G. (1996). Validation of a quality of life questionnaire for critically ill patients. *Intensive Care Med.*, **22**, 1034–1042.

and reduced sexual activity than community controls. Reliability analysis performed on the 13 scales within this instrument yielded Cronbach's alpha values between 0.71 and 0.93 with test-retest correlations ranging from 0.61 to 0.85 in healthy individuals. Further studies to demonstrate the construct validity of this instrument have not been performed. Finally, in the last study employing a third unvalidated instrument, a smaller evaluation of 13 patients demonstrated mostly minor complaints related to physical condition in 54%, an increase in anxiety in 46% but a return to living at home in 100% of respondents (Rustom and Daly, 1993).

In summary, although the PQOL scale has demonstrated some responsiveness to change in the HRQL of ICU populations, its construct validity has not been firmly established. Initial studies using the QOL-IT instrument have demonstrated good reliability and validity; however, further studies demonstrating the construct validity of this instrument are required before it can be recommended for widespread use. The QOL-SP appears to have the best reliability and construct validity for use in critically ill patients. As this instrument is used in different ICU populations, its construct validity should increase. The three remaining ICU-specific instruments cannot be recommended for routine use because of the limited information regarding their psychometric properties.

HRQL after ICU has not been shown to correlate with illness severity such as the APACHE II score. ICU-specific HRQL measures display an element of autocorrelation before and after admission to the ICU; patients who have better HRQL prior to ICU admission appear to suffer the greatest deterioration in their HRQL following critical care, compared to those with worse HRQL prior to their admission to the ICU. However, it is important to note that only a minority of patients appear to suffer major deterioration in HRQL after ICU discharge.

Generic and disease-specific HRQL instruments

Of the 17 studies that have utilized validated generic or disease-specific HRQL instruments not initially designed for critical care, the greatest experience has been with the use of the EuroQol 5D (EuroQol Group, 1990), the Sickness Impact Profile (SIP) (Bergner et al., 1981), and the SF–36 (Ware, 1993).

The EuroQol is a generic HRQL instrument composed of three parts. The first section is descriptive, defining health states in terms of five areas (mobility, personal care, usual activities, pain/discomfort, anxiety/depression) which are divided into three levels (1: without problems, 2: moderate problems, 3: very severe problems). The second part is a visual analogue scale where individuals rate their own health state from a minimum of 0 to a maximum of 100. In the third part, respondents are asked to value, on a visual analogue scale from 0 to 100, each of 14 health states of varying degrees of impairment (Table 7.8).

Finally, respondents are asked to mark on the same scale where 'being dead' is scored.

Table 7.8 The five domains (with main activities and social relationships considered as one domain and excluding being dead) of the EuroQol and four examples of the health states described in the final questionnaire that the patients are asked to score on a visual analogue scale ranging from 0 to 100

Domains	Combinations of domains	Examples of final combinations (n = 16)
Mobility 1 No problem walking about 2 Unable to walk about without a stick, crutch or walking frame 3 Confined to bed **Self care** 1 No problems with self care 2 Unable to dress self 3 Unable to feed self **Main activity** 1 Able to perform main activity (e.g. work, study, housework) 2 Unable to perform main activity **Social relationships** 1 Able to pursue family and leisure activities 2 Unable to pursue family and leisure activities **Pain** 1 No pain or discomfort 2 Moderate pain or discomfort 3 Extreme pain or discomfort **Mood** 1 Not anxious or depressed 2 Anxious or depressed **Being dead**	With 16 descriptions of differing health state within all domains, there are 216 possible combinations. The developers wanted to cover health states that were both common and yet encompassed a wide range of severity. They reduced the possible combinations to 16 (with being dead appearing twice to check internal consistency)	No problem walking about No problems with self care Unable to perform main activity Able to pursue family and leisure activities Moderate pain or discomfort Not anxious or depressed Unable to walk about without a stick, crutch or walking frame No problems with self care Unable to perform main activity Unable to pursue family and leisure activities Extreme pain or discomfort Anxious or depressed Confined to bed Unable to dress self Unable to perform main activity Unable to pursue family and leisure activities Extreme pain or discomfort Anxious or depressed Being dead

The agreement between patient and surrogate measures of HRQL, and the change in HRQL before the onset of critical illness as compared to that prior to discharge from a step down unit, has been described using the EuroQol in a Spanish population of mostly cardiac surgical patients (Badia *et al.*, 1996). Agreement between patients and surrogates regarding their prior health state was moderate to good in physical and pain areas (kappa values between 0.43 and 0.58) and fair for mood (kappa value 0.38). Also, there was no statistically significant difference between mean scores for prior health states between patients and their proxies. However, after ICU, patients produced lower scores in all physical domains and the mean overall score, but with no significant differences in scores for pain/discomfort and anxiety/depression.

In a subsequent Spanish study, perceived health status assessed by proxy 3 months prior to hospital admission was compared with the status of patients surviving ICU (Diaz-Prieto *et al.*, 1998). Trauma patients were noted to have the best prior health status scores as measured by proxy answers to the EuroQol. Elective surgical patients had the worst. A strong positive correlation between proxy EuroQol scores and Karnofsky scale has been demonstrated, thereby enhancing the construct and criterion validity of the EuroQol. However, neither the EuroQol nor Karnofsky instrument was predictive of hospital mortality, whereas SAPS II (Le Gall *et al.*, 1993) was a strong predictor of mortality. The EuroQol instrument has also been evaluated in a Spanish population of ICU patients suffering from multiple organ failure, of whom only 28% survived (Garcia Lizana *et al.*, 2000). Fifty-nine percent of the survivors either improved or recovered their previous HRQL with 18% remaining severely debilitated.

The SIP consists of 136 items that describe specific sickness-related behavioural dysfunction grouped into 12 subscales (body care and movement, mobility, ambulation, emotional behaviour, social interaction, alertness behaviour, communication, sleep and rest, eating, recreation and pastimes, home management, work) (Table 7.9).

The SIP is scored by summing the weights for each item as an aggregate score expressed as a percentage of the maximum possible score of 100; a higher score indicates greater dysfunction. Profile scores may also be calculated for each of the 12 subscales and are reported as percentages. In a Dutch study of 3655 respondents 1 year after discharge from ICU, mean SIP scores ranged from 5.8 for patients aged between 17 and 29 to 10.5 for those over 70 years of age; the overall mean SIP score was 8.5. This was mainly due to dysfunction in the physical dimension, with the exception of those patients aged between 30 and 49 years in whom the psychosocial changes were responsible for approximately 50% of the total score differences (Tian and Reis Miranda, 1995). More optimistic results were reported 1 year after admission to a multidisciplinary ICU in Hong Kong. The median SIP score was 5.1 (Short *et al.*, 1999). In this study, age, cardiorespiratory arrest, intracranial haemorrhage and trauma were identified as independent predictors of higher SIP scores. Neither the Dutch nor the Hong Kong studies found a strong correlation between SIP score and the severity of illness, as measured by APACHE II system, nor was there a correlation

Table 7.9 The domains and a selection of questions pertaining to those domains

Domains	Selected Items
Sleep and rest	I sit during much of the day I sleep or nap during the day
Eating	I am eating no food at all, nutrition is taken through tubes or intravenous fluids I am eating special or different food
Work	I am not working at all I often act irritably toward my work associates
Home Management	I am not doing any of the maintenance or repair work around the house that I usually do I am not doing heavy work around the house
Recreation and pastimes	I am going out for entertainment less I am not doing any of my usual physical recreation or activities
Ambulation	I walk shorter distances or stop to rest often I do not walk at all
Mobility	I stay within one room I stay away from home only for brief periods of time
Body care and movement	I do not bathe myself at all, but am bathed by someone else I am very clumsy in body movements
Social interaction	I am doing fewer social activities with groups of people I isolate myself as much as I can from the rest of the family
Alertness behaviour	I have difficulty reasoning and solving problems, for example, making plans, making decisions, learning new things I sometimes behave as if I were confused or disoriented in place or time, for example, where I am, who is around, directions, what day it is.
Emotional behaviour	I laugh or cry suddenly I act irritable and impatient with myself, for example, talk badly about myself, swear at myself, blame myself for things that happen
Communication	I am having trouble writing or typing I do not speak clearly when I am under stress

Modified from Bergner, M., Bobbitt, R. A., Kressel, S., Pollard, W. E., Gibson, B. S., Morris, J. R. (1981). The Sickness Impact Profile: development and final revision of a health status measure. *Med. Care*, **19**, 787–805.

between the SIP score, Therapeutic Intervention Score System (TISS), and length of ICU stay.

The use of the SIP in the ICU population has been limited by the lack of information regarding its reliability and validity in this population and also by its length. Previous investigators have demonstrated that response rates after the distribution of the SIP to survivors of critical illness varied from 56% in those to whom the instrument was mailed, to 77% of patients who were telephoned with an invitation to participate prior to distribution of the questionnaire (Hulsebos et al., 1991). Significant differences in SIP scores were noted between patients who were mailed the questionnaire and those personally interviewed. However, the differences in scores may have been attributed to sample characteristics and it is difficult to comment on the possible influence of different application methods.

The best studied generic HRQL instrument in the ICU setting has been the SF–36. The SF–36 has 36 questions grouped into eight domains (physical functioning, role-physical, bodily pain, general health, vitality, social functioning, role-emotional, and mental health). The eight domains are further aggregated into two higher-order domains, physical health and mental health (Table 7.10).

With respect to its reliability and validity just prior to discharge from a general ICU, internal consistency and reliability as measured by Cronbach's alpha exceeded 0.85 for seven domains but not for the mental health domain (Chrispin et al., 1997). In a retrospective study of 30 septic patients, internally consistent reliability (Cronbach's alpha) ranged from 0.65 (general health domain) to 0.94 (physical functioning) whereas test-retest reliability ranged from 0.56 (physical and social functioning domains) to 0.94 (mental health summary) (Heyland et al., 2000). Surrogate responses using the SF–36 at ICU discharge and 6 months later produced Cronbach's alphas greater than 0.85 and reliability coefficients over 0.70 suggesting acceptable reliability (Rogers et al., 1997). Surrogate responses using the SF–36 agreed moderately with patient responses at ICU discharge (kappa values of between 0.21 and 0.6) but improved at 6 months with 50% of kappa values exceeding 0.6 (good agreement). Surrogate responses also tended to underestimate patient scores in physical health domains, vitality and social functioning and overestimate emotional role and mental health at ICU discharge.

Construct validity for the SF–36 is supported by a difference in the distribution of scores by age and gender and content validity is strengthened by the broad distribution of scores throughout the range of answers (Chrispin et al., 1997). In a subsequent study of the same ICU population, the SF–36 was distributed to 166 patients at ICU discharge and 6 months later. Overall, the patients' pre-morbid scores at discharge were lower than normal for all eight domains of the SF–36, while 6 months later there were significant increases in the mental health, vitality, social functioning domains and a reduction in bodily pain scores (Ridley et al., 1997). The lower overall mean score (i.e. worsening HRQL) at 6 months was recorded in patients admitted with acute problems while patients with chronic co-morbidities maintained their HRQL. This is consistent with a previous study which used a composite instrument of several HRQL measures (Ridley and Wallace, 1990) as well as studies utilizing the QOL-SP (Vazquez Mata et al., 1992) and the PQOL (Perrins et al., 1998). A validated Finnish version of the

SF–36 has also been used in a population of 307 critically ill individuals (43% diagnosed with multiple organ dysfunction) and compared with a general Finnish population of age- and gender-matched controls. At 12 months after ICU discharge 59.6% of the ICU patients assessed their HRQL as measured by the SF–36 to be better than or similar to that before their intensive care admission (Pettila *et al.*, 2000). Compared to the population control, impairment was greatest in the domains of social functioning, mental health and role limitations because of emotional problems and vitality. Moreover, patients diagnosed with multiple organ dysfunction syndrome scored significantly worse than the remaining ICU population in the domains of vitality, emotional role limitations, physical functioning and bodily pain.

Six additional studies have used either individual quality of life scales (Ridley *et al.*, 1994; Hurel *et al.*, 1997; Perrins *et al.*, 1998), or composite instruments of previously validated scales (Ridley and Wallace, 1990; Ridley *et al.*, 1994; Ortiz *et al.*, 1998). Both the Nottingham Health Profile and the PQOL are well correlated, providing some evidence for criterion validity (Hurel *et al.*, 1997). However, good HRQL, as measured by the Nottingham Health Profile, was present in only 38.8% of respondents, and a high PQOL score was recorded in only 23.7% of respondents. Variability in HRQL appeared to be dependent on the admitting diagnosis, with attempted suicide and chronic obstructive pulmonary disease demonstrating the worst HRQL using these measures. In a separate study assessing psychological dysfunction after an ICU admission, the General Health Questionnaire 28-item version, the Rosenberg Self-Esteem Scale and the Impact of Events Scale were given to 72 patients at 6 weeks, 6 and 12 months after ICU discharge (Perrins *et al.*, 1998). Changes in the scores of these instruments were found to be dependent on the indication for admission to the ICU, the mode of admission (e.g. elective, postoperative versus unconscious from the ward) and patient recall. As a result, these factors must be considered when validating any future HRQL instruments in critical care.

One study, which utilized Spitzer's Quality of Life Index on admission to the ICU and at 6 and 12 months after the initial survey, found reduced Activities of Daily Living at 6 and 12 months (Konopad *et al.*, 1995). However, perceived health improved over the year, which agreed with the findings of the study using the SF–36 (Ridley *et al.*, 1997). In a further study of 536 Spanish patients utilizing an aggregate instrument composed of the Karnofsky Scale, the Daily Life Activities Index and PQOL, the composite score prior to ICU admission was an independent predictor of both hospital mortality and the degree of deterioration after ICU admission (Ortiz *et al.*, 1998).

In the only study to assess a composite quality of life measure with a cost-utility analysis, the quality of life for the majority of patients remained the same following critical care, except for survivors who previously perceived a good quality of life or were admitted with respiratory problems, in which case their quality of life diminished (Ridley *et al.*, 1994). Furthermore, the hospital cost per quality adjusted life year (QALY) was approximately £7500.

With respect to generic HRQL measures in ICU, several generalizations may be made. The EuroQol is supported by a sound theoretical framework (i.e. good

Table 7.10 Questions 7 (bodily pain), 8 (bodily pain) and 9 (vitality and mental health) of the SF–36 modified slightly to emphasize that the patient's quality of life prior to their acute illness was being assessed. The answers to the 36 questions should be transformed and weighted according to instructions produced by the questionnaire's designer. Summary scores were calculated for each of the eight groups of domains and expressed as a percentage from 0 to 100, with the higher scores indicating better perceived health or functioning

7. How much <u>bodily pain</u> have you had during the <u>4 weeks</u> prior to your hospital admission?

(circle one)

None	1
Very mild	2
Mild	3
Moderate	4
Severe	5
Very severe	6

8. In the <u>4 weeks</u> prior to <u>your</u> hospital admission, how much did <u>pain</u> interfere with your normal work (including both work outside the home and housework)?

(circle one)

Not at all	1
A little bit	2
Moderately	3
Quite a bit	4
Extremely	5

9. These questions are about how you feel and how things have been with you in the <u>4 weeks prior to your hospital admission</u>.

For each question, please give the one answer that comes closest to the way you have been feeling. How much of the time during the <u>4 weeks prior to your hospital admission</u>:

(circle one number on each line)

	All of the time	Most of the time	A good bit of the time	Some of the time	A little of the time	None of the time
a. Did you feel full of life?	1	2	3	4	5	6
b. Have you been a very nervous person	1	2	3	4	5	6
c. Have you felt so down in the dumps that nothing could cheer you up?	1	2	3	4	5	6
d. Have you felt calm and peaceful?	1	2	3	4	5	6
e. Did you have a lot of energy?	1	2	3	4	5	6
f. Have you felt downhearted and low?	1	2	3	4	5	6
g. Did you feel worn out?	1	2	3	4	5	6
h. Have you been a happy person?	1	2	3	4	5	6
i. Did you feel tired?	1	2	3	4	5	6

Reproduced from Chrispin, P. S., Scotton, H., Rogers, J., Lloyd, D., Ridley, S. A. (1997). Short Form 36 in the intensive care unit: assessment of acceptability, reliability and validity of the questionnaire. *Anaesthesia*, **52**, 15–23.

content and construct validity) and the facility for patients to value various health states, so permitting the calculation of QALYs. However, data published about the reliability of this instrument in the ICU population are limited, apart from being a reliable instrument for use by patient proxies. It does, however, hold promise for future use in the ICU. The SIP also possesses sound content validity. However, it is limited by its length (136 items) and infrequent reports of its reliability and construct validity in the general ICU population. Of the three most widely used generic measures in critical care, the SF–36 appears to be best studied, possessing good reliability, content, construct and criterion validity across several studies.

Important generalizations can be made regarding the relationship between HRQL before and after ICU admission and severity of illness and hospital mortality. Most studies utilizing either ICU-specific or generic HRQL measures have demonstrated that previously healthy patients who suffer critical illness tend to suffer greater deterioration in their HRQL than individuals who had lower HRQL status prior to ICU admission. Moreover, studies utilizing the QOL-SP, EuroQol, SIP, SF–36 and Karnofsky instruments have failed to demonstrate a correlation with illness severity scoring systems such as the APACHE II, SAPS II and TISS systems. The breadth of these findings does not support the theoretical construct that HRQL of patients requiring critical care is either positively or negatively associated with the degree of physiological derangement at ICU admission. These differences probably result from different theoretical constructs underlying HRQL and illness severity measurement. Finally, based on the present literature, it is unclear whether retrospective measurement of HRQL prior to ICU admission predicts subsequent hospital mortality. One study utilizing the EuroQol and Karnofsky instruments failed to demonstrate an association, whereas another study which utilized a composite measure did demonstrate a positive correlation with hospital mortality (Ortiz et al., 1998; Diaz-Prieto et al., 1998).

HRQL in subgroups of critically ill patients

Acute respiratory distress syndrome (ARDS)

Studies of HRQL in patients who have suffered from ARDS have used the SIP (Grose McHugh et al., 1994), SF–36 (Schelling et al., 1998, 2000; Davidson et al., 1999) and St George's Respiratory Questionnaire (Davidson et al., 1999). Three studies have found good criterion validity in the SIP and SF–36, as reflected by the correlation between decrements in standard tests of pulmonary function and poorer HRQL. Pulmonary function as measured by forced expiratory volume in one second (FEV_1), forced vital capacity (FVC), total lung capacity (TLC) and diffusing capacity (D_{Lco}) appears to improve significantly during the first 6 months after discharge and then stabilize (Grose McHugh et al., 1994). At a median of 5.5 years following ICU discharge, approximately 50% of patients had normal pulmonary function (defined as $\geq 80\%$ of the predicted value of FVC, FEV_1, TLC, D_{Lco} or capillary PO_2 during exercise), whereas less than 15% had impairments in two or more parameters of pulmonary function defined as $< 80\%$ of predicted values (Schelling *et al.*, 2000). Patients with impairments in at least two parameters of pulmonary function described significantly worse HRQL as measured by the SF–36. Irrespective of the HRQL instrument used, the majority of survivors of ARDS appear to have a moderate decline in HRQL within the first year after ICU discharge, followed by long-term improvement. When using the SF–36, a more serious impairment in HRQL was noted in the physical profiles as opposed to the mental profiles. However, in one study, 20% of ARDS survivors met standard self-reported criteria for post-traumatic stress disorder (Schelling *et al.*, 1998). The St George's Respiratory Questionnaire appeared to be better than the SF–36 at discriminating between subgroups of ARDS survivors; patients with ARDS triggered by sepsis having worse HRQL as compared to ARDS patients following trauma (Davidson *et al.*, 1999). This finding illustrates the advantage of using disease-specific instruments when trying to discriminate between patient groups suffering from the same general illness.

Long-stay patients

The importance of measuring non-mortality outcomes in patients with prolonged ICU stays is accentuated by their high mortality and resource consumption. This is exemplified by a recent study of 1960 admissions to a Canadian medical-surgical ICU. Patients staying on ICU for less than 2 days accounted for 60.3% of all admissions but 16.4% of all ICU days. On the other hand, patients with an ICU stay exceeding 2 weeks accounted for 7.3% of admissions, but 43.5% of total patient-days (Wong *et al.*, 1999).

Studies of ICU patients with prolonged stays have concentrated on cardiac surgical (Trouillet *et al.*, 1996), general surgical (Fakhry *et al.*, 1996), elderly (Montuclard *et al.*, 2000) and general populations of ICU patients (Heyland *et al.*, 1998b). These studies have used heterogeneous instruments to evaluate HRQL in small numbers of survivors. In those patients with a prolonged ICU stay after cardiac surgery, only a modest worsening of the physical mobility score of the Nottingham Health Profile has been demonstrated (Trouillet *et al.*, 1996). In a study of 83 patients requiring more than 14 days in a surgical ICU, 70% of respondents reported less than 50% functional recovery (using a non-validated HRQL instrument). The average 'charge' to achieve one long-term survivor was US $247 812 (Fakhry *et al.*, 1996).

Using several validated instruments in French patients over 70 years old and treated for more than 30 days on ICU, slight to moderate declines in HRQL were recorded using the Nottingham Health Profile and PQOL. However, larger decreases in functional autonomy as measured by Katz's Activities of Daily Living Scale have been reported (Montuclard *et al.*, 2000). In this population of patients, only 47% survived to hospital discharge with an estimated cost per survivor of US $60 246. For critically ill patients requiring more than 2 weeks intensive care, HRQL at 12 months has been shown to be comparable to that of short-stay patients; the incremental cost-effectiveness ratio was Canadian $4350 per life year saved (Heyland et al., 1998b).

The elderly

Depending on the type and location of ICU, the elderly may account for 26–51% of admissions. Interest in critically ill elderly patients has prompted at least seven studies and two review articles since 1989; each examined the impact of age on outcome following critical care (Lawton, 1969, 1971; Katz et al., 1970; Rubins, 1989; Mahul et al., 1991; Chelluri et al., 1992, 1993; Kass et al., 1992; Rockwood et al., 1993; Broslawski et al., 1995; Chelluri and Grenvik, 1995; Montuclard et al., 2000). Overall, this work suggests that age alone has little or no important effect on outcome from critical illness, with some exceptions such as severe closed head injury and out-of-hospital cardiac arrest. Outcome is most strongly influenced by severity of illness and, to a varying extent, prior health status and ICU length of stay.

With respect to the 'very old', two studies of patients over the age of 85 years concluded that advanced age was not an appropriate contraindication for allocation of ICU resources, and was less important than acute severity of illness (Chelluri et al., 1992; Kass et al., 1992). Other data suggest that advanced age cannot be used to predict functional ability.

Follow-up studies of the elderly after critical care have evaluated quality of life in a variety of ways, using several instruments (Table 7.11).

Table 7.11 Quality of life instruments used in studies of elderly patients

Perceived Quality of Life Scale (PQOL)
Nottingham Health Profile (NHP)
Katz and Downs Activity of Life Scale
Lawton and Brody Instrumental Activities of Daily Living
Geriatric Depression Scale (Sheikh and Yesavage, 1986)
Mini-mental state (Folstein et al., 1975)
Centre for Epidemiologic Studies Depression Score (Weissman et al., 1977)

Less robust data have also come from personal and telephone interviews, collecting data on subjective perceptions of quality of life.

While our present understanding suggests that age is not a major factor influencing either quantity or quality of survival following critical care, this generalization requires further evaluation in relation to specific diseases and interventions.

Longitudinal changes in HRQL after critical care

Although several studies have followed cohorts of patients for extended periods of time after ICU discharge, few comparable studies have repeatedly measured HRQL. Such studies are needed to characterize the rate of recovery of HRQL in critically ill patients. This information would better inform survivors of critical illness of their non-mortality outcomes and improve understanding of the effectiveness of rehabilitation on non-mortality outcomes (Ridley, 2000).

Important issues to be considered in future cohort studies are the duration of follow-up after hospital discharge, the appropriateness of the instrument selected in terms of validity and reliability, and the use of appropriate statistical methods. These considerations are vital to avoid incorrect inferences from the data. It has been suggested that critically ill patients should be followed-up until their survival curves match those of comparable populations (i.e. those with a comparable propensity to enter the ICU) (Ridley, 2000). Estimates of the time taken for the survival curves of a cohort of critically ill patients to parallel that of the general population vary from 1 (Zaren and Bergstrom, 1998) to 4 years (Ridley and Plenderleith, 1994). In the largest cohort studied to date of 12 180 patients, approximately 2 years was needed for survival to parallel that of the general population (Niskanen *et al.*, 1996).

Based on these studies and recommendations, future studies describing longitudinal measurements of HRQL in patients discharged from an ICU should probably follow patients for at least 2 years, with longer follow-up depending upon the critical illness itself and the country in which intensive care is provided.

In order to address responsiveness of generic instruments, possible sub-optimal performance of disease-specific measures and reliability and validity over time, the simultaneous use of both generic and disease-specific measures together with measures of physiological functioning is recommended. Utilizing disease-specific tools should provide improved responsiveness to longitudinal changes of HRQL. The concurrent collection of physiological data should add to the criterion validity of any instrument used. If proxy respondents are to be enrolled in such studies, care should be taken to measure the reliability of their responses over time, as the reliability of proxies changes with time after hospital discharge.

Finally, valid conclusions about changes in HRQL can only be made when the correct statistical methods are used to distinguish between individuals and their baseline HRQL (cohort effects) and from HRQL changes over time following hospital discharge (time effects). Longitudinal observations on individual subjects tend to be intercorrelated and this must be considered in any longitudinal analysis. The QOL-SP and other instruments have demonstrated that previous HRQL measurements were predictive of later results using the same measurement. Consequently, sophisticated statistical models such as random-effects linear regression and general estimating equations, which explore and account for the correlation structure within and between individuals over time, have been developed. These should probably be used in future longitudinal studies involving serial HRQL measurements (Diggle *et al.*, 1994; Burton *et al.*, 1998).

Economic considerations in HRQL

John von Neuman and Oscar Morgenstern (1944) published an extension of economic utility theory dealing with rational decision making under uncertainty. This theory supports the 'standard gamble', which is the conventional method for measuring utilities. The standard gamble method is a paired comparison between two health states, whereby the subject may either choose to take one health state with certainty (e.g. chronic disease) or gamble on a therapy that has the potential for either improving or worsening health status (e.g. a high-risk operation) (Torrance and Feeny, 1989). Decisions based on the standard gamble technique may be measured in terms of QALYs. A QALY is defined as the equivalent of a completely healthy year of life or a year of life free of symptoms or health-related disabilities. QALYs provide a standard to compare the effect of technologies and therapies within and across diseases (Torrance and Feeny, 1989; Fabian, 1994; Torrance, 1986). Although utility measures have been evaluated in neonatal intensive care units, similar measures have not been applied to adult ICU populations.

Unfortunately, there is a potential disparity between functional ability and measures of utility. For example, patients with coronary artery disease, which produced similar functional limitations as measured by the classification of the Canadian Cardiovascular Society, varied considerably in their perception and tolerance of symptoms as measured by utilities (Nease et al., 1995). Consequently, relying solely on functional or physiological measures (such as illness severity scores) may not capture all the benefits of providing specific medical therapies.

One of the scales used to calculate QALYs is the Quality of Well-being Scale (Kaplan et al., 1998; Andersen et al., 1998). The Quality of Well-being Scale measures observable levels of function pertaining to mobility and physical and social activity. A 'quality' rating of preferences for health states between 0 for death and 1.0 for complete health has been determined for the Quality of Well-being Scale and is used to calculate QALY values. A recent review has outlined the strengths and limitations of both the SF–36 and the Quality of Well-being Scale and their complementary nature (Kaplan et al., 1998). In general, the Quality of Well-being Scale avoids the problem of floor or ceiling effects (as with the SF–36) and has been designed as an integral measure of cost-utility. However, the Quality of Well-being Scale does not provide as much information on health profiles as the SF–36.

Although there are accepted instruments for HQOL assessment, there are no standard tools for measuring ICU costs in cost-utility studies. Several methods for costing intensive care have been proposed; however, a recent review has pointed out that most of these methods are flawed and fail to provide accurate information (Gyldmark, 1995). There have been few attempts at cost accounting at the individual patient level (Noseworthy et al., 1996). The majority of methods sum total ICU costs and attribute cost as an average daily cost per patient. This may be inappropriate because of the heterogeneity of illness severity and the variability in requirements for care encountered within the ICU. The best method for costing ICU resources should permit an accurate comparison of the patient-specific costs of therapy with the outcome measure of interest in terms of mortality, HRQL or functional outcome. Such a method requires recording resource use of each patient rather than calculations that assume homogeneity of ICU patients. This approach would enable investigations of the influence of different patient characteristics or novel therapies on the cost of ICU care.

Edbrooke *et al.* (1997, 1999) have described and utilized an activity-based costing methodology at patient level and has shown the advantages of such a method over the use of traditional measures of costing. This method has demonstrated the difference in ICU costs of caring for critically ill patients with severe sepsis or septic shock. However, to date, no rigorous large scale studies have attempted to link the cost of providing intensive care with both validated measures of HRQL and utilities, in order to provide an estimate of the cost-utility of providing care to the critically ill. Such information is crucial for informed allocation of resources in the ICU and as such is an important area for future research.

Conclusion

As the discipline of critical care medicine has evolved over the past quarter century, so too have the methods used to measure the outcomes of the process of caring for the critically ill. Initial enthusiasm and advancements in the measurement of the severity of illness and its relationship to mortality have given way to new measurements, whether they be of physiological outcomes such as pulmonary function, or multidimensional analyses of quality of life. Much of the latter advancement in the knowledge pertaining to HRQL in critically ill populations has come from the application of psychometric theory to the development of validated generic and disease-specific instruments used in these populations. Several validated HRQL instruments are now available to ICU clinicians and researchers for use in observational and experimental studies for which a difference in HRQL is an important outcome. Areas of future research should focus on better defining the cost-utility of caring for various subgroups of critically ill patients and mechanisms for minimizing declines in HRQL.

References

Andersen, E. M., Rothenberg, B. M., Kaplan, R. M. (1998). Performance of a self-administered mailed version of the Quality of Well-Being (QWB-SA) questionnaire among older adults. *Med. Care*, **36**, 1349–1360.

Badia, X., Diaz-Prieto, A., Rue, M., Patrick, D. L. (1996). Measuring health and health state preferences among critically ill patients. *Intensive Care Med.*, **22**, 1379–1384.

Bergner, M. (1985). Measurement of health status. *Med. Care*, **23**, 696–704.

Bergner, M., Bobbitt, R. A., Kressel, S., Pollard, W. E., Gibson, B. S., Morris, J. R. (1981). The Sickness Impact Profile: development and final revision of a health status measure. *Med. Care*, **19**, 787–805.

Bindman, A. B., Keane, D., Lurie, N. (1990). Measuring health changes among severely ill patients. The floor phenomenon. *Medical Care*, **28**, 1142–1151.

Brooks R., with the EuroQol Group. (1996). EuroQol: the current state of play. *Health Policy*, **37**, 53–72.

Brooks, R., Bauman, A., Daffurn, K., Hillman, K. (1995). Post-hospital outcome following intensive care. *Clin. Intensive Care*, **6**, 127–135.

Brooks, R., Kerridge, R., Hillman, K., Bauman, A., Daffurn, K. (1997). Quality of life outcomes after intensive care: comparison with a community group. *Intensive Care Med.*, **23**, 581–586.

Broslawski, G. E., Elkins, M., Algus, M. (1995). Functional abilities of elderly survivors of intensive care. *J. Am. Osteopath. Assoc.*, **92**, 712–717.

Burton, P., Gurrin, L., Sly, P. (1998). Tutorial in biostatistics. Extending the simple linear regression model to account for correlated responses: An introduction to generalized estimating equations and multi-level mixed modeling. *Stat. Med.*, **17**, 1261–1291.

Capuzzo, M., Bianconi, M., Contu, P., Pavoni, V., Gritti, G. (1996). Survival and quality of life after intensive care. *Intensive Care Med.*, **22**, 947–953.

Capuzzo, M., Grasselli, C., Carrer, S., Gritti, G., Alvisi, R. (2000a). Quality of life before intensive care admission: agreement between patient and relative assessment. *Intensive Care Med.*, **26**, 1288–1295.

Capuzzo, M., Grasselli, C., Carrer, S., Gritti, G., Alvisi, R. (2000b). Validation of two quality of life questionnaires suitable for intensive care patients. *Intensive Care Med.*, **26**, 1296–1303.

Carmenes, E. G., Zeller, R. A. (1981). *Reliability and Validity Assessment*. Sage Publications.

Chelluri, L., Grenvik, A. (1995). Intensive care for critically ill elderly: mortality, costs, and quality of life. *Arch. Intern. Med.*, **155**, 1013–1022.

Chelluri, L., Pinsky, M. R., Donahoe, M. P., Grenvik, A. (1993). Long-term outcome of critically ill elderly patients requiring intensive care. *JAMA*, **269**, 3119–3123.

Chelluri, L., Pinsky, M. R., Grenvik, A. N. A. (1992). Outcomes of intensive care of the 'oldest-old' critically ill patients. *Crit. Care Med.*, **20**, 757–761.

Chrispin, P. S., Scotton, H., Rogers, J., Lloyd, D., Ridley, S. A. (1997). Short Form 36 in the intensive care unit: assessment of acceptability, reliability and validity of the questionnaire. *Anaesthesia*, **52**, 15–23.

Clancy, M., Eisenberg, J. M. (1998). Outcomes research: Measuring the end results of health care. *Science*, **282**, 245–246.

Cronbach, L. J., Meehl, P. E. (1955). Construct validity in psychological tests. *Psychol. Bull.*, **52**, 281–302.

Daffurn, K., Bishop, G. F., Hillman, K. M., Bauman, A. (1994). Problems following discharge after intensive care. *Intensive Crit. Care Nurs.*, **10**, 244–251.

Davidson, T. A., Caldwell, E. S., Randall Curtis, J., Hudson, L. D., Steinberg, K. P. (1999). Reduced quality of life in survivors of acute respiratory distress syndrome compared with critically ill control patients. *JAMA*, **281**, 354–360.

Diaz-Prieto, A., Gorriz, M. T., Badia, X. *et al.* (1998). Proxy-perceived prior health status and hospital outcome among the critically ill: is there any relationship? *Intensive Care Med.*, **24**, 691–698.

Diggle, P. J., Liang, K., Zeger, S. L. (1994). *Analysis of Longitudinal Data*. Oxford University Press.

Dupuy, H. (1984). The Psychological General Well-being (PGWB) Index. In: *Assessment of Quality of Life in Clinical Trials of Cardiovascular Therapies* (N.K. Wenger, M.E. Mattson, C.D. Furberg, J. Elinson eds). LeJacq.

Edbrooke, D. L., Hibbert, C. L., Kingsley, J. M., Smith, S., Bright, N. M., Quinn, J. M. (1999). The patient-related costs of care for sepsis patients in a United Kingdom adult general intensive care unit. *Crit. Care Med.*, **27**, 1760–1767.

Edbrooke, D. L., Stevens, V. G., Hibbert, C. L., Mann, A. J., Wilson, A. J. (1997). A new method of accurately identifying costs of individual patients in intensive care: the initial results. *Intensive Care Med.*, **23**, 645–650.

EuroQol Group. (1990). EuroQol-a new facility for the measurement of health-related quality of life. *Health Policy*, **16**, 199–208.

Fabian, R. (1994). Qualy Approach. In: *Valuing Health for Policy* (G. Tolley, D. Kenkel, R. Fabian, eds) pp 118–136, University of Chicago Press.

Fakhry, S. M., Kercher, K. W., Rutledge, R. (1996). Survival, quality of life, and charges in critically ill surgical patients requiring prolonged ICU stays. *J. Trauma*, **41**, 999–1007.

Feeny, D. H., Torrance, G. W. (1989). Incorporating utility-based quality-of-life assessment measures in clinical trials: Two examples. *Med. Care*, **27**, S190–S204.

Feeny, D. H., Torrance, G. W., Furlong, W. J. (1996). Health utilities index. In: *Quality of Life and Pharmacoeconomics in Clinical Trials*, 2nd edn. (B. Spiker, ed.) pp 239–252, Lippincott-Raven.

Folstein, M. F., Folstein, S. E., McHugh, P. R. (1975). 'Mini-mental state': a practical method for grading the cognitive state of patients for the clinician. *J. Psychiat. Res.*, **12**, 189–198.

Garcia Lizana, F., Manzano Alonso, J. L., Gonzalez Santana, B., Fuentes Esteban, J., Saavedra Santana, P. (2000). Survival and quality of life of patients with multiple organ failure one year after leaving an intensive care unit. *Med. Clin. (Barc.)*, **114** Suppl 3, 99–103.

Gill, T. M., Feinstein, A. R. (1994). A critical appraisal of the quality of quality-of-life measurements. *JAMA*, **272**, 619–626.

Goldberg, D. P., Hillier, V. F. (1979). A scaled version of the General Health Questionnaire. *Psychol. Med.*, **9**, 139–145.

Grieco, A., Long, C. J. (1984). Investigation of the Karnofsky Performance Status as a measure of quality of life. *Health Psychol.*, **3**, 129–142.

Grose McHugh, L., Milberg, J. A., Whitcomb, M. E. *et al.* (1994). Recovery of function in survivors of the acute respiratory distress syndrome. *Am. J. Respir. Crit. Care Med.*, **150**, 90–94.

Guyatt, G. H., Feeny, D. H., Patrick, D. L. (1993). Measuring health-related quality of life. *Ann. Intern. Med.*, **118**, 622–629.

Guyatt, G., Feeny, D., Patrick, D. (1991). Issues in quality-of-life measurement in clinical trials. *Controlled Clinical Trials*, **12**, 81S–90S.

Gyldmark, M. (1995). A review of cost studies of intensive care units: Problems with the cost concept. *Crit. Care Med.*, **23**, 964–972.

Heyland, D. K., Guyatt, G., Cook, D. J. (1998a). Frequency and methodologic rigor of quality-of-life assessments in the critical care literature. *Crit. Care Med.*, **26**, 592–598.

Heyland, D. K., Konopad, E., Noseworthy, T. W., Johnston, R., Gafni, A. (1998b). Is it 'worthwhile' to continue treating patients with a prolonged stay (> 14 days) in the ICU? An economic evaluation. *Chest*, **114**, 192–198.

Heyland, D. K., Hopman, W., Coo, H., Tranmer, J., McColl, M. (2000). Long-term health-related quality of life in survivors of sepsis. Short Form 36: A valid and reliable measure of health related quality of life. *Crit. Care Med.*, **28**, 3599–3605.

Hillers, T. K., Guyatt, G. H., Oldridge, N. *et al.* (1994). Quality of life after myocardial infarction. *J. Clin. Epidemiol.*, **47**, 1287–1296.

Horowitz, M., Wilner, N. (1979). The impact of event scale: a measure of subjective stress. *Psychosom. Med.*, **41**, 209–218.

Hulsebos, R. G., Beltman, F. W., Reis Miranda, D., Spangenberg, J. F. A. (1991). Measuring quality of life with the Sickness Impact Profile: a pilot study. *Intensive Care Med.*, **17**, 285–288.

Hunt, S. M., McKenna, S. P., McEwen, J., Williams, J., Rapp, E. (1981). The Nottingham Health Profile: subjective health status and medical consultations. *Soc. Sci. Med.*, **15A**, 221–229.

Hurel, D., Loirat, P., Saulnier, F., Nicolas, F., Brivet, F. (1997). Quality of life 6 months after intensive care: results of a prospective multicenter study using a generic health status scale and a satisfaction scale. *Intensive Care Med.*, **23**, 331–337.

Juniper, E. F., Guyatt, G. H., Jaeschke, R. (1996). How to develop and validate a new health-related quality of life instrument. In: *Quality of Life and Pharmacoeconomics in Clinical Trials*, 2nd edn. (B. Spiker, ed.) pp 49–56, Lippincott-Raven.

Kaplan, R. M., Ganiats, T. G., Sieber, W. J., Anderson, J. P. (1998). The Quality of Well-Being Scale: critical similarities and differences with SF–36. *Int. J. Qual. Health Care*, **10**, 509–520.

Kass, J. E., Castriotta, R. J., Malakoff, F. (1992). Intensive care unit outcome in the very elderly. *Crit. Care Med.*, **20**, 1666–1671.

Katz, S., Downs, T. D., Cash, H. R. *et al.* (1970). Progress in development of the index of ADL. *Gerontologist*, **10**, 20–30.

Kind, P., Rosser, R. M., Williams, A. (1982). Valuation of quality of life: some psychometric evidence. In: *The Value of Life and Safety* (M. W. Jones-Lee, ed.) pp 159–170, North Holland Publishing Co.

Konopad, E., Noseworthy, T. W., Johnston, R., Shustack, A., Grace, M. (1995). Quality of life measures before and one year after admission to an intensive care unit. *Crit. Care Med.*, **23**, 1653–1659.

Lawton, M. P. (1969). Assessment of older people: Self-maintaining and instrumental Activities of Daily Living. *Gerontologist*, **9**, 179–186.

Lawton, M. P. (1971). The functional assessment of elderly people. *J. Am. Geriatr. Soc.*, **19**, 465–481.

Le Gall, J. R., Lemeshow, S., Saulnier, F. (1993). A new Simplified Acute Physiology Score (SAPS II) based on a European/North American multicenter study. *JAMA*, **270**, 2957–2963.

Mahul, P. H., Perrot, D., Tempelhoff, G. *et al.* (1991). Short and long-term prognosis, functional outcome following ICU for elderly. *Intensive Care Med.*, **17**, 7–10.

McCusker, J., Stoddard, A. (1984). Use of a surrogate for the Sickness Impact Profile. *Med. Care*, **22**, 789–795.

McDowell, I., Newell, C. (1996). The theoretical and technical foundations of health measurement. In: *Measuring Health: A Guide to Rating Scales and Questionnaires*, 2nd edn. (I. McDowell, C. Newell, eds) pp 10–46, Oxford University Press.

Montuclard, L., Garrouste-Orgeas, M., Timsit, J., Misset, B., De Jonghe, B., Carlet, J. (2000). Outcome, functional autonomy, and quality of life of elderly patients with a long-term intensive care unit stay. *Crit. Care Med.*, **28**, 3389–3395.

Munn, J., Willatts, S. M., Tooley, M. A. (1995). Health and activity after intensive care. *Anaesthesia*, **50**, 1017–1021.

Nease, R. F., Kneeland, T., O'Connor, G. T. *et al.* for the Ischemic Heart Disease Patient Outcomes Research Team. (1995). Variation in patient utilities for outcomes of the management of chronic stable angina. *JAMA*, **273**, 1185–1190.

Niskanen, M., Kari, A., Halonen, P. (1996). Five-year survival after intensive care – comparison of 12 180 patients with the general population. Finnish ICU Study Group. *Crit. Care Med.*, **24**, 1926–1967.

Noseworthy, T. W., Konopad, E., Shustack, A., Johnston, R., Grace, M. (1996). Cost accounting of adult intensive care: Methods and human capital inputs. *Crit. Care Med.*, **24**, 1168–1172.

Nunnally, J. C., Bernstein, I. H. (1994). *Psychometric Theory.* McGraw-Hill.

Ortiz, D., Galguera, F., Jam, M. R., Vilar, S., Castella, X., Artigas, A. (1998). Quality of life and mortality of patients in intensive care. Indices of quality of life. *Enferm. Intensiva*, **9**, 141–150.

Osoba, D. (1995). Measuring the effect of cancer on health-related quality of life. *PharmacoEconomics*, **7**, 308–319.

Patrick, D. L., Danis, M., Southerland, L. I., Hong, G. (1988). Quality of life following intensive care. *J. Gen. Intern. Med.*, **3**, 218–223.

Perrins, J., King, N., Collings, J. (1998). Assessment of long-term psychological well-being following intensive care. *Intensive Crit. Care Nurs.*, **14**, 108–116.

Pettila, V., Kaarlola, A., Makelainen, A. (2000). Health-related quality of life of multiple organ dysfunction patients one year after intensive care. *Intensive Care Med.*, **26**, 1473–1479.

Ridley, S. A. (2000). Quality of life and longer term outcomes. In *Evaluating Critical Care. Using Health Services Research to Improve Quality* (W. J. Sibbald, J. F. Bion, eds) pp 104–118, Springer.

Ridley, S. A., Plenderleith, L. (1994). Survival after intensive care. Comparison with a matched normal population as an indicator of effectiveness. *Anaesthesia*, **49**, 933–935.

Ridley, S. A., Wallace, P. G. M. (1990). Quality of life after intensive care. *Anaesthesia*, **45**, 808–813.

Ridley, S., Biggam, M., Stone, P. (1994). A cost-utility analysis of intensive therapy. *Anaesthesia*, **49**, 192–196.

Ridley, S. A., Chrispin, P. S., Scotton, H., Rogers, J., Lloyd, D. (1997). Changes in quality of life after intensive care: comparison with normal data. *Anaesthesia*, **52**, 195–202.

Rivera Fernandez, R., Sanchez Cruz, J. J., Vazquez Mata, G. (1996). Validation of a quality of life questionnaire for critically ill patients. *Intensive Care Med.*, **22**, 1034–1042.

Rivera Fernandez, R., Vazquez Mata, G., Gonzalez Carmona, A. *et al.* (1991). Description de una encuesta de calidad de vida en medicina intensiva. *Med. Intensiva*, **15**, 313–318.

Rockwood, K., Noseworthy, T. W., Gibney, R. T. N. *et al.* (1993). One-year outcome of elderly and young patients admitted to intensive care units. *Crit. Care Med.*, **21**, 687–691.

Rogers, J., Ridley, S., Chrispin, P., Scotton, H., Lloyd, D. (1997). Reliability of the next of kins' estimates of critically ill patients' quality of life. *Anaesthesia*, **52**, 1137–1143.

Rosenberg, M. (1965). *Society and the Adolescent Self-Image.* Princeton University Press.

Rothman, M. L., Hedrick, S. C., Bulcroft, K. A., Hickam, D. H., Rubenstein, L. Z. (1991). The validity of proxy generated scores as measures of patient health status. *Med. Care*, **29**, 115–124.

Rubins, H. B. (1989). Intensive care and the elderly. *Hospital Practice*, **30**, 9–12.

Rustom, R., Daly, K. (1993). Quality of life after intensive care. *Br. J. Nurs.*, **2**, 316–320.

Sawdon, V., Woods, I., Proctor, M. (1995). Post-intensive care interviews: implications for future practice. *Crit. Care Nurs.*, **11**, 329–332.

Schelling, G., Stoll, C., Haller, M. *et al.* (1998). Health-related quality of life and post-traumatic stress disorder in survivors of acute respiratory distress syndrome. *Crit. Care Med.*, **26**, 651–659.

Schelling, G., Stoll, C., Vogelmeier, C. *et al.* (2000). Pulmonary function and health-related quality of life in a sample of long-term survivors of the acute respiratory distress syndrome. *Intensive Care Med.*, **26**, 1304–1311.

Sheikh, J. I., Yesavage, J. A. (1986). Geriatric Depression Scale (GDS): Recent evidence and development of a shorter version. *Clin. Gerontol.*, **4**, 165–173.

Short, T. G., Buckley, T. A., Rowbottom, M. Y., Wong, E., Oh, T. E. (1999). Long-term outcome and functional health status following intensive care in Hong Kong. *Crit. Care Med.*, **27**, 51–57.

Spitzer, W. O., Dobson, A. J., Hall, J. *et al.* (1981). Measuring the quality of life of cancer patients: A concise Quality of Life Index for use by physicians. *J. Chronic Dis.*, **34**, 585–597.

Streiner, D. L., Norman, G. R. (1989). *Health Measurement Scales. A Practical Guide to their Development and Use.* Oxford University Press.

Suter, P., Armaganidis, A., Beaufils, F. *et al.* (1994). Predicting outcome in ICU patients. *Intensive Care Med.*, **20**, 390–397.

Thiagarajan, J., Taylor, P., Hogbin, E., Ridley, S. (1994). Quality of life after multiple trauma requiring intensive care. *Anaesthesia*, **49**, 211–218.

Tian, Z. M., Reis Miranda, D. (1995). Quality of life after intensive care with the Sickness Impact Profile. *Intensive Care Med.*, **21**, 422–428.

Torrance, G. W. (1986). Measurement of health state utilities for economic appraisal. A review. *J. Health Economics*, **5**, 1–30.

Torrance, G. W., Feeny, D. (1989). Utilities and quality-adjusted life years. *Int. J. Tech. Ass. Health Care*, **5**, 559–575.

Trouillet, J. L., Scheimberg, A., Vuagnat, A., Fagon, J. Y., Chastre, J., Gibert, C. (1996). Long-term outcome and quality of life of patients requiring multidisciplinary intensive care unit admission after cardiac operations. *J. Thorac. Cardiovasc. Surg.*, **112**, 926–934.

Vazquez Mata, G., Rivera Fernandez, R., Gonzalez Carmona, A. *et al.* (1992). Factors related to quality of life 12 months after discharge from an intensive care unit. *Crit. Care Med.*, **20**, 1257–1262.

von Neumann, J., Morgenstern, O. (1944). *Theory of games and economic behaviour.* Princeton University Press.

Ware, J. E. (1993). *SF–36 Health Survey Manual and Interpretation Guide.* The Medical Outcomes Trust.

Weissman, M. M., Sholomskas, D., Pottenger, M., Prusoff, B. A., Locke, B. (1977). Assessing depressive symptoms in five psychiatric populations: a validation study. *Am. J. Epidemiol.*, **106**, 203–214.

Wong, D. T., Gomez, M., McGuire, G. P., Kavanagh, B. (1999). Utilization of intensive care unit days in a Canadian medical-surgical intensive care unit. *Crit. Care Med.*, **27**, 1319–1324.

Zaren, B., Bergstrom, R. (1998). Survival of intensive care patients. I: prognostic factors from the patient's medical history. *Acta Anaesthesiol. Scand.*, **32**, 93–100.

Practical aspects after intensive care

Richard Griffiths and Christina Jones

Introduction

To some, the follow-up of patients after a stay in intensive care is an anathema of how their practice has developed within the walls of an intensive care unit (ICU). Yet for others, it represents the professional maturity of a modern specialty and the completion of the full cycle of care. We are often asked what is the benefit of long-term follow-up care to the ICU and its practice but our principal objective has always been to focus on helping the patients in their recovery. This chapter condenses a number of issues from several authors published in a parallel book *Intensive care after care* (Griffiths and Jones, 2002).

The methods discussed in previous chapters are exercises in population description and outcome, which have resulted in the development of the illness severity measures we routinely use today. Much of the impetus for these developments in the late 1970s and early 1980s was directed towards being able to assess how ill patients were and to relate this to their ICU and hospital survival. This impetus partly resulted from concerns over spiralling costs. Unlike our colleagues in neonatal care who, from the start, have concentrated on the functional outcome of their infant patients, adult intensive care has only tried to examine broad descriptions of patient outcome and to count those who died. The neonatal specialists established elaborate follow-up programmes, but the usual practice following adult intensive care has been for patients to be returned to their referring specialty. This means that their follow-up concentrated on the admitting diagnosis that might not reflect the problems developed as a consequence of being critically ill.

In 1988 in response to a request from the Kings Fund (1989), a collaboration with the University of York (Centre for Health Economics) resulted in the first exploration of the costs and outcome from adult intensive care in terms of mortality and morbidity in the UK (Shiell *et al.*, 1990). Using quality of life measures, this preliminary study identified a significant degree of morbidity across a range of patient types. At 6 months over two-fifths of patients still found that their health restricted their daily activities and one-fifth reported serious disability or distress. It also confirmed the futility of assessing survival at ICU discharge alone. Indeed, many similar questionnaire studies have explored the relationship between pre-morbid health, age, illness severity and length of stay and outcome in terms of broad measures of function. While such studies have a role, their weakness is that the choice of questionnaire used and the questions asked have to be guided by some knowledge of the anticipated problems and consequently may miss new or unexpected problems. It is only through clinical interview and physical examination with critical questioning and analysis that unexpected problems can surface.

The experience of a number of ICU physicians who followed-up patients in routine medical outpatients suggested that ICU patients had particular problems and a prolonged convalescence. So, in 1990, as part of a research programme, a dedicated ICU follow-up clinic was set up at Whiston Hospital in Merseyside, UK. By seeing patients on the wards a few days after discharge from intensive care and in outpatients at 2 months and 6 months, we found a core of both physical and psychological problems that characterized patients recovering from critical illness (Griffiths, 1992). While some of these problems were closely related to particular diagnoses, others, such as profound muscle weakness, were more generic and reflected extremes of critical illness and the pathophysiological challenges of a prolonged intensive care stay.

Recovery is heavily influenced by pre-morbid health status, diagnosis and age as well as the ICU variables and patient perceptions. Furthermore, because of the wide range of patients' case-mix, interpretation of data to inform intensive care locally or help individual patients recover was extremely limited. However, recently, with data drawn from thousands of patients, it is possible to start unravelling some of the confounding variables that influence recovery.

Should ICU staff be involved?

If intensive care is to develop further as a specialty the complete path of critical illness needs to be understood. This is why the responsibility for after intensive care support must in part lie with the ICU doctors and nurses. The specialty needs to understand the outcome of its patients if it is to improve its care within ICU. This process will inevitably identify problems after intensive care that can be solved in partnership with other specialties and the general practitioner. Leaving this responsibility to other specialties that have a variable understanding of intensive care is unrealistic and is unlikely to improve care. In many areas of medicine, the primary pathology leads to disturbance in only one organ system and this is reflected in the development of organ-based specialties. Many such single organ specialists may have limited expertise and experience of other system disorders.

However, intensive care doctors and nurses who have developed the knowledge and skills to deal with multisystem disorders in the most severely ill patients have the expertise to contribute to the multisystem recovery that is required. Understandably, most general practitioners will have little or no knowledge of what transpired in ICU and, with only a few patients who have been in ICU in their practice, they cannot be expected to deal with the likely problems.

Research and development of our technologies and therapies in intensive care need robust measures of survival and morbidity. Outlining the common problems encountered by patients during their recovery and then designing studies that can test interventions to prevent such problems or improve recovery is a way forward. For example, our early experience of follow-up of 292 ICU patients suggested that 87 and 92% of their 5-year mortality occurred at 6 months and 1 year respectively. In addition, most patients had shown good recovery by 6 months suggesting that this would be an appropriate end point to examine the survival effect of a nutritional intervention. This knowledge of outcome provided the framework for a randomized controlled study of glutamine supplementation of parenteral nutrition within ICU with survival and morbidity outcome measured at 6 months (Griffiths *et al.*, 1997). We have recently completed a study examining a self-help rehabilitation package that was able to enhance physical recovery (Griffiths and Jones, 2002).

Is there a demand for intensive care after care?

Society is now developing a new relationship with the medical profession that incorporates full understanding and agreement by the patient. Perhaps the most compelling reason for patients to expect follow-up care after critical illness is for them to discover what was done to them while they were unaware and hence unable to consent to their treatment. Although a few patients may not wish to know what happened as part of a denial strategy, there is a need to rebuild lost autobiographical information (Griffiths *et al.*, 1996). The importance of patient follow-up has been recognized by the Audit Commission's survey of UK critical care services (Audit Commission, 1999). Similarly the UK Government's white paper, Comprehensive Critical Care (Department of Health, 2000), made it clear that all ICUs in England and Wales should be following-up their patients. Our experience suggests it is not only patients but also relatives who request the follow-up because many patients do not remember that they have been in intensive care. With 10 years of experience we can now catalogue many problems of both a physical and psychological nature. However, this alone is not justification unless the identified problems need treatment or the new problems lead to better care within the ICU.

The cost of such a service is frequently put forward as a bar to setting up a follow-up clinic. Yet when compared to the costs of caring for individual ICU patients (approximately £1000–2000 per day and £1000–30 000 per admission), such costs are put into perspective and become less significant (Table 8.1).

Table 8.1 Annual costing for clinic run twice a month (courtesy of Dr Carl Waldmann, Royal Berkshire Hospital, UK)

Nursing G Grade salary for $37\frac{1}{2}$ hours per week. • Time to visit patients on the ward and at home • Two or more clinics per month • Counselling • Teaching and feeding back information to other staff	£18,000
Medical One consultant session per week	£6,000
Administration 10 hours per week • Appointments • Coordinating clinic appointments • Gathering hospital notes	£4,000
Laboratory tests and X-rays • Methicillin-resistant *Staph. aureus* screening • Magnetic resonance imaging • Blood tests • Pulmonary function tests	£2,000
Total	£30,000

Problems on discharge to the ward

Although patients discharged from the ICU to the general ward can breathe unaided, they may still have several active physical problems. Although not serious enough to keep the patient in the ICU, if left untreated, they could lead to re-admission. This is a particular problem if a patient has returned to the care of a specialty for further management (e.g. orthopaedic surgery for a multiple trauma victim) when the dominant medical problems are recovering respiratory and renal function. Ideally the decision to discharge a patient from intensive care should be taken when it is clear that the patient is ready. In the UK the number of intensive care beds is limited and hence ICUs are often under pressure to discharge patients prematurely to allow admission of a more critically ill patient. However, 9–16% of discharges may require re-admission to intensive care (Rubins and Moskowitz, 1988; Goldhill and Sumner, 1998).

Once they are transferred to the general ward, patients may require input from the critical care team. Educating ward staff about the unique needs of patients after prolonged and debilitating illness may encourage patience and forbearance as the patient painstakingly struggles to full recovery. It may also be possible, because of familiarity with these patients, to help forestall re-admission through earlier recognition of re-emergence of old problems. Whether this service is provided by experienced ICU nurses or doctors will depend on local circumstances.

Table 8.2 lists the physical problems reported by patients after critical illness. Breathlessness, sexual dysfunction, poor sleep and taste changes are common. Skeletal muscle weakness and fatigue, predominantly due to muscle wasting will be present in nearly all patients and is more marked the longer the ICU stay (Jones and Griffiths, 2000). The incidence of other problems is difficult to cite. Our own observations suggest that tracheal stenosis identified at 6 months is relatively rare, at about 3%, and tends not to occur in tracheostomized patients, yet develops in patients who are intubated more than twice (Jones *et al.*, 1997). Joint pain and stiffness is more common and at 8 weeks 12% of 148 patients complained of shoulder problems (Jones and Griffiths, 2000). Significant numbness and paraesthesia of limbs seems to be less common in recent years, although minor abnormalities can be found on close inspection or questioning.

The necessity for a prolonged period of convalescence after a serious illness, particularly in the days before antibiotics, has long been known. Florence

Table 8.2 Examples of physical disorders occurring after critical illness

---

Recovering organ failure (e.g. lung, kidney, liver, etc.)
Muscle wasting and weakness
  • Reduced cough power
  • Pharyngeal weakness

Joint pain and stiffness (particularly the shoulders)

Numbness, paraesthesia (peripheral neuropathy)

Taste changes resulting in favourite foods being unpalatable

Itching, dry skin

Disturbances of sleep rhythm and pattern
  • Waking at night, poor sleep, not rested
  • Muscle aches and stiffness during day

Cardiac and circulatory decompensation
  • postural hypotension (autonomic neuropathy)
  • heart failure

Reduced pulmonary reserve
  • breathlessness on mild exertion
  • increased work of breathing

Disturbed sexual function

Iatrogenic
  • Tracheal stenosis (e.g. repeated intubations)
  • Nerve palsies (needle injuries)
  • Scarring (needle and drain sites)

Nightingale (1859) understood clearly the kind of physical weakness left by such illness and the strain it puts upon a patient during their recovery:

> *Do not meet or overtake a patient who is moving about in order to speak to him, or to give him any message or letter. You might just as well give him a box on the ear. . . . You do not know the effort it is to a patient to remain standing for even a quarter of a minute to listen to you.*

Severe sepsis results in catabolism of protein reserves in skeletal muscle. The loss of muscle mass sustained during critical illness is both large and rapid, about 2% per day of the illness (Helliwell *et al.*, 1998). This is due to a combination of primary muscle catabolism and atrophy secondary to neuropathic degeneration. This can mean that an elderly patient may lose half his or her remaining muscle mass resulting in severe physical disability. Rebuilding such muscle loss can take more than a year. Initially, while on the general ward, patients may be so weak that they struggle to feed themselves; their cough is greatly reduced and they may have poor control of their swallowing and upper airway. If these patients can stand, they are prone to falls because of autonomic disturbances leading to postural hypotension. Many patients report taste changes and complain that the nutritional supplements available on the wards taste too sweet. Favourite foods may seem unappetizing. Coupled with their difficulty in eating properly, this may further compromise their nutritional state. Body mass is a poor indicator of muscle wasting since many ICU patients are salt and water overloaded and will lose weight when they first return to the wards as they start to recover and undergo a diuresis.

When patients leave ICU, they may appear to be completely orientated and to understand what information they are given about their illness. Yet when asked on the ward a few days later, a high proportion of patients have little or no memory of their stay in the ICU (Jones *et al.*, 1994) remembering only pain, suctioning, or lack of sleep. A recent review discusses the theories behind the possible cognitive deficits following a stay in intensive care but firm research evidence is currently lacking (Jones *et al.*, 2000). For some patients, memories of intensive care are nightmares, often of a persecutory nature involving torture or paranoid delusions (Brooks *et al.*, 1995). These nightmares and delusions can be partially attributed to their illness process, opiates and other sedative drugs and the unnatural environment of the ICU with its lack of a proper day and night and constant noise (Jones *et al.*, 2000).

Some patients have difficulty accepting that the nightmares and hallucinations were not real. In addition, patients are reticent about telling the ward staff about the nightmares in case they are considered mad. Recognition of such problems through discussion allows patients to build a coherent story rather than chaotic, intrusive memories and so put the experience behind them (Harber and Pennebacker, 1992). There seems to be a high incidence of post-traumatic stress disorder (PTSD) following ICU (Koshy *et al.*, 1997; Schelling *et al.*, 1998). PTSD is characterized by a range of symptoms such as re-experiencing the event (i.e. flashbacks), avoidance of situations that remind one of the event, a numbed reaction and symptoms of increased arousal, such as sleeplessness. Recent work suggests that it is those patients who have no recall of events or vivid distorted memories who are more likely to suffer PTSD-related symptoms than those who have some real recall of intensive care (Jones *et al.*, 2001).

Without memory of their illness, delusions can appear real and subsequent events, such as their dramatically changed appearance can be frightening if there is no explanation. In addition, the lack of recall of ICU makes it hard for the patient to understand why they feel so awful (Griffiths *et al.*, 1996). Keeping an ICU diary (Bäckman and Walter, 2001) is an innovative way of conveying to patients exactly what has happened during their time on ICU. Working together, staff and relatives build a record in colour photographs and hand-written text of the important daily events and milestones during a patient's stay. Patients and relatives have positively received this innovation. Photographs of the patient at various stages of their ICU illness is concrete proof that the diary is factually correct. It also relieves the family of repeatedly reliving their own trauma about events in ICU. However, formal studies of whether the diary allows patients to fill the memory gaps and provide a context to explain the frightening memories are required. Information written by the patients' family as well as ICU staff may help patients overcome their delusional memories and, in turn, lower the risk of developing PTSD and other psychological problems.

Discharge home

Occasionally only on return home do patients first realize how debilitated they have become. Commonly, climbing stairs is beyond their physical capacity and they are forced to use their hands and knees. Relatives take on the care of the patients. For example, they report sleeplessness and anxiety about whether the patient is still breathing! Relatives frequently complain that patients are very hard to live with because of irritability and impatience with the slowness of their recovery.

The family may tell the patient what has happened in ICU but for the relatives their own memories of ICU can be sufficiently disturbing that they find this difficult. Without memories, patients fail to understand how ill they have been and how long it will take them to recover. Consequently, patients may have unrealistic expectations of recovery and think in terms of weeks instead of months or years (Griffiths *et al.*, 1996). The most important predictors of impaired outdoor mobility are the length of ICU stay and hours of ventilation. Age, APACHE II score and pre-morbid health appear less important (Jones and Griffiths, 2000).

Except for the very elderly, some trauma victims and patients with neurological problems, the majority of intensive care patients will not receive physiotherapy once they are able to walk unaided in hospital. However, due to muscle loss and peripheral neuropathies their balance may be compromised and their ability to right themselves can be poor. Walking unaided outside in icy conditions or in a wind is potentially dangerous and frightening for the patient. In addition, minor physical problems like hair loss, skin dryness, or fingernail ridges, that frequently occur following critical illness, can be particularly distressing to patients, often simply because of the lack of an adequate explanation.

Two months to one year

Physical problems related to muscle weakness are still common at 2 months after intensive care and can still be seen 6 months later. Of 148 patients attending their 2-month outpatient appointment at Whiston Hospital, 44% either could not manage stairs or had difficulty climbing more than a few steps at a time; 29% were still using a wheelchair outside the house (Jones and Griffith, 2000). These problems often affect other activities such as getting out of the bath, turning off taps, driving a car and returning to work. Fear of falling and being unable to get up again is common. This prolonged recovery period leads to a number of other problems such as depression and anxiety in about 20–30% of patients (Table 8.3). PTSD may develop in 15–25% of patients but recurrent nightmares are rarer.

Table 8.3 Examples of psychological disorders occurring after critical illness

---

Depression
- Anger and conflict with the family
- Anger with themselves

Anxiety
- Are they going to get back to normal?
- Panic attacks
- Fear of dying
- Agoraphobia

Post traumatic stress disorder

Guilt

Recurrent nightmares

Patients often avoid company and show less affection to their partners. Coupled to this social isolation is a dependence on others to make decisions and a tendency towards being obstinate. Some also report feeling overwhelmed in crowded places, or being afraid to go out alone, with some patients describing panic attacks in these situations, although not necessarily recognizing them as such. These can occur at night; their sleep is disturbed leaving them feeling physically tired during the day with associated aches and stiffness. The longer this situation continues uncorrected, the more refractory these panic attacks are likely to become. Long-term treatment is needed by 36–40% of panic attack sufferers presenting for help (Keller and Hanks, 1993). An example of therapy would be a gradual desensitization to the precipitating cause or situation if known; patients are taught to cope with the physiological effects of panic under controlled conditions. Patients understandably feel that the recovery phase of their critical illness is the most stressful period as they try to come to terms with how ill and close to death they have been (Compton, 1991).

Social isolation and conflict between couples is common following critical illness. In one study, 45% of patients questioned at 6 months reported going out less often, 41% taking part in fewer social activities, with a quarter reporting being irritable with their relative (Jones et al., 1994). It is now established that the presence of social support, in the form of someone to confide in and to supply physical and psychological support increases tolerance to stressful situations and has a beneficial effect on health. Social isolation appears to act as a source of chronic stress. It has been suggested that much of the impact caused by life events is due to the profound changes produced in social relationships.

Rehabilitation following critical illness

With this combination of physical and psychological problems, early intervention to reduce their consequences and aid recovery is needed. This should start as the patients move to the general ward. Physical activity is a key to recovery, but the overwhelming weakness that patients report as they start to recover and the length of convalescence requires considerable determination on their part to exercise. Most patients have little idea how and when to start exercising or how to pace themselves. Simply giving intensive care patients a discharge booklet outlining possible problems they might encounter during their recovery has proved unsuccessful (Jones and O'Donnell, 1994). Despite using this booklet 25% of patients attending an ICU follow-up clinic scored highly for anxiety and depression at 2 months after intensive care. The information in the booklet should be regarded as the initial part of a rehabilitation package. Integrated physical and psychological care is ideal, in partnership with the general practitioner, ICU and other hospital doctors. Clear information about the patient's illness needs to be provided to the patient, their family and their general practitioner. Patients need to be given estimates of recovery times. Both the patients and their families need the opportunity to talk about the illness and the time in the ICU, preferably with staff who were involved in their care. Such discussions should tackle not only what brought the patient into ICU and the events while they were there, but also any distorted memories. For those patients still distressed by these memories, particularly those too upset to talk about them, other methods can be tried. Current recommendations suggest that patients who continue to experience high levels of PTSD symptoms at 1–3 months after ICU discharge should be actively treated because of the high risk of developing chronic PTSD (Foa et al., 1999). Under these circumstances, it is also much more likely that associated disorders such as substance abuse, depression, panic disorders and generalized anxiety disorder will be present. Alcohol is frequently used as self-medication by PTSD sufferers, but this can progress into alcohol dependence (Warsaw *et al.*, 1993). Opiate and benzodiazepine dependence are also reported in disaster victims, particularly if they sustained severe injuries (Sturgeon, 1993). For this reason monitoring symptoms of PTSD and offering therapies, such as exposure therapy, anxiety management and psychoeducation about the normality of PTSD symptoms to those at high risk of PTSD is now thought to be the most effective first line psychological intervention (Foa *et al.*, 1999). Returning to normal allows the patient to understand that their agitation, hypervigilance and sleeplessness are all part of the symptoms of an acute stress reaction so making them less frightening. The next step in the healing process involves reworking the story of the traumatic event. The memory is transformed using exposure therapy to reduce the sense of insecurity experienced by the patient.

It is helpful to outline a plan with the patient and their family for their convalescence and rehabilitation. There should be referral to other specialties including clinical psychologists and dieticians as required. Preliminary results suggest a structured programme of rehabilitation could aid recovery. Improvements in physical recovery can be demonstrated but the effect of delusional memories confounds psychological recovery.

Intensive care outpatient clinic

Without a better picture of the problems and consequences that these patients suffer it is hard to place a value on support after ICU. Initial general ward care may prevent problems and reduce re-admissions to intensive care. In the outpatient clinic, most of the benefits are patient specific and are related to the identification of evolving pathology or problems relating to treatment. A common issue is the continued inappropriate use of a drug first started in intensive care. Amiodarone use is a good example and is a particular problem in the elderly where bradycardia can be symptomatic.

Lessons gained from a follow-up programme have important consequences. For example, a clinical follow-up of tracheal stenosis showed that it was associated with multiple repeated intubations (Jones *et al.*, 1997). This promoted the move to earlier tracheostomy when intubation had occurred more than once. Skin tethering at the tracheostomy scar is appearing with the introduction of percutaneous methods. In a few patients this results in distressing chest sensations with swallowing and has required surgery for correction. The use of starch products is associated with severe itching lasting for some months (Sharland *et al.*, 1999). This itching can be generalized or localized to the arms and legs. The symptoms can be distressing requiring specialist dermatological therapy for up to 6 months. The advent of nursing the patient prone has raised new pressure-related problems, such as neuropraxias, the consequence of which may only become evident in follow-up.

One of the least recognized benefits of ICU follow-up is the educational and outcome feedback that is directly personal and easily understood by all the staff. For staff, intensive care can at times be oppressively grim. The highlight for many staff is to have a visit from a former patient well on the way to recovery. The patient also finds this supportive. It helps confirm their recall and allows them the chance to thank the staff involved in their care at a time when they were extremely vulnerable.

Conclusion

The recognition of problems, some possibly unique, following intensive care is creating a demand for a more integrated and thorough approach to the care of patients after intensive care. We are only starting to understand the links between what we do in ICU and the effect on patients' physical and psychological recovery. Although large follow-up studies with questionnaires have had a role to play, it is clinical interviews with patients and their relatives that have allowed the recognition of unanticipated problems. To complete the cycle of care the intensive care professional must have some involvement in the recovery of patients to inform, advise, treat and support.

References

Audit Commission. (1999). *Critical to Success. The place of efficient and effective critical care services within the acute hospital.* Audit Commission Publications.

Bäckman, C. G., Walther, S. M. (2001). Use of a personal diary written on the ICU during critical illness. *Intensive Care Med.*, **27**, 426–429.

Brooks, R., Bauman, A., Daffurn, K., Hillman, K. (1995). Post-hospital outcome following intensive care. *Clin. Intensive Care,* **6**, 127–135.

Compton, P. (1991). Critical Illness and Intensive Care: What it means to the Client. *Crit. Care Nurse,* **11**, 50–56.

Department of Health. (2000). *Comprehensive Critical Care. A review of adult critical care services.* Department of Health.

Foa, E. B., Davidson, J. R. T., Frances, A. (1999). The expert consensus guideline series: Treatment of post traumatic stress disorder. *J. Clin. Psychiatr.*, **60**, S16.

Goldhill, D. R., Sumner, A. (1998). Outcome of intensive care patients in a group of British intensive care units. *Crit. Care Med.,* **26**, 1337–1345.

Griffiths, R. D. (1992). Development of normal indices of recovery from critical illness. In *Intensive Care Britain* (M. J. Rennie, ed.) pp 134–137, Greycoat Publishing.

Griffiths, R., Jones, C. (2002). *Intensive Care After Care.* Butterworth-Heinemann.

Griffiths, R. D., Jones, C., Macmillan, R. R. (1996). Where is the harm in not knowing? Care after intensive care. *Clin. Intensive Care,* **7**, 144–145.

Griffiths, R. D., Jones, C., Palmer, T. E. A. (1997). Six month outcome of critically-ill patients given glutamine supplemented parenteral nutrition. *Nutrition,* **13**, 295–302.

Harber, K. D., Pennebaker, J. W. (1992). Overcoming traumatic memories. In: *The Handbook of Emotion and Memory* (S.-A. Christianson, ed.) pp 359–87, Lawrence Erlbaum Associates.

Helliwell, T. R., Wilkinson, A., Griffiths, R. D., McClelland, P., Palmer, T. E. A., Bone, M. J. (1998). Muscle fibre atrophy in patients with multiple organ failure is associated with the loss of myosin filaments and the presence of lysosomal enzymes and ubiquitin. *Neuropathol. Appl. Neurobiol.,* **24,** 507–517.

Jones, C., Griffiths, R. D. (2000). Identifying post intensive care patients who may need physical rehabilitation. *Clin. Intensive Care,* **11,** 35–38.

Jones, C., O'Donnell, C. (1994). After Intensive Care, what then? *Intensive Crit. Care Nurse,* **10,** 89–92.

Jones, C., Griffiths, R. D., Humphris, G. (2000). Disturbed memory and amnesia related to intensive care. *Memory,* **8,** 79–94.

Jones, C., Griffiths, R. D., Humphris, G. (2001). Acute Post Traumatic Stress Disorder: a new theory for its development after intensive care. *Crit. Care Med.,* **29,** 573–580.

Jones, C., Griffiths, R. D., Macmillan, R. R., Palmer, T. E. A. (1994). Psychological problems occurring after intensive care. *Br. J. Intensive Care,* **4,** 46–53.

Jones, C., Macmillan, R. R., Harris, C., Griffiths, R. D. (1997). Severe tracheal stenosis associated with reintubations. *Clin. Intensive Care,* **8,** 122–125.

Keller, M. B., Hanks, D. L. (1993). Course and outcome in panic disorder. *Prog. Neuropsychopharmacol. Biol. Psychiatry,* **17,** 551–570.

Kings Fund Panel (1989). Intensive care in the United Kingdom. *Anaesthesia,* **44,** 428–431.

Koshy, G., Wilkinson, A., Harmsworth, A., Waldmann, C. S. (1997). Intensive care unit follow-up program at a district general hospital. *Intensive Care Med.,* **23,** S160.

Nightingale F. (1859). *Notes on nursing: what it is, and what it is not.* Harrison and Sons.

Rubins, H. B., Moskowitz, M. A. (1988). Discharge decision making in a medical intensive care unit. *Am. J. Med.,* **84,** 863–869.

Schelling, G., Stoll, C., Meier, M. *et al.* (1998). Health-related quality of life and post-traumatic stress disorder in survivors of acute respiratory distress syndrome. *Crit Care Med.,* **26,** 651–659.

Sharland, C., Huggett, A., Nielsen, M. (1999). Persistent pruritus after hydroxyethyl starch (HES) infusions in critically ill patients. *Crit. Care,* **3,** S150.

Shiell, A. M., Griffiths, R. D., Short, A. I. K., Spiby, J. (1990). An evaluation of the costs and outcome of adult intensive care in two units in the UK. *Clin. Intensive Care,* **1,** 256–262.

Sturgeon, D. (1993). Post Traumatic Stress Disorder. In: *Stress – from synapse to syndrome* (S. C. Stanford, P. Salmon, eds) pp 421–31, Academic Press.

Warsaw, M. G., Fierman, E., Pratt, L. *et al.* (1993). Quality of life and dissociation in anxiety disorder patients with histories of trauma or PTSD. *Am. J. Psychiatr.,* **150,** 1512–1516.

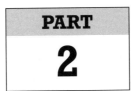

PART

2

Healthcare workers' perspective

Chapter

9

Complications and adverse events

Dinis Reis Miranda

'Complications' and 'adverse events' are terms commonly used to describe unfavourable changes in the course of illness; they may or may not be expected. However, these terms may be interpreted differently; for example, *complication* can be used to describe a combination, complexity, aggravation, difficulty, drawback, problem, obstacle or snag, etc. Similarly, *adverse* may be interpreted as antagonistic, conflicting, detrimental, hostile, inopportune, negative, unfavourable or unlucky, etc.

In medicine, the term complication is usually applied to a newly diagnosed secondary condition that slows or prevents the clinical recovery of a patient. For example, nosocomial pneumonia in a critically ill trauma victim may be listed as a complication. Pneumonia in this case is an additional obstacle in a potentially uneventful recovery. On the other hand, pneumonia could also be viewed as a barrier to future essential therapeutic measures such as weaning from mechanical ventilation. Thus, a 'complication' may vary in its significance on the intensive care unit (ICU).

The term adverse event is more commonly applied to an unexpected additional illness or other ill health that is a direct consequence of a therapeutic intervention. It is the therapeutic intervention that is classified as the adverse event and the resulting ill health as a complication. For example, if pneumonia is caused by contaminated equipment such as a bronchoscope or ventilator tubing, pneumonia is the complication and cross-infection is the adverse event.

Assessment of care

Outcome can be qualified as the final degree of derangement (functional, physiological, etc.), after one or more courses of care are applied. In the last 20 years, the science of predicting the outcome of critically ill patients has been and continues to be developed (Knaus *et al.*, 1991). However, the prediction models were all directed at estimating survival or death at discharge from the hospital. Comparisons of predicted risk versus observed outcome have been used to evaluate care throughout the hospital stay including the ICU admission. Unfortunately, hospital survival or death is too remote for evaluation of critical care services. While final outcomes measured at hospital discharge are useful for administrative and/or global comparative purposes, they are not suitable for understanding (and improving) the effectiveness of critical care. Measuring the incidence of complications and adverse events may be a more valid reflection of ICU care.

The return of 'health', or the adequate functioning of all organs and systems, results from the appropriate and timely correction of any functional or physiological derangement (Figure 9.1).

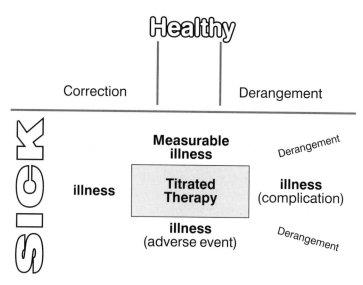

Figure 9.1 Titrated therapy

All physiological variables oscillate within a range of normality. In health when these values deviate from normality, they are usually 'automatically' corrected by homeostatic mechanisms. The difference between health and illness may therefore depend upon the appropriate and timely correction of physiological derangement. If the corrective care is insufficient to correct the derangement, measurable illness ensues. At this stage, external organ support is often required to preserve the internal milieu. For this reason 80% of ICU activity is directed towards clinical evaluation and supportive correction of physiological derangement (e.g. correcting hypokalaemia, instituting mechanical ventilation, providing parenteral nutrition). This continuous bedside cycle of observation, registration, comparison, decision making, action and observation is called the cycle of 'titrated' therapy. Complications and adverse events may be regarded as the result of additional physiological derangement. If the derangement is successfully corrected, further complications and adverse events may not appear.

Complications in the ICU

Complications are not frequently reported on ICU. This may relate to the very nature of critical illness and the difficulty in distinguishing between a complication recognized as part of the disease or as a consequence of an adverse event. Complications on ICU are not always well described in textbooks of intensive care medicine. When they are included, they are listed in separate chapters in the classical organ system fashion (Pingleton and Hall, 1992; Arroliga, 1999). Complications are often presented as a newly diagnosed illness as if appearing unexpectedly in the course of the primary critical illness. In these cases, the most frequent or life-threatening complications are included in the description of that illness. Unfortunately, the same complication can be listed among the complications of different critical conditions, implying that complications are independent clinical entities.

The timing of presentation of a complication is important for its correct recognition and classification. By definition, a complication is a secondary illness (or condition) emerging during the course of a primary illness. For example, sepsis can be listed as a complication of pneumonia. However, on occasions, the sequence of events can be reversed, as pneumonia can complicate sepsis originating outside the respiratory tract.

The clinical relevance is also an important element in the definition of complications. For example, pulmonary aspergillosis after near-drowning in a ditch, or sepsis with anaerobic beta-haemolytic streptococci after a small finger wound acquired while fishing are serious potentially life-threatening diseases and should be considered the primary illnesses. Trauma (near-drowning and finger wound) is the causal vector or factor. Possible subsequent clinical events, such as acute respiratory distress syndrome (ARDS) and bronchopleural fistulae should be listed as complications of the infectious diseases and not as complications of trauma.

The most frequently listed complications in the intensive care unit are briefly summarized below. It is important to emphasize that the lists in the following subsections are by no means comprehensive.

Cardiovascular complications

Cardiovascular complications – pulmonary emboli; ischaemia; occult hypoperfusion; arrhythmias (whether or not drug induced); complications following therapeutic interventions such as cardiopulmonary bypass, pulmonary artery catheterization, intra-aortic balloon pump, cardioversion and defibrillation, transoesophageal echocardiography and pericardiocentesis.

It is important to note that many of the complications are not necessarily caused by improperly performed therapeutic interventions and hence not consequences of adverse events. Such complications represent an inherent risk associated with effective and appropriate therapies or procedures. For example, this is the case in complications associated with the use of cardiopulmonary bypass (Quinlan *et al.*, 2000). It was recently shown that coronary artery grafting, performed without cardiopulmonary bypass, had a lower incidence of complications, such as atrial fibrillation and low output syndrome (Boyd *et al.*, 1999; Iacó *et al.*, 1999). However, for certain cardiac surgical procedures bypass is an essential manoeuvre without which surgery could not be contemplated.

Pulmonary complications

Pulmonary complications – arterial oxygen desaturation, hypoventilation; ARDS; pneumonia; atelectasis and collapse; fibrosis; complications following therapeutic interventions such as airway management and mechanical ventilation, introduction of catheters, barotrauma, pneumothorax, bronchopleural fistula, pleural effusion, haemothorax, chylothorax, empyema (Strange, 1999).

Of those listed, ARDS (Ware and Matthay, 2000) can be a lethal pulmonary complication in ICU. Infection is often associated with ARDS either as a precipitating cause or as a complication. The causal relation of ARDS to therapeutic interventions is well established. For example, cardiopulmonary bypass is a documented risk factor for developing ARDS (Quinlan *et al.*, 2000). The incidence of ARDS is also associated with the general condition of the patient. For example, the severity of metabolic acidosis after trauma is a predictor of ARDS and other complications (Eberhard *et al.*, 2000). Similarly, occult hypoperfusion is associated with infection after trauma (Claridge *et al.*, 2000) and can be anticipated when there is an increase in serum lactate (Blow *et al.*, 2000). The increase in serum lactate may be the first symptom in a chain of events leading to ARDS.

Digestive tract complications

Digestive tract complications – mesenteric ischaemia; intra-abdominal hypertension; abdominal compartment syndrome; haemorrhage; intra-abdominal sepsis; acute pancreatitis; liver failure; altered motility (Lidios *et al.*, 1999).

Gastrointestinal complications are common in critical illness (Afessa and Kubilis, 2000). Liver failure is perhaps the most frequent exception. Liver failure, developing after ICU admission, is almost invariably related to the patient's severity of illness. Conditions such as shock, multiple organ failure or sepsis often precede a variable degree of liver insufficiency (Shakil *et al.*, 2000). As the primary metabolizing organ where biotransformation of drugs takes place, the liver is sensitive to the toxic effect of drugs, particularly isoniazid, alpha-methyldopa, oestrogens, antibiotics (e.g. tetracycline, erythromycin) and chlorpromazine (Albertson *et al.*, 1992).

Renal complications

Renal complications – acute renal failure; complications associated with therapeutic interventions, such as dialysis (Briglia and Paganini, 1999), technique related (e.g. haemorrhage, electrolyte disturbances), circuit related (e.g. disconnection, air embolism), access related (e.g. embolism, infection, arterial occlusion).

Acute tubular necrosis is the most frequent cause of renal failure on ICU and if the patient had pre-morbid normal renal function, the chances of them requiring long-term renal replacement therapy is very low (<3%) (Noble *et al.*, 2001). However, acute tubular necrosis may represent the natural progression of the disease or could be considered an adverse event because of failure by the ICU staff to maintain satisfactory renal perfusion pressures. Acute renal failure is a very important complication because it adversely affects ICU and hospital mortality.

Neurological complications

Neurological complications – psychosis; stupor and coma; metabolic encephalopathy (following sepsis and/or organ failure); ischaemia or anoxic induced encephalopathy; seizures; stroke; complications related to therapeutic interventions such as lumbar punctures and intracerebral catheters.

Besides those originating from primary neurological pathology, the neurological complications are usually a consequence of serious physiological derangement in another organ system. Among them, psychosis in relation to intensive care deserves a special mention. Often designated as 'ICU psychosis', this term covers all symptoms of unclear psychological derangement appearing during or after intensive care admission. These symptoms may range from mild and temporary (Pirraglia *et al.*, 1999; Jones *et al.*, 2000) to very severe (Richman, 2000). Unfortunately, little is known about psychological derangement during and after intensive care (McGuire *et al.*, 2000). Metabolic derangements caused by physiological derangement in another organ system may precipitate a neurological deficit (Pirraglia *et al.*, 1999; Perlman, 1999). There is also substantial evidence indicating that the ICU environment (noise, constant light, loss of day-night rhythm) affects the sleep pattern of patients (Gelling, 1999); the magnitude and duration of sleep disturbances may be the start of psychological illness after ICU admission.

Severe neuromuscular disturbances have been observed after the continuous use of muscle relaxing drugs (Hund, 1999; Aranda and Hanson, 2000). Pancuronium entered clinical practice in the ICU in the 1980s. These new drugs allowed easy and controllable paralysis. The continuous infusion of muscle relaxants for periods up to several weeks became usual practice. More recently, reports of muscular weakness and/or prolonged muscular paralysis after the use of muscle relaxants have appeared frequently in the literature (Walting and Dasta, 1994). Attributing these complications to the use of muscle relaxants remains controversial, as myopathy and neuropathy are common complications of several clinical conditions (e.g. sepsis and multiple organ failure) where muscle relaxation is not used (Latronico et al., 1996).

Endocrine complications

Endocrine complications – adrenal insufficiency; calcium disorders; thyroid dysfunction; disorders of glucose metabolism (Martinez and Lash, 1999).

As with neurological complications, most endocrine complications are secondary to a serious physiological derangement in another organ system. It is important to note that these complications often trigger other organ dysfunction. For example, disordered glucose metabolism increases the risk of renal failure (Weisberg et al., 1999) and infection (Morricone et al., 1999).

Skin complications

Skin complications – pressure ulcers are by far the most frequent skin-related complication in ICU. Occasionally they occur within 24 h of admission to ICU (Allman et al., 1999; Peerless et al., 1999). The clinical relevance of pressure ulcers is important as they are quite often associated with severe life-threatening disease. Pressure ulcers may become the 'primary illness' in some patients, particularly when large and infected with multiresistant pathogenic bacteria.

Infective complications

Infective complications – infection is perhaps the single most frequent complication in the ICU. Several factors predispose the occurrence of infections (Wallace et al., 2000) of which nosocomial pneumonia is the most frequent (Georges et al., 2000). The extensive use of antibiotics in the ICU can play an important role in promoting the development of nosocomial infections (Weber et al., 1999). However, changes in the epidemiology of infections (Rangel-Frausto et al., 1999; Bowton, 1999) or changes in the population of patients admitted (Afessa and Gree, 2000) should be closely monitored. Several studies indicate that the use of specific protocols and guidelines reduces the incidence of nosocomial infections in the ICU (Price et al., 1999). The systemic inflammatory response syndrome (SIRS) is a clinical entity which may represent a non-infectious 'septic condition' (Brun-Buisson, 2000).

Drug interactions

Drug interactions – every patient in the ICU receives many drugs. The usual daily number is around five but many exceed ten. These drugs are usually administered as intravenous boluses or infusions. The use of other routes of administration (e.g. oral, subcutaneous, intramuscular) decreases with the severity of the clinical condition of the patients because of altered bioavailability. The drugs most commonly administered fall into three categories (Romac and Albertson, 1999):

1. support functioning of vital organs and systems (e.g. vasoactive, bronchodilation, diuretic drugs)
2. anti-infection drugs (e.g. antibiotics)
3. drugs for reducing pain and distress (e.g. sedatives, analgesics).

Drug interaction is common on ICU and may involve the following mechanisms:

1. absorption alterations – related to the dysfunction of the digestive tract. This is one of the reasons why this route of administration is seldom used in the ICU
2. distribution alterations – drugs can compete for transport sites in the serum, depending on pH and plasma albumin level
3. metabolism alterations – the enzymatic biotransformation (oxidation, reduction, hydrolysis) of the majority of the drugs occurs in the liver. Competition between drugs for these processes may exist, resulting in prolonged drug half-life (with ensuing drug accumulation), or in active intermediate metabolites (with toxic or other unexpected properties)
4. excretion changes – particularly in the presence of reduced kidney function.

Clinicians are quite often not aware of the existence of drug interactions. Yet, this is one of the more frequent causes of adverse events in the ICU (see below). The avoidance and the control of drug interactions should therefore be part of daily clinical ICU practice.

Studies on adverse events

It is important to identify adverse events on ICU. Detailed study of adverse events enhances insight to the processes of illness while, at the same time, improving the processes of care. Also, by monitoring the incidence and nature of such events it is possible to ensure that professional standards are maintained. The number of adverse events is also an indirect measure of clinical competence.

Unfortunately, despite their importance, adverse events have only recently been studied on ICU.

The Harvard Medical Practice study

This retrospective study analysed the incidence of adverse events in hospitals in New York State; 30 121 hospital records were randomly selected for analysis. Adverse events were defined as injury caused by medical management that prolonged hospital stay and/or disability. The research was performed by a team of medical records analysts, assisted by two physicians specially trained for the study (Brennan *et al.*, 1991).

About 1300 adverse events were identified (in 3.7% of the hospital admissions). Of these, 56.8% caused minor impairment, 16.5% caused important disability and 6.5% caused permanent disability; 13.6% of the adverse events were connected with the patient's death. The incidence of adverse events appeared to be significantly and positively associated with the age of the patients: 27% of the patients were older than 64 years of age but accounted for 43% of all adverse events recorded. In all categories, patients older than 45 years had two to three times more adverse events than patients below this age. After stratifying the patients into four categories with increasing risk of dying using the Diagnosis Related Groups classification, there was a clear and significant increase in the incidence of adverse events: from 1.82% in category one (low risk), up to 7.13% in category four (higher risk of dying). The results of the study suggest that the incidence of adverse events is strongly associated with the severity of illness of the patients. Although 27.6% of the overall adverse events were caused by negligence, negligence was not associated with increasing severity of illness but rather ICU workload.

Forty-eight percent of the adverse events were related to a surgical procedure (e.g. wound infection, technical complication or surgical failure). The non-operative adverse events (52.3%) encompassed more varied causes (e.g. drug related, diagnostic or therapeutic mishaps, fall) (Leape *et al.*, 1991). As could be expected, most adverse events occurred in the operating theatre (41%) and the ward (26.5%), where most hospital activities take place. Only 2.7% of the adverse events occurred in the ICU.

More than 70% of errors were related to human factors, such as inadequate preparation of patient before procedure, avoidable delay of treatment, failure to use indicated tests or to act on their results, error in drug dose or method of use. The type of error could not be identified in about 20% of the adverse events. Only a small portion of the adverse events were related to the systems in use or clinical environment (e.g. defective equipment, inadequate monitoring system, inadequate staffing). Because of the high percentage of human errors involved, one of the authors concluded 'that more or less all adverse events could have been avoided' (Leape *et al.*, 1991).

The incidence of adverse events in relation to the severity of illness and human factors should be stressed. The direct relation between workload and adverse events suggests analysis and control of the processes of ICU care may be important.

The AIMS-ICU study

The Australian Incident Monitoring Study was a national study developed by the Australian and New Zealand Intensive Care Society (ANZICS), together with the Australian Patient Safety Foundation. The aim of this study was the development of a national incident report system 'to improve quality of care in the intensive care units by accumulating experience of incidents that may affect patient safety'.

An 'incident' was defined as 'any unintended event or outcome which could have, or did, reduce the safety margin for the patient'.

After the preliminary development of the recording system, and the performance of a pilot study for testing its feasibility in three ICUs (Beckmann *et al.*, 1996a), the final reporting form was tested in seven ICUs (Beckmann *et al.*, 1996b). The reporting form included: patient demographic details, data on severity of illness and major therapeutic interventions, patient outcome in relation to the reported incident, a detailed description of the incident and the possible factors involved. The incident was described in a 'narrative fashion' by whom it was detected. Information concerning the place where the incident occurred (e.g. ICU, in/outside the hospital), the time elapsed before detection and how it was detected (routine or incidental check), and the method of detection (e.g. visual, monitoring) was also registered on the form. Later, all the described incidents were clustered into five categories:

1. airway/ventilation
2. drugs/therapeutics
3. procedures/lines/equipment systems
4. patient management/environment
5. ICU management.

Three groups of factors (n = 59) contributing to the incident were defined: *system-base* (22 possible entries): physical environment (e.g. lack of space, excessive noise, staff mealtime, ward round), equipment (e.g. unavailable or inadequate, poor maintenance, failure), work practices (e.g. communication problem, inadequate assistance, lack of supervision); *human* (34 possible entries): knowledge-based error (e.g. judgement, charting, prescription, interpretation), rule-based error (e.g. patient assessment, unfamiliar equipment, labelling, calculation); *chance* or unforeseeable problem (three possible entries), such as allergic reaction. These factors were defined after six group interviews (conducted by the principal researchers) with a total of 29 staff members. It is important to note that the study used a deductive methodology (from description to definition) for identifying the incidents occurring in the ICUs, whereas an inductive methodology (from definition to description) was used for identifying the causal factors of each incident.

Five hundred and six reporting forms identified a total of 610 incidents (mean 1.14 incidents per report/patient) (Beckman *et al.*, 1996b). Unfortunately, the published material does not provide information concerning the total number of patients admitted to the seven units during the study period. However, extrapolating from data of a national report (Anderson and Hart, 2000), we estimate that a total of about 4900 patients were involved in the study. Accordingly, the incidence of adverse events in the AMI-ICU study was 12.5%. This assumes that all admitted patients were submitted to the systematic surveillance of incidents.

The distribution of adverse events in the five categories was:

1. 20% were included in the category 'airway/ventilation'
2. 28% in 'drugs/therapeutics'
3. 23% in 'procedures'
4. 21% in 'patient management and environment'
5. 9% in the category 'management'.

A total of 1896 contributing factors (3.5 factors per incident) was recorded by those detecting the incidents: 33% were attributed to 'system-based factors', 66% to 'human factors' and 1% to 'chance'. Most incidents (91%) did not result in an adverse event or complication. However, in 3% morbidity such as physical and psychological injuries, prolonged hospital stay and patient or family dissatisfaction were reported. No deaths were associated with any of the incidents.

The Lori Andrews' study

This was a 9-month prospective study examining adverse events in three units (two ICUs and one general ward) (Andrews *et al.*, 1997). Trained researchers attended all scheduled meetings, ward rounds and shift changes during which exchange of information between professionals took place. The two assumptions behind the research were that, first, all adverse events are identified by the professionals before any formal reporting takes place and second, not all adverse events are formally reported.

One thousand and forty-seven patients were enrolled in the study and 2183 adverse events were observed in 46% of the patients (on average 4.5 adverse events per patient). In 185 patients (17.7%) the adverse event was classified as serious and ranged from temporary physical disability to death.

The researchers identified 368 specific categories of adverse events. These categories were divided into nine broad groups as follows: diagnosis (48 categories), surgery (38), anaesthesia (11), treatment (25), nutrition (5), drugs (20), monitoring and daily care (97), complications (112) and others (12). A few examples of adverse events include:

1. *Diagnosis*: failure to order indicated tests, incorrect conclusion from test information

2. *Surgery*: inadequate preparation of patient, surgery not indicated
3. *Anaesthesia*: improper dosage or improper monitoring
4. *Treatment*: delay in undertaking treatment, unnecessary treatment
5. *Complications*: leaking of anastomosis due to inappropriate healthcare decisions.

Two important conclusions can be drawn from this study. First, the prospectively observed incidence of adverse serious events that caused harm (17.7%) was five times higher than the incidence of similar events reported in the Harvard study (3.7%). Therefore, it appears that retrospective analysis of adverse events, registered in the patients' records, seriously underestimates the overall incidence. Second, the study did not succeed in defining meaningful and mutually exclusive categories of adverse events. This is important as the 368 categories of adverse events were defined in close collaboration with the healthcare professionals participating in the study. This suggests that healthcare professionals focus preferentially on global activities (e.g. surgery, anaesthesia) rather than on the various professional elements or activities making up each process of care.

The incidence of complications and adverse events is often used as one of the measures of performance of ICUs. Experience shows that individual physicians, or groups of physicians within one ICU, are consistent in their interpretations of primary and secondary conditions; this does not lead to bias in the performance comparison. However, different interpretations will confound comparisons of performance when undertaken by different groups of physicians or researchers (Rowan, 1996; Reis Miranda and Moreno, 1997).

The EURICUS-II study

The Euricus-II study entitled 'the effect of harmonising and standardising the nursing tasks in the ICUs of the European Community' was a Concerted Action included in the Biomed–2 research programme of the European Commission (Contract: BMH4-CT96–0817). This 3-year study (1996–99) was implemented in 41 European ICUs by the Foundation for Research on Intensive Care in Europe (FRICE). The study has just ended and the final results are being prepared for publication. An interested reader might want to visit the website 'www.frice.nl' for further information on the design and methodology of the study.

The study tested the hypothesis that improvements in collaborative practice between nurses and physicians in the ICU would decrease the incidence of adverse events, morbidity and mortality. The study also examined the relationship between adverse events and intermediate (morbidity) and final outcomes (vital status at hospital discharge).

The adverse events studied focused on the stability or derangement of four commonly but continuously measured physiological variables (i.e. systolic blood pressure, heart rate, oxygen saturation and urinary output). The nurses were instructed to register at least hourly, on special study-forms, each time the physiological parameters were out of an accepted range set daily by the physicians. Ranges of normality were developed by a panel of intensive care professionals so that a common baseline was created in the survey. The range of values accepted as normal were usually the threshold values that trigger alarms in the monitoring systems. However, the ICUs were allowed to deviate from the suggested values under special circumstances when normal values were no longer appropriate (e.g. in chronic obstructive airways disease, anuria). The recommended ranges were a systolic blood pressure of 90–180 mmHg; a heart rate between 60 and 120 bpm, an oxygen saturation above 90% and at least 30 ml/h of urine. The study surveyed the incidence and the duration of real-time adverse events. In order to avoid alarms due to technical error, the 'out-of-range-measurements' were registered only if the 'alarm' condition persisted for at least 10 minutes. Two types of out-of-range-measurements were defined:

1. an 'event' if the out-of-range-measurement lasted for more than 10 minutes but less than 1 h except for urine output where 1 h or more was allowed
2. a 'critical event' where the out-of-range-measurements lasted for more than 1 h or 2 h or more for urine output.

During the 10-month research, data for 16 848 patients and 86 726 patient-days were collected; 294 884 out-of-range measurements were registered. At least one out-of-range measurement was observed in 75% of patients. On average, 23 out-of-range measurements were registered per patient during ICU admission, of which 17 were of short duration (events), and 6 lasted for more than 1 h (critical events). Of the total out-of-range measurements, 217 017 (73.6%) were events, and 77 867 (26.4%) were critical events. The distribution of both types of event among the four variables measured was similar for both types of out-of-range measurements: 30% for systolic blood pressure, 23% for heart rate, 12% for oxygen saturation and 35% for urine output. The incidence of all events, indexed to the number of patient-days, is shown in Table 9.1. The incidence of events in the

Table 9.1 Incidence and duration of events (Mean/patient-day (standard deviation))

Events	Survived	Died
Systolic blood pressure	0.50 (1.04)	1.73 (2.16)
Heart rate	0.36 (0.99)	1.19 (1.96)
Oxygen saturation	0.18 (0.70)	0.79 (1.57)
Urine output	0.57 (1.33)	1.66 (2.69)
Critical events (hours)		
Systolic blood pressure	2.58 (1.99)	3.95 (2.98)
Heart rate	3.40 (2.80)	4.05 (3.33)
Oxygen saturation	2.55 (2.43)	3.48 (2.99)
Urine output	3.03 (2.57)	5.94 (4.57)

group of non-survivors was at least three times higher than in survivors. Taking the example of systolic blood pressure, survivors had on average one event every second day; whereas those who died had almost two events every day. The mean duration of each critical event was also significantly longer in the non-survivors (Table 9.1). For example, the mean duration of a systolic blood pressure critical event was about 2.5 h in the survivors but almost 4 h in the non-survivors.

A more detailed analysis of the data has shown that the incidence and the duration of out-of-range measurements is associated with mortality after controlling for Simplified Acute Physiology Score II (SAPS II) (Le Gall *et al.*, 1993) and for age (Blow *et al.*, 1999). In contrast to the SAPS II score that loses predictive power over time (Sicignano *et al.*, 1996), the incidence and the duration of out-of-range measurements over time increases the reliability of predicted outcome in the ICU. This is logical, as the persistence of out-of-range measurements indicates continued physiological derangement. Another important finding is that the incidence and particularly the duration of out-of-range measurements during the first days in the ICU influence outcome. The median duration of out-of-range measurements during the first 5 days of ICU admission was 3.2 h. After the fifth day, mortality was significantly higher in patients for whom the duration of out-of-range measurements in the first 5 days was above the median.

The significant association between organ system failure as measured by SOFA (sequential organ failure score) (Vincent *et al.*, 1996) and mortality has been shown on several occasions (Vincent *et al.*, 1998; Moreno *et al.*, 1999). SOFA measures failure (or persistent physiological derangement) of six organ systems: respiratory, cardiovascular, renal, neurological, hepatic, haematological. The EURICUS-II study has shown a significant association between the incidence and the duration of out-of-range measurements and SOFA. The SOFA score was significantly dependent on the values of out-of-range measurements in the previous days. Similar to the score for mortality, the SOFA score of the patients who stayed in the ICU longer than 5 days was significantly higher in the patients for whom the duration of out-of-range measurements in the first 5 days was above the median (3.2 h) (preliminary results). This suggests that the subsequent physiological disturbance may be dependent upon adverse physiological trends in the preceding 24 h.

The EURICUS-II study has clearly shown that the incidence of abnormal values of the four measured physiological variables is significantly associated with the incidence of morbidity (complications) of patients in the ICU.

There is a large difference between the studies, concerning both the incidence of adverse events in the populations studied and their frequency of occurrence in those affected (Table 9.2).

These differences may be related to the different methodologies employed in these four observational studies. Furthermore, the studies addressed different adverse events, with regard to both nature and clinical relevance. In the Harvard Medical Practice study, adverse events were regarded as injury caused by medical management and analysed retrospectively using information available in the medical records. The study analysed only those cases where adverse events

Table 9.2 Incidence of adverse events in three different studies

Study	Incidence adverse events (%)	Number of adverse events per patient
Harvard Medical Practice	3.7	1.2
AIMS-ICU	12.4	1.1
Lori Andrews	46	4.5
EURICUS-II	76	23

were both identified and recorded. This was possibly one of the reasons why a relatively large percentage (13.6%) of the adverse events could be connected to the patient's death. In the AIMS-ICU study, no patient died following the incidents identified and 91% of these incidents had no measurable effect on the outcome of the patients. This might be related to the imprecise definition of adverse event used (an event 'eventually reducing the safety margin for patients'). The raw data collected in this study on only 536 incidents are rather meagre bearing in mind that those reporting had a choice of a possible 59 risk factors. In comparison to the Harvard study, the AIMS-ICU study found more system-based factors at the origin of the incidents. However, several 'system-based' factors could also be listed as human factors (e.g. communication, excessive noise, staff mealtime, ward round, inadequate assistance). Furthermore, the methodology for defining the causal factors of incidents was perhaps strongly influenced by the researchers who used centrally guided interviews rather than a less biased Delphi method. Also, the professional involved with the adverse occurrence was responsible for simultaneously reporting it; this would tend to lower the reporting rate. Similarly in the Andrews' study, the recognition and recording of an adverse event was dependent upon it being identified, recalled and mentioned by the professionals during those occasions when they met each other. One important aspect was that in this study the adverse events reported were not previously defined and did not follow any particular structure. In the EURICUS-II study the out-of-range measurements were systematically screened (for presence or absence) each day. Therefore, the study focused on the real-time precursors of adverse events and complications. The out-of-range measurements are simply symptoms of approaching physiological derangement and imminent organ dysfunction.

Processes of care

One aim of care is to counter illness by correcting physiological derangement. This requires knowledge of the sequential elements in the chain of illness as well as the role of each element of care itself. This chapter focused on the importance of monitoring and recording physiological derangement and the necessary action for correction. Although this rather symptomatic approach for handling derangement is important, a thorough understanding of the process of illness is obviously required. A non-symptomatic approach to illness is not as rigorous at correcting the derangement. Until now, the non-symptomatic approaches are similar to 'prepared expectancy', which involves corrective action after a confirmed change in clinical condition. The rationale supporting this approach is that, often, 'superficial' symptoms of derangement (e.g. low systolic blood pressure) do not sufficiently reflect a more profound problem. Eliminating the symptom might, therefore, reduce appreciation of ongoing illness (e.g. shock due to sepsis). The limitations of this approach are clear in that one has to wait for the adverse events to develop. Severity of illness scoring systems could be modified by including appropriate variables for predicting complications. In other words, if the derangement of today is the precursor of the further illness tomorrow, we should be able to predict it.

The process of care, however, should also be seen from a managerial perspective: the collection of interrelated tasks (grouped into interventions) such that both avoid disorder (Hitchins, 1992). The Harvard Medical Practice study (Brennan et al., 1991) showed clearly that the incidence of adverse events was related to human factors. It has also suggested subsequently that the incidence of events was related to intensity or volume of work, implying that more severely ill patients would experience more adverse events. The EURICUS-studies appear to confirm these findings: human factors, such as collaborative practice and organization commitment, are significantly associated with intermediate (adverse events and complications) and final (mortality) outcomes.

Besides human factors, these studies have shown that variables of the organization of the ICUs, such as elementary organization framework, standardization of procedures and interventions, a team-like structure (e.g. decentralization of decision making), were also associated with final outcomes (Reis Miranda et al., 1998). In other words, ICUs that were better organized had better outcomes (thus performed better) after controlling for case-mix (i.e. SAPS II score, age and origin of patients). Moreover, factors outside the organization in the ICU, but influencing the work organization in the unit, such as task and work flow predictability (resulting from labile clinical conditions, emergency admissions, difficult transfer negotiations with the wards) were also significantly associated with the performance of the ICU (Goldfrad and Rowan, 2000).

Conclusion

In brief, the major goal of care in the ICU is to reverse the critical condition of patients so that 'regular care' may be resumed in the general ward. Sometimes the patient becomes sicker instead of improving because the primary disease worsens or an additional disease is present. These additional diseases are often called complications. I have suggested in this chapter that, in principle, the clinical conditions 'complicating' the primary illness should not be interpreted independently of the primary disease nor of the process of care in the ICU. The so-called complications can be the result of:

1. aggravation of disease due to further physiological derangement, in which the process of illness overrules the process of care. Therefore, the importance of reversing physiological derangement was underlined.
2. inappropriateness of activities of care leading to the (iatrogenic) aggravation of disease.

The importance of adverse events in the deterioration of the clinical condition of ICU patients is well documented in published studies. The mastering of complications and adverse events in the intensive care unit should therefore be based on two courses of professional activities: better understanding of processes of illness and better description and control of processes of care.

References

Afessa, B., Gree, B. (2000). Bacterial pneumonia in hospitalized patients with HIV infection: the pulmonary complications, ICU support, and prognostic factors of hospitalized patients with HIV (PIP) study. *Chest*, **117**, 1017–1022.

Afessa, B., Kubilis, P. S. (2000). Upper gastrointestinal bleeding in patients with hepatic cirrhosis: clinical course and mortality prediction. *Am. J. Gastroenterol.*, **95**, 484–489.

Albertson, T. E., Foulke, G. E., Tharratt, S., Allen, R. (1992). Pharmacokinetics and iatrogenic drug toxicity in the intensive care unit. In: *Principles of Critical Care* (J. B. Hall, G. A. Schmidt, L. D. H. Wood, eds) pp 2061–2079, McGraw-Hill Inc.

Allman, R. M., Goode, P. S., Burst, N. *et al.* (1999). Pressure ulcers, hospital complications, and disease severity: impact on hospital costs and length of stay. *Adv. Wound Care*, **12**, 22–30.

Anderson T., Hart G. (2000). *ANZICS intensive care survey 1998: an overview of Australian and New Zealand critical care resources.* ANZICS Research Centre for Critical Care Resources.

Andrews, L. B., Stocking, C., Krizek, T. H. *et al.* (1997). An alternative strategy for studying adverse events in medical care. *Lancet*, **349**, 309–313.

Aranda, M., Hanson, C. W. 3rd. (2000). Anesthetics, sedatives, and paralytics. Understanding their use in the intensive care unit. *Surg. Clin. North Am.*, **80**, 933–947.

Arroliga, A. C. (1999). *Intensive care unit complications. Clinics in Chest Medicine, Volume 20.* Saunders Company.

Beckmann, U., West L. F., Groombridge G. J. *et al.* (1996a). The Australian Incident Monitoring Study in intensive care: AIMS-ICU. The development and evaluation of an incident reporting system in intensive care. *Anaesth. Intens. Care*, **24**, 314–319.

Beckmann, U., Baldwin I., Hart G. K., Runciman W. B. (1996b). The Australian Incident Monitoring Study in intensive care: AIMS-ICU. An analysis of the first year of reporting. *Anaesth. Intens. Care*, **24**, 320–329.

Blow, O., Magliore, L., Claridge, J. A. *et al.* (1999). The golden hour and the silver day: detection and correction of occult hypoperfusion within 24 hours improves outcome from major trauma. *J. Trauma*, **47,** 964–969.

Bowton, D. L. (1999). Nosocomial pneumonia in the ICU – year 2000 and beyond. *Chest,* **115,** 28S–33S.

Boyd, W. D., Desai, N. D., Del Rizzo, D. F. *et al.* (1999). Off-pump surgery decreases postoperative complications and resource utilization in the elderly. *Ann. Thorac. Surg.,* **68,** 1490–1493.

Brennan, T. A., Leape, L. L., Laird, N. M. *et al.* (1991). Incidence of adverse events and negligence in hospitalized patients: results of the Harvard Medical Practice Study I. *N. Engl. J. Med.,* **324,** 370–376.

Briglia, A., Paganini, E. P. (1999). Acute renal failure in the intensive care unit: therapy overview, patient risk stratification, complications of renal replacement, and special circumstances. *Clin. Chest Med.,* **20,** 347–366.

Brun-Buisson, C. (2000). The epidemiology of the systemic inflammatory response. *Intensive Care Med.,* **26,** S64–S74.

Claridge, J. A., Crabtree, T. D., Pelletier, S. J. *et al.* (2000). Persistent occult hypoperfusion is associated with a significant increase in infection rate and mortality in major trauma patients. *J. Trauma*, **48,** 8–14.

Eberhard, L. W., Morabito, D. J., Matthay, M. A. *et al.* (2000). Initial severity of metabolic acidosis predicts the development of acute lung injury in severely traumatized patients. *Crit. Care Med.,* **28,** 125–131.

Gelling, L. (1999). Causes of ICU psychosis: the environmental factors. *Nurs. Crit. Care,* **4,** 22–26.

Georges H., Leroy O., Guery B. *et al.* (2000). Predisposing factors for nosocomial pneumonia in patients receiving mechanical ventilation and requiring tracheostomy. *Chest,* **118,** 767–774.

Goldfrad, C., Rowan, K. (2000). Consequences of discharges from intensive care at night. *Lancet,* **355,** 1138–1142.

Hitchins, D. K. (1992). *Putting Systems to Work*. Wiley and Sons.

Hund, E. (1999). Myopathy in critically ill patients. *Crit. Care Med.,* **27,** 2544–2547.

Iacó, A. L., Contini, M., Teodori G. *et al.* (1999). Off or on bypass: what is the safety threshold? *Ann. Thorac. Surg.,* **68,** 1486–1489.

Jones, C., Griffiths, R. D., Humphris, G. (2000). Disturbed memory and amnesia related to intensive care. *Memory,* **8,** 79–94.

Knaus, W. A., Wagner, D. P., Draper, E. A. *et al.* (1991). The APACHE III prognostic system; risk prediction of hospital mortality for critically ill hospitalised adults. *Chest,* **100,** 1619–1636.

Latronico, N., Fenzi, F., Recupero, D. *et al.* (1996). Critical illness myopathy and neuropathy. *Lancet,* **347,** 1579–1582

Le Gall, J. R., Lemeshow, S., Saulnier, F. (1993). A new Simplified Acute Physiology Score (SAPS II) based on an European/North America multicenter study. *JAMA,* **270,** 2957–2963.

Leape, L. L., Brennan, T. A., Laird, N. M. *et al.* (1991). The nature of adverse events in hospitalized patients: results of the Harvard Medical Practice Study II. *N. Engl. J. Med.,* **324,** 377–384.

Liolios, A., Oropello, J. M., Benjamin, E. (1999). Gastrointestinal complications in the intensive care unit. *Clin. Chest Med.,* **20,** 329–345.

Martinez, F. M., Lash, R. W. (1999). Endocrinologic and metabolic complications in the intensive care unit. *Clin. Chest Med.,* **20,** 401–421.

McGuire, B. E., Basten, C. J., Ryan, C. J., Gallagher, J. (2000). Intensive care unit syndrome: a dangerous misnomer. *Arch. Intern. Med.*, **160**, 906–909.

Moreno, R., Vincent, J. L., Matos R. *et al.* (1999). The use of maximum SOFA score to quantify organ dysfunction/failure in intensive care. Working Group on Sepsis related Problems of the ESICM. *Intensive Care Med.*, **25**, 686–696.

Morricone, L., Ranucci, M., Denti, S. *et al.* (1999). Diabetes and complications after cardiac surgery: comparison with a non-diabetic population. *Acta Diabetol.*, **36**, 77–84.

Naik-Tolani, S., Oropello, J. M., Benjamin, E. (1999). Neurologic complications in the intensive care unit. *Clin. Chest Med.*, **20**, 423–434.

Noble, J. S., MacKirdy, F. N., Donaldson, S. I., Howie, J. C. (2001). Renal and respiratory failure in Scottish ICUs. *Anaesthesia*, **56**, 124–129.

Peerless, J. R., Davies, A., Klein, D., Yu, D. (1999). Skin complications in the intensive care unit. *Clin. Chest. Med.*, **20**, 453–467.

Perlman, J. M. (1999). Maternal fever and neonatal depression: preliminary observations. *Clin. Pediatr. (Phila)*, **38**, 287–291.

Pingleton, S. K., Hall, J. B. (1992). Prevention and early detection of complications of critical care. In: *Principles of Critical Care* (J. B. Hall, G. A. Schmidt, L. D. H. Wood, eds) pp 587–611, McGraw-Hill Inc.

Pirraglia, P. A., Peterson, J. C., Williams-Russo, P. *et al.* (1999). Depressive symptomatology in coronary artery bypass graft surgery patients. *Int. J. Geriatr. Psychiatr.*, **14**, 668–680.

Price, J., Ekleberry, A., Grover, A. *et al.* (1999). Evaluation of clinical practice guidelines on outcome of infection in patients in the surgical intensive care unit. *Crit. Care Med.*, **27**, 2118–2124.

Quinlan, G.J., Mumby, S., Lamb, N. J. *et al.* (2000). Acute respiratory distress syndrome secondary to cardiopulmonary bypass: do compromised plasma iron-binding anti-oxidant protection and thiol levels influence outcome? *Crit. Care Med.*, **28**, 2271–2276.

Rangel-Frausto, M. S., Wiblin, T., Blumberg, H. M. *et al.* (1999). National epidemiology of mycoses survey (NEMIS): variations in rates of bloodstream infections due to Candida species in seven surgical intensive care units and six neonatal intensive care units. *Clin. Infect. Dis.*, **29**, 253–258.

Reis Miranda, D., Moreno R. (1997). Intensive care unit models and their role in management and utilization programs. *Curr. Opin. Crit. Care*, **3**, 183–187.

Reis Miranda, D., Ryan, D. W., Schaufeli, W. B., Fidler V. (1998). *Organisation and Management of Intensive Care: a Prospective Study in 12 European Countries.* Springer-Verlag.

Richman, J. (2000). Coming out of intensive care crazy: dreams of affliction. *Qual. Health Res.*, **10**, 84–102.

Romac, D. R., Albertson, T. E. (1999). Drug interactions in the intensive care unit. *Clin. Chest Med.*, **20**, 385–399.

Rowan, K. (1996). The reliability of case-mix measurement in intensive care. *Curr. Opin. Crit. Care*, **2**, 209–213.

Shakil, A. O., Kramer, D., Mazariegos, G. V. *et al.* (2000). Acute liver failure: clinical features, outcome analysis, and applicability of prognostic criteria. *Liver Transpl.*, **6**, 163–169.

Sicignano, A., Carozzi, C., Giudicu, D. *et al.* (1996). The influence of length of stay in the ICU on power of discrimination of a multipurpose severity score (SAPS). *Intensive Care Med.*, **22**, 1048–1051.

Strange, C. (1999). Pleural complications in the intensive care unit. *Clin. Chest Med.*, **20**, 317–327.

Vincent, J. L., de Mendonça, A., Cantraine, F. *et al.* (1998). Use of the SOFA score to assess the incidence of organ dysfunction/failure in intensive care units: results of a multicenter, prospective study. Working Group on 'sepsis-related problems' of the European Society of Intensive Care Medicine. *Crit. Care Med.*, **26**, 1793–1800.

Vincent, J. L., Moreno, R., Takala, J. *et al.* (1996). The SOFA (Sepsis-related Organ Failure Assessment) score to describe organ dysfunction/failure. On behalf of the Working Group on Sepsis-Related Problems of the European Society of Intensive Care Medicine. *Intensive Care Med.*, **22**, 707–710.

Wallace, W. C., Cinat, M. E., Nastanski F. *et al.* (2000). New epidemiology for postoperative nosocomial infections. *Am. Surg.*, **66**, 874–878.

Walting, S. M., Dasta, J. F. (1994). Prolonged paralysis in intensive care unit patients after the use of neuromuscular blocking agents: a review of the literature. *Crit. Care Med.*, **22**, 884–893.

Ware, L. B., Matthay, M. A. (2000). The acute respiratory distress syndrome. *N. Engl. J. Med.* **342**, 1334–1349.

Weber, D. J., Raasch, R., Rutala, W. A. (1999). Nosocomial infections in the ICU: the growing importance of antibiotic-resistant pathogens. *Chest*, **115**, 34S–41S.

Weisberg, L. S., Allgren, R. L., Kurnik, B. R. (1999). Acute tubular necrosis in patients with diabetes mellitus. *Am. J. Kidney Dis.*, **34**, 1010–1015.

Chapter 10

Economic outcomes

Clare Hibbert and Dave Edbrooke

Introduction

An estimated £800 million is spent each year providing intensive care services in the UK. Intensive care is reported to cost between four and six times more than care on a general hospital ward (Wagner *et al.*, 1983; Royal College of Anaesthetists and Royal College of Surgeons, 1996); it is thus generally considered an expensive specialty. The average six-bedded general intensive care unit (ICU) has 47 nurses (33.5 whole-time equivalents), three consultants with fixed commitments to the unit and three more taking part in the on-call rota (Audit Commission, 1999). A multidisciplinary team of clinicians and professionals allied to medicine is required, as critically ill patients admitted to an ICU are in, or at imminent risk of, organ failure. In the UK, ICU survival is approximately 75%.

Demand for intensive care is perceived as exceeding the available supply. In the UK, the average number of designated beds for intensive care patients is just over 10 for every 500 acute hospital beds, representing just 2% of the total number of all hospital beds; however, there is wide variation about this average (Audit Commission, 1999). The number of designated intensive care beds varies not only between hospitals, but also between countries (Table 10.1).

The UK has one of the lowest percentages of hospital beds allocated to intensive care but a similar workload to other European countries (Table 10.2).

The USA devotes between 5 and 10% of hospital beds to critical care patients (Chalfin *et al.*, 1995), which is much higher than other countries. Despite the fact that the USA spends considerably more money on intensive care than others, there is little information regarding the added benefits accrued with this additional expenditure (Angus *et al.*, 1997).

Many factors are thought to influence ICU expenditure; some of the most important are:

1. The size of the ICU (number of staffed beds)
2. The case-mix of patients (their severity of illness and level of organ support required), which will affect the use of and, hence, expenditure on special

Table 10.1 The number of hospital beds allocated to the ICU in 10 European countries (Reis Miranda, 1986)

Country	Mean (standard deviation) of ICU beds expressed as a percentage of total hospital beds	Mean (standard deviation) of number of beds per ICU
Austria	2.8 (1.3)	10 (3)
Belgium	3.7 (2.0)	19 (16)
Denmark	4.1 (2.0)	14 (4)
France	3.3 (2.9)	11 (6)
Germany	3.4 (1.6)	12 (5)
Holland	3.6 (1.3)	10 (7)
Spain	3.0 (1.5)	14 (11)
Sweden	3.3 (1.8)	13 (5)
Switzerland	3.8 (1.4)	14 (8)
UK	2.6 (2.0)	6 (2)

treatment modalities, such as extracorporeal membrane oxygenation (ECMO) and haemodialysis

3. The ratio of emergency to elective patients
4. Patients' lengths of stay influenced not only by case-mix but also the number of available beds on the hospital wards and skill-mix of nurses working on those wards

Table 10.2 Workload and number of nurses in 10 European countries (Reis Miranda, 1986)

Country	Mean (standard deviation) admissions per bed per year	Average length of ICU admission	Average occupancy rate (%)	Average number of nurses per bed
Austria	46 (10)	5.3	67.6	2.2
Belgium	67 (18)	4.6	88.6	2.4
Denmark	74 (7)	2.9	59.0	1.2
France	58 (35)	5.6	83.3	1.9
Germany	83 (38)	4.4	94.8	2.1
Holland	93 (40)	3.5	78.0	3.0
Spain	50 (17)	5.9	72.6	2.2
Sweden	124 (54)	3.0	99.0	1.9
Switzerland	74 (21)	3.0	60.2	3.1
UK	65 (47)	3.5	67.6	4.2

5. The organizational structure of the critical care services (presence of a separate high-dependency unit (HDU) or combined ICU/HDU)
6. Whether the ICU is located in a university or non-university hospital
7. The grade-mix of nurses and seniority of medical staff.

A British study of 21 ICUs examined the causes of variation in expenditure (Edbrooke *et al.*, 2001). Using staff as an example, the study found that variations in expenditure on nursing staff could be explained by the number of ICU beds ($r_s = 0.79$), the number of patient days ($r_s = 0.66$), the number of admissions ($r_s = 0.56$) and hospital type (university versus non-university, $r_s = 0.68$). Regression analysis selected the number of ICU beds as being the most important determinant of cost, explaining 89% of the variation in nursing costs. If the ICU was supported by an HDU, the presence of the HDU and nursing staff together explained 92% of the cost variation.

The link between case-mix and cost has not been adequately explored because of difficulties in quantifying case-mix. Previous research has shown that critically ill patients are very heterogeneous with regard to the precipitating cause of their illness; for a significant number of patients, a diagnosis, even retrospectively, cannot always be made (Stevens *et al.*, 1998). These factors have made describing patient costs in terms of clinical groupings difficult. However, two of the most important causes of variation in individual patient's total costs of care are their length of stay in the ICU and their need for and duration of organ support (Hibbert *et al.*, 1999).

Meaningful comparison of expenditure on intensive care between countries requires careful adjustments for case-mix and for economic and organizational factors. Despite comparative data on overall health expenditure for 24 countries from the Organization for Economic Cooperation and Development (OECD, 1989), there were few data on ICU expenditure. Gross national product has been used in the past to compare overall expenditure on health. However, as gross national product varies enormously between countries, a direct comparison of the percentage of expenditure allocated to health care is of limited value. Expenditure on a per capita basis is a more meaningful measure but its translation into a common currency, such as euros, does not explain the quantities of healthcare resources that can be purchased within each country. For example, the increase in health spending per capita from 1985 to 1991 was 9% in the USA, 7.5% in Canada, 7.3% in the UK and France, and 6.5% in the Netherlands (Battista and Hodge, 1995). However, these figures are difficult to put into the context of critical care because an increase in healthcare expenditure does not necessarily equate to a similar increase in intensive care expenditure.

Factors that confound direct comparison of ICU expenditure between different countries are:

1. Demographic characteristics of the country, such as population size
2. Economic factors such as gross domestic product and social deprivation
3. Differences in socioeconomic distribution between countries

4. Health status such as major causes of death, mortality and morbidity rates, accident rates and life expectancy
5. The structure of the healthcare system, such as the funding and entitlement arrangements for healthcare and the methods of rationing
6. Measurement of health care expenditure.

Little is known about how intensive care resources are distributed and no useful economic information exists to help decision makers maximize efficiency of critical care services (Heyland *et al.*, 1996).

Why measure costs?

The costs of critical care are expected to rise significantly over the next decade as a result of doctors' and patients' expectations and the projected increases in life expectancy. Finite resources for healthcare mean that cost-effective use of resources is mandatory. Increasing pressure is being placed on clinicians to practice evidence-based medicine that achieves optimal outcomes for patients, but within the constraints of limited resources. Thus the use of appropriate methods to measure both costs and outcomes are important for critical care.

History of costing studies

Economic evaluation is being increasingly used to study the clinical and economic ramifications of medical interventions and to enable more rational decisions about resource use in intensive care (Chalfin *et al.*, 1995). However, there are difficulties using cost-effectiveness analyses to guide decision making. These include:

1. The lack of accurate estimates of treatment effectiveness and reliable measurement of cost
2. Variation in assumptions used in different cost-effectiveness analyses
3. No ethical or regulatory mandate to ensure that any decisions reached will be carried out fairly (Rubenfeld, 1998).

Controversy surrounding the costs of adult intensive care is not new (Gapen, 1983; Birnbaum, 1986). The first papers highlighting the problems of costs and rationing within intensive care were published in the 1970s (Martin, 1972; Phillips, 1977). The first studies of ICU costs originated from France (Nedey, 1980; Beurton, 1980; Cara-Beurton, 1985). One of the first costing studies in the UK was performed by Gilbertson (1991) who estimated (using a bottom-up method) the costs of patients admitted to the ICU at the Royal Liverpool Hospital. In this prospective study, the daily costs for patients with severe combined acute respiratory and renal failure who required mechanical ventilation and renal replacement therapy were significantly higher than other patients. Approximately 44% of the total cost of treatment was related to staff (28% for the provision of nurses and 16% on other staff) (Gilbertson et al., 1991). These findings were confirmed by Singer et al. (1994) who, by conducting a combined retrospective and prospective audit of expenditure, found staff costs were by far the largest single item of expenditure.

A prospective study of costs, severity of illness and patient outcomes was published by Slatyer et al. (1986). They measured direct clinical costs such as nurses' time, diagnostic tests, drug and fluid costs, oxygen costs and light and power costs in a sample of 100 consecutive patients. The majority of costs for ICU patients and the running of ICUs were the staff and drugs costs and not those associated with buildings and equipment.

Ridley et al. (1991) calculated the costs of individual patients consecutively admitted to an ICU in Glasgow, Scotland, dividing the costs into three main categories, fixed, semi-fixed and marginal costs. The fixed costs consisted of equipment, services and land opportunity cost and were calculated as £82.29 per patient-day. The semi-fixed costs consisted of nursing and medical staff. The costs of these were apportioned by dependency points allocated on a daily basis. Marginal costs consisted of treatment costs such as mechanical ventilation, drugs and fluids. The total costs per patient were calculated from the sum of the fixed, semi-fixed and marginal costs. The results from this study suggested that the costs of intensive care patients was dependent upon severity of illness, the level of intervention and ICU mortality, as non-survivors incurred significantly more expense than survivors.

The review of cost studies by Gyldmark (1995) made a significant contribution to highlighting the problems associated with cost measurement in the intensive care setting. This review of 20 published cost studies of adult intensive care identified many different approaches to costing. This meant that it was not always possible to make valid comparisons between the studies. The most damning conclusion from this review was that the methods studied were flawed and failed to provide correct answers. The review concluded that 'standardizing the cost model would lead to better, faster, and more reliable costing'.

A prospective 1-year cost accounting study was performed by Noseworthy et al. (1996) in Canada. They found no relationship between age and costs but reported costs per patient-day (about $1500) (1992 Canadian dollars) to be constant across most diagnoses, which was an interesting find as this contradicts other findings (Ridley et al., 1991; Stevens et al., 1998). The mean (± standard deviation) cost per patient was $7520 (± $11 606). Median cost per stay for all patients was $2600. Cost per ICU admission was less than $5000 for 66% of patients; these patients had an ICU survival of 85%. High cost was not associated with poor survival.

A study by Havill et al. (1997) looked for a relationship between direct nursing time and the costs of critically ill patients. In this study of 139 patients, they collected data on the hours of nursing care applied to each patient, cost and the daily Therapeutic Intervention Scoring System (TISS) scores (Cullen et al.,

1974; Keene and Cullen, 1983). In broad terms, the TISS score measures the number and types of interventions (and hence workload required) for ICU patients. Nurses assign a TISS score to their patients on a daily basis, which is meant to reflect the treatment requirements incurred over the previous 24-h period. The list is comprehensive in so far that it covers a wide range of therapeutic procedures, but it may not accurately reflect the nursing components of care. Havill found a strong correlation between the nursing hours of care and the total cost per patient ($r^2 = 0.98$) (total cost = 54 × nursing hours + 344). They also reported strong correlations between patients' total TISS scores and their total costs ($r^2 = 0.96$) (total cost = 67.13 × total TISS).

In France, Sznajder et al. (1998) attempted to estimate the direct costs of intensive care patients using the Omega Nursing Workload System. This measures activity allocated to one of three task groupings, based upon 47 therapeutic and diagnostic manoeuvres weighted with a score between 1 and 10 according to the workload involved. Omega 1 includes 28 procedures such as enteral feeding for more than 9 days or the insertion of a uretheral catheter, and these are recorded only once during a patients' stay (regardless of their frequency). Omega 2 is based on 11 interventions, e.g. gastrointestinal endoscopy and an ultrasonic procedure and these are noted every time they occur. Omega 3 includes eight treatments recorded on a daily basis, such as mechanical ventilation and continuous monitoring in the ICU. A total score is then calculated by adding all the points together at the end of a patient's ICU stay. This study found the Omega score was strongly correlated to total direct costs, medical direct costs and nursing requirements. In general, workload scoring systems have been found to be effective, as a proxy for costs, when studying groups of patients but ineffective when estimating the costs of individual patients.

Present costing methods

Top-down method

Top-down costing is a retrospective costing method (Gyldmark, 1995) that produces an average cost per patient-day by dividing the total expenditure of the critical care unit over a given time period by the number of patient-days of care provided within the same time period. It is frequently used for reimbursement purposes (in the absence of reliable diagnosis-related groups or healthcare resource group classifications). The cost per patient is generated by multiplying the derived cost per day by patient's length of stay.

Top-down costing has provided overall estimates of intensive care costs in different countries (Jacobs and Noseworthy, 1990; Halpern et al., 1994; Clermont et al., 1998) and has been particularly useful for benchmarking purposes in the UK (Edbrooke et al., 1999a). Although costing with the top-down method is comparatively easier to use than more patient-focused methods, it is important that the components of cost are specified and measured rigorously using standard definitions. This is to ensure that the costs can be reproduced and valid comparisons made between different studies.

Over the years, researchers have used top-down costing to allocate costs to patients according to their TISS scores (Reis Miranda *et al.*, 1996). This 'weighted' approach attempts to compensate for the potential differences in individual patient costs, which are ignored using a cost per day for all patients. Although ICUs continue to use this type of scoring system as a proxy for costing their patients, there are a number of problems. The elements that make up a TISS score are related to the care delivered. Unfortunately, a wide variety of combinations of care with different resource implications can give the same score. A TISS based costing system assumes a certain degree of homogeneity with respect to the resources required to deliver each TISS point; this may not be the case.

To use TISS for costing, the following theoretical method would apply. If the ICU spent £1.4 million in the previous year treating patients who required a total of 40 000 TISS points of care, then the cost per TISS point would be £1.4 million divided by 40 000, namely £35. Thus, if a patient has been in the ICU for 3 days and has daily TISS scores of 25, 32 and 17, the total costs of care will be:

$$(25 \times £35) + (32 \times £35) + (17 \times 35) = £2590.$$

In practice, however, it is not so straightforward. If the patient is admitted to ICU at 13:00 and the nurses routinely score all patients at 11:00, the patient will not have a TISS score for the day of admission. Even if the patient had arrived at 11:00, then the nurses would still not be able to score the patient because the TISS score should relate to the previous 24 hours of care. Thus TISS scores for day one may be difficult to generate. Another problem relates to discharge from the ICU when a patient leaves before the score is routinely collected. Unless special attention is paid to data collection before discharge, then the final day's score will be missing. The costs of patients staying less than 24 h will also be missed. Overall, there is potential to underestimate expenditure using TISS scoring, unless the cost per TISS point is inflated to compensate for both missing data and short-stay patients. The results of one study (Havill *et al.*, 1997) found that 10 patients' total costs were underestimated by at least $984 while another 10 patients' costs were overestimated by at least $1496 (New Zealand dollars) using the TISS scoring system.

Cost blocks

The cost block method uses a top-down method and was developed by a National Working Group on Intensive Care Costs in the UK between 1994 and 1999 (Edbrooke *et al.*, 1999a). The Working Group was charged with reviewing the methods for costing intensive care and, if possible, developing a standard method that would overcome differences in accounting practices employed by individual hospitals. At the time of the group's formation, comparing the results of studies was difficult because different methods had been used. This made the development of a standard method desirable. The Working Group produced ten questions of common interest that they felt warranted answers from any costing method (Table 10.3). Having searched the literature to no avail for an appropriate system, the group developed a new method.

Table 10.3 Top ten questions of common interest (Edbrooke *et al.*, 1999a)

---

1 What is the cost of opening another ICU bed?
2 What is the daily cost per patient?
3 How does cost per category of patient vary with throughput?
4 How do we include quality?
5 What are the budgetary requirements for an ICU?
6 Can we link with healthcare resource groups, the Therapeutic Intervention Scoring System (TISS) and the Acute Physiology And Chronic Health Evaluation (APACHE)?
7 How can we define fixed, non-fixed and marginal costs?
8 How can we weight costs to take into account teaching and research?
9 Exactly what should be included in costing?
10 Can daily costs be multiplied by length of stay to produce total costs?

The 'cost block' method identified the six major components of resource use in intensive care:

1. Current cost of using equipment (e.g. purchase price modified using linear standard depreciation; total maintenance and annual lease or hire charges)
2. Estates (e.g. value of buildings taking into account depreciation; water, sewerage, waste disposal and energy; building maintenance, engineering maintenance and decoration; rates)
3. Non-clinical support services (e.g. administration; management and cleaning)
4. Clinical support services (e.g. pharmacy; physiotherapy; radiology; dieticians; cardiology; renal support from another ICU; clinical neuroservices and laboratory services)
5. Consumables (e.g. drugs, fluids and nutrition; blood and blood products and disposables)
6. Staff (e.g. medical staff, nursing staff and technicians).

After refining the definitions relating to the collection of the above blocks, the method was piloted in 11 ICUs when retrospective costs, ICU size and workload data were collected for two financial years. The pilot study highlighted difficulties in the collection of the first three cost blocks (current cost of using equipment, estates and non-clinical support services) because of the availability

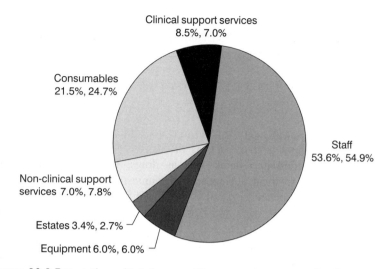

Figure 10.1 Proportion of total expenditure over two years distributed by each cost block (Edbrooke *et al.*, 1999a).

and reliability of the data. These three cost blocks accounted in all for only 15% of total expenditure (Figure 10.1).

By apportioning total expenditure on each cost block to the number of ICU beds and the number of patients and patient-days, it was possible to answer seven of the ten original questions posed by the group. The method was adapted to focus primarily on the latter three cost blocks, which were directly related to patient care. A larger pilot study was conducted before the method was introduced for national use in November 1999. By March 2001, approximately 75 hospitals in the UK were using the cost block method.

Bottom-up method

'Extremely time consuming ... very labour intensive ... and not free from difficulties' were the words used by Gilbertson *et al.* (1991) after calculating the costs of patients in their ICU in detail. Such detailed costing of individual patients is recognized as a complex undertaking.

The bottom-up method produces a cost per patient-day by adding together the individual patient's use of resources. Each resource is broken down into its smallest unit and multiplied by the number of units used. For example, if a patient requires a nurse for 10 minutes then a cost per minute of a nurse's time is required in order to produce an accurate total cost. 'Micro-costing' or 'activity-based' are terms frequently used to describe such bottom-up costing principles.

Activity-based costing ascribes a cost to individual patients based upon their actual use of resources (Edbrooke *et al.*, 1995, 1997). Activities of care have been used for costing individual intensive care patients since 1995 at the Royal Hallamshire Hospital, Sheffield, UK. The concept behind activity-based costing is that the clinical care delivered to patients is partitioned into discrete elements or activities. The cost of patient care is then quantified by allocating resources (and therefore costs) to each activity. The total patient-related cost of care is the sum of the costs of the activities delivered to that patient. Currently, over 300 activities of care are included in the system. They cover all drugs, treatments and major monitoring procedures used on ICU and also the 'background' nursing care, such as discussions with relatives. Since the resources are classified into items such as drugs, fluids, disposable items, equipment, nursing, medical, technical and administrative staff, it is possible to analyse and compare the costs of delivering different types of treatment.

Since the implementation of this system, it has been used in many ways. First, to calculate accurate costs per case for recharging other departments within and outside of the hospital for their use of intensive care services (following the mandate of the White Paper 'Working for Patients') (Department of Health, 1989). Secondly, it has been used to help the development of healthcare resource groups (HRGs) by classifying patients into homogeneous groups with respect to cost (Stevens *et al.*, 1998). Thirdly, it has been used to cost patients recruited into clinical trials. This is a useful application as it can detect the differences in treatment requirements and costs between patients in either arm of a trial. Data from the costing system were used to study the costs of treating sepsis and found that in one centre, 15% of patients who had sepsis consumed 50% of the ICU budget (Edbrooke *et al.*, 1999b). Activity-based costing has several advantages when undertaking economic evaluations. It captures the nursing time spent with patients and, as such, can be used to identify ways of optimizing this resource. For example, if a senior nurse is performing tasks such as hygiene and patient repositioning, data from the costing system can estimate the cost of this and calculate the cost implications of a more junior nurse performing these tasks. It can be used to perform simple cost-minimization studies by measuring the differential costs of treatments producing clinically identical outcomes. Such calculations are simple to perform without a computerized costing system, but an automated system dispenses with laborious time and motion studies. A disadvantage of an activity-based method of costing is that it requires a patient data management system with a computer terminal at each patient's bed-side for staff to record the clinical procedures and interventions performed on each patient. Table 10.4 provides a summary of the Sheffield patient data management system's main functions (Edbrooke *et al.*, 1995).

These data are collected prospectively and have to be checked against the medical records for any omissions. Commitment of all ICU staff is mandatory to ensure accurate recording of data. Collection of unit costs to assign against the activities of care takes time, as there are more than 3000 costs to be entered each year. As a result, activity-based systems tend to be used primarily for research, but as experience grows, such systems may be introduced into routine practice.

Table 10.4 Patient data management system characteristics (Edbrooke *et al.*, 1995)

- Basic demographic data (e.g. age, gender, weight and home address)
- Admission data (e.g. source of admission, emergency/elective/re-admission (<6 weeks), postoperative status, referring team, referring consultant, Acute Physiology And Chronic Health Evaluation (APACHE II) score, primary reason for admission, International Classification of Disease codes for admitting pathology (ICD9) and principal diagnosis)
- Cardiovascular data acquisition (e.g. heart rate, arterial, central venous pressure and pulmonary capillary wedge pressures)
- Respiratory and other physiological data acquisition (e.g. oxygen saturation and respiratory rate)
- Nursing care plans
- Therapeutic Intervention Scoring System (TISS) data
- Patient procedures (e.g. tracheal intubation, continuous veno-venous haemofiltration (CVVH) and percutaneous tracheostomy)
- Drug and fluid administration
- Relatives information summaries
- Patient discharge summaries (e.g. procedures performed, tubes/lines, complications for any reason using ICD9 codes and ICU survival)

Economic definitions

Once ICU costs have been determined, it is important to consider how they can be used to improve efficiency and resource allocation within the ICU. Economics evaluation is important. There are four basic categories of economic evaluation, namely cost-minimization, cost-utility, cost-benefit and cost-effectiveness analyses. These can be used to investigate the economic value of the various interventions used on ICU (Rittenhouse, 1996). It is worth stating that many different definitions exist for economic evaluation. A selection is presented here.

Cost-effectiveness analysis

Drummond *et al.* (1987) defined cost-effectiveness analysis as a form of full economic evaluation, where both costs and consequences of health programmes or treatments are examined. In cost-effectiveness analysis the incremental cost of a programme is compared to the incremental health effects of that programme, where the health effects are measured in natural units, e.g. cases found, cases of disease averted, lives saved, life-years gained. The results are usually expressed as a cost per unit of effect.

Folland *et al.* (1997) defined cost-effectiveness analysis as a method that tries to find the least costly method of achieving desired objectives; these are not necessarily measured in monetary terms, e.g. the ability to walk without a cane.

Bowling's (1997) definition, while similar to that of Drummond, links the analysis to efficiency describing cost-effectiveness analysis as 'an approach to the assessment of efficiency which is concerned with the measurement of outcomes in "natural" units (e.g. improvement in health status), which are compared with the monetary costs of the health care'.

Cost-minimization analysis

Drummond *et al.* (1987) state that this type of analysis looks at the consequences of two or more alternatives alongside their costs, when the consequences are known to be equivalent. The cheapest intervention is deemed optimal assuming there are no other relevant non-economic considerations such as a higher incidence of side effects (Rittenhouse, 1996). Bowling (1997) warns that cost-minimization should be undertaken only where the outcomes are guaranteed to be identical because if they are actually different, the analysis will give misleading results.

Rittenhouse (1996) emphasizes that both cost-minimization analysis and cost-effectiveness analysis can only indicate relative superiority. They can answer questions such as 'Which is better?' or 'What does it cost to bring about a certain effect?' from an economic point of view. They do not claim that what is better is necessarily worth doing.

Cost-utility analysis

Drummond *et al.* (1987) define cost-utility analysis as a form of economic appraisal that focuses particular attention on the quality of health caused or averted by health programmes or treatments. 'Utility' is a term used by economists to signify what a person expects to gain from the consumption of goods or services and is applied to healthcare to mean the individual's preference for different states of well-being after healthcare interventions (Jefferson *et al.*, 2000). In cost-utility analysis, the incremental cost of a programme is compared to the incremental health improvement and can be quantified in different ways. The most common method is quality-adjusted life-years (QALYs) gained. QALYs are calculated simply by multiplying the value of preference of being in a certain state by the length of time of being in that state. The EuroQol is another utility that measures health status in different domains, such as mobility, self-care, usual activities, pain/discomfort, anxiety/depression and applies preferences from large population based studies. Another method is the healthy year equivalent (HYE) which uses a two-stage lottery method and is thought better to represent individual preferences (Jefferson *et al.*, 2000). Bowling (1997) considers cost-utility analysis as providing one approach to addressing issues of efficiency of resource allocation in relation to the setting of health priorities. All the requirements and considerations for cost-effectiveness apply equally to cost-utility analysis (Torrance, 1996).

There are two important advantages to using cost-utility analysis. First, the QALY is a general measure of health outcome that captures changes in both mortality and morbidity and is applicable to all diseases and conditions. Thus, it provides a common mechanism for comparing all types of programmes. Second, it includes the preferences of individuals for the choices of outcomes. Clearly any approach that wishes to be responsive to individuals must incorporate their preferences (Torrance, 1996).

Cost-benefit analysis

Cost-benefit analysis attempts to value the beneficial consequences of programmes in monetary terms. While in theory it is a broad form of evaluation, in practice cost-benefit analysis is usually more restricted than cost-utility or cost-effectiveness analysis because it is limited to a comparison of those costs and consequences than can easily be expressed in monetary units (Drummond et al., 1987). Cost-benefit analyses often restrict themselves to narrowly defined economic changes brought about by treatments and programmes, such as changes in healthcare costs and the productive output of patients (or those caring for them) (Drummond et al., 1987). McGuire et al. (1988) defined cost-benefit analysis as an economic appraisal that seeks to determine whether particular projects, involving the use of resources available for healthcare, are socially efficient and equitable. Folland et al. (1997) added that the rationale for a formal cost-benefit analysis rests on the premise that a project or policy will improve social welfare if the benefits associated with the project or policy exceed the costs. The benefits and costs include not only direct benefits and costs to patients and healthcare organizations but also any indirect benefits or costs to third parties, such as relatives, employers or carers. Patrick and Erickson (1996) believe that cost-benefit analysis has not been widely used in health policy making because of the difficulty of using monetary units (dollars) to value life. Although willingness-to-pay, human capital and revealed-preference methods are useful for assigning monetary value to human life in selected studies, the conceptual and practical concerns have prevented any single method becoming widely accepted (Patrick and Erickson, 1996).

Health economic studies within intensive care

The first study of the cost and benefit of intensive care was published by Loes et al. (1987). The researchers performed a detailed descriptive study of 961 patients treated in the general ICU of Akershus Central Hospital in Norway from 1978 to 1981. They found that intensive care improved 81.4% of the patients, 5.2% were unchanged, and 13.4% died. The ICU survivors discharged between 1978 and 1979 ($n = 363$) were followed on average for 20 months after ICU admission. Of these ICU survivors, 28 (8%) died later during the same stay in the hospital, and another 47 (13%) died after discharge from the hospital, leaving 288 (79%) alive.

Ridley *et al.* (1993) performed a cost-benefit analysis of 90 patients. Considerable variation in cost was found between diagnoses. Renal failure, sepsis and pneumonia were found to be some of the most expensive conditions to treat while postoperative respiratory failure was the least expensive. The mean daily cost of non-survivors was almost £300 greater than the cost of survivors. The cost per survivor at 1 year was low (<£5000) in those conditions where the survival rate exceeded 80% (chronic obstructive airways disease, recovery after respiratory arrest, postoperative observation and monitoring, aortic aneurysm repair, gastrointestinal bleeding and trauma). Whereas the cost of 1-year survivors of pneumonia, haemorrhagic and septic shock, conditions associated with a high mortality, was over £10 000.

Studies of respiratory failure

Byrick *et al.* (1980) studied the cost-effectiveness of intensive care for patients with respiratory failure. This study did not fulfil the definition of cost-effectiveness, as the researchers did not compare the costs and outcomes of patients who did not receive intensive care as a control group. However, the study did find that a major determinant of outcome was the patient's age.

Studies of cardiogenic pulmonary oedema

Holt *et al.* (1994) compared admitting patients with severe cardiogenic pulmonary oedema for mask continuous positive airway pressure (CPAP) with admitting only patients failing conventional non-CPAP treatment who required mechanical ventilation. They showed that mask CPAP reduced the need for mechanical ventilation from 35 to 0%. The mean cost of a mask CPAP treatment was $1156 (1991 Australian dollars) and the patients had a mean stay of 1.2 days; in ventilated patients, the mean cost was $5055 and mean duration of stay 4.2 days. The researchers concluded that mask CPAP for severe cardiogenic pulmonary oedema was cost-effective.

Studies of infection

de Clercq *et al.* (1983) examined the additional costs incurred by patients with nosocomial infection. They found infected patients stayed in the ICU twice as long as non-infected patients; the mean cost of antibiotics prescribed was four times higher and the mean expenditure of other drugs and infusion fluids was approximately one and a half times higher. A further study of the costs of nosocomial infection was performed in Spain (Diaz Molina *et al.*, 1993). They also found significant additional hospital costs due to ICU acquired infection. As a result of their infection, infected patients stayed for 14.2 days on ICU compared to 9.9 days for non-infected patients.

A study from San Francisco looked at the cost and outcome of intensive care for acquired immune deficiency syndrome (AIDS) patients with *Pneumocystis carinii* pneumonia causing severe respiratory failure; by studying patients over time Wachter *et al*. (1995) found intensive care was not cost-effective. For example, it cost on average $174 781 per year of life saved for survivors, which was significantly more costly than those patients who died before discharge. This expense remained high during the three periods studied. During the period 1981–85, the cost was $305 795 (US dollars), between 1986 and 1988, it was $94 528 and between 1989 and 1991 the cost was $215 233 (Wachter *et al*., 1995).

A study by Edbrooke *et al*. (1999b) found patients with severe sepsis and/or early septic shock spent prolonged periods of time in the ICU and were significantly more expensive to treat than patients without sepsis. This study showed that the cost of treating a septic patient varied from twice to eleven times that of a non-septic patient.

Studies on prolonged stay in the ICU

Becker *et al*. (1984) performed a study of the cost and outcome of 50 surgical patients who required more than 2 weeks of care in the ICU. The researchers found that patients' quality of life following discharge was poor. Their results suggested that increased mortality was associated with multiple organ failure, age, sepsis, cancer, a combination of infection and failure of a major organ system, requirement for a tracheostomy for prolonged respiratory support and haemodialysis for renal failure. The total hospital charge for these patients was $1 094 056 (US dollars). A significant correlation between length of stay and total cost was found with an average cost per day of approximately $1000. The most expensive patients to treat were those with sepsis, costing on average, $35 039 per stay, while the least expensive were observation and congestive heart failure patients ($23 187 and $19 507 respectively).

Studies on patients with cancer

Schapira *et al*. (1993) undertook a study of survival and costs of treating critically ill cancer patients (i.e. patients with solid tumours or lymphoma admitted for non-postoperative care) in the ICU at the H. Lee Moffitt Cancer Center and Research Institute in Tampa between July 1988 and June 1990. A higher percentage of patients from the haematological group died during their ICU admission (32 of 64 (50%) versus 34 of 86 (41%)); however, overall survival was similar in the two groups (60% survival in the solid tumour group and 50% in the haematological group). Mean survival after ICU discharge for patients with solid tumours was 4.8 months, and mean time spent at home was 4.2 months. However, 68 (79%) patients in this group spent less than 3 months at home before they died. Mean survival of patients with haematological cancers was 5 months, but 50 (78%) of these 64 patients spent less than 2.5 months at home. The cost per life year gained for patients with solid tumours was $82 845 while for patients with haematological cancers it was considerably more at $189 339 (1991 US dollars).

Studies on sedative regimens

Economic evaluations of pharmaceutical agents are becoming increasingly common. A study by Cernaianu *et al.* (1996) examined the cost-efficiency of sedation and anxiolysis with lorazepam against continuous midazolam infusions. This study found sedation and anxiolysis with both agents was safe and clinically effective. However, the dose of midazolam required for sedation was much larger than that of lorazepam, so the researchers concluded that midazolam was less cost-efficient than lorazepam. These findings were confirmed by another study from the Netherlands (Swart *et al.*, 1999) which favoured lorazepam on economic grounds for the long-term sedation of patients.

Studies on management strategies

A retrospective cost-effectiveness analysis was performed by Cohen *et al.* (1991) to evaluate whether having a management team could reduce the duration and cost of mechanical ventilation. All patients requiring mechanical ventilation in the ICU were included; patients admitted 1 year before the introduction of the ventilatory management team were compared with those patients admitted in the following year. The team consisted of a senior ICU physician, nurse and respiratory therapist and they conducted rounds regularly to supervise the ventilatory management of ICU patients. A total of 236 patients required 250 episodes of mechanical ventilation in the earlier group, and 211 patients required 229 episodes of mechanical ventilation after the team's introduction. The two study groups were similar in terms of their demographic characteristics; however, there were significant reductions in resource use following the introduction of the team. The number of days on mechanical ventilation decreased by 3.9 days per episode of mechanical ventilation (95% confidence interval: 0.3–7.5 days), as did days in the ICU by 3.3 days per episode of mechanical ventilation (95% confidence interval: 0.3–6.3 days). The number of arterial blood gas measurements fell by 23.2 per episode of mechanical ventilation as did the number of indwelling arterial catheters by one per episode of mechanical ventilation. The estimated cost savings from these reductions was US $1303 per episode of mechanical ventilation. They concluded that a ventilatory management team could significantly and safely expedite weaning patients from mechanical ventilation.

A study from France by Chaix *et al.* (1999) compared the costs and benefits of a methicillin-resistant *Staphylococcus aureus* control programme in ICU. They performed a case-control study of 27 randomly selected patients who had methicillin-resistant *Staphylococcus aureus* with 27 controls who did not. ICU costs attributable to methicillin-resistant *Staphylococcus aureus* infection were computed from excess therapeutic intensity using a cost model derived in the same ICU. The results of this study recommended selective screening and isolation of methicillin-resistant *Staphylococcus aureus* carriers at ICU admission because of the costs attributable to methicillin-resistant *Staphylococcus aureus* treatment.

Glance *et al.* (1998) studied the cost-effectiveness of using prognostic scoring systems to reduce costs in non-survivors. They used decision analysis to evaluate the cost-effectiveness of withdrawing care from patients in the ICU who were predicted to have a high probability of death (greater than 90%) after 48 hours using a mortality risk estimate based on daily Acute Physiology And Chronic Health Evaluation (APACHE) III scores. The researchers concluded that the predictive power of the scoring system was not sufficiently good for reliably predicting death, and as such its potential for reducing costs was limited.

Conclusion

The future of intensive care research will certainly incorporate economic evaluations that consider both the costs and benefits of treatments. It will not be possible to ignore the pressures that an increasing demand for services will place on limited financial resources. Standardization of costing methods will improve meaningful comparison of the published literature, which should help researchers to synthesize cost data from different studies. The use of costing methods described (e.g. top-down and bottom-up) will increase, as will studies that reconcile the two methods so making patient related costing easier. Through the collection of cost block data, those factors thought to influence expenditure on an ICU will be better understood, leading to an improved understanding of where resources are allocated. The difficult problem of patient classification is likely to continue, which will necessitate new methods for categorizing patients into homogeneous groups on cost as well as clinical grounds.

Studies that make the association between costs and outcomes will need to be performed so that the true effectiveness and cost-effectiveness of intensive care can be measured. The principles behind analytical methods for economic evaluation, such as cost-effectiveness analysis and cost-benefit analysis will need to be understood so that researchers select the most appropriate method for their studies. Unfortunately, the full cost-effectiveness of intensive care services will never be measured without the randomized allocation of patients to ICU (with organ support) or to the general ward (without advanced organ support), as the ethical problems are insurmountable. However, studies that, for example, evaluate the cost-effectiveness of new treatments for sepsis and the acute respiratory distress syndrome will be particularly welcome, in light of the high costs and poor outcomes associated with these conditions.

The question facing clinicians will no longer be 'does intensive care work' but 'intensive care for whom?' (Knaus, 1987). The most probable route for the future endeavour will be a combination of triage policies and economic evaluations to identify patients who are most likely to benefit from intensive care. This is probably the only way that we can hope to provide intensive care in the future in an affordable way.

References

Angus, D. C., Sirio, C. A., Clermont, G., Bion, J. (1997). International comparisons of critical care outcome and resource consumption. *Crit. Care Clin.*, **13**, 389–407.

Audit Commission. (1999). *Critical to Success. The place of efficient and effective critical care services within the acute hospital.* Audit Commission.

Battista, R. N., Hodge, M. J. (1995). The development of health technology assessment. *Int. J. Technol. Assess. Health Care*, **11**, 287–300.

Becker, G. J., Strauch, G. O., Saranchak, H. J. (1984). Outcome and cost of prolonged stay in the surgical intensive care unit. *Arch. Surg.*, **119**, 1338–1342.

Beurton, M. C. (1980). Cost price analysis for intensive care services within the framework of the total budget. (Saint-Germain-en-Laye Hospital Center. 2 years' experience: 1977–1978). *Ann. Anesthesiol. Fr.*, **21**, 335–340.

Birnbaum, M. L. (1986). Cost-containment in critical care. *Crit. Care Med.*, **14**, 1068–1077.

Bowling, A. (1997). *Research Methods in Health, Investigating Health and Health Services.* Open University Press.

Byrick, R. J., Mindorff, C., McKee, L., Mudge, B. (1980). Cost-effectiveness of intensive care for respiratory failure patients. *Crit. Care Med.*, **8**, 332–327.

Cara-Beurton, M. (1985). Analysis of the net cost of intensive care in the framework of the global budget. Attempt at determining the cost of infection over a 5-year period (1978–1984). *Agressologie.*, **26**, 177–179.

Cernaianu, A. C., Del Rossi, A. J., Flum, D. R. *et al.* (1996). Lorazepam and midazolam in the intensive care unit: a randomized, prospective, multicenter study of hemo-dynamics, oxygen transport, efficacy, and cost. *Crit. Care Med.*, **24**, 222–228.

Chaix, C., Durand-Zaleski, I., Alberti, C., Brun-Buisson, C. (1999). Control of endemic methicillin-resistant *Staphylococcus aureus*: a cost-benefit analysis in an intensive care unit. *JAMA*, **282**, 1745–1751.

Chalfin, D. B., Cohen, I. L., Lambrinos, J. (1995). The economics and cost-effectiveness of critical care medicine. *Intensive Care Med.*, **21**, 952–961.

Clermont, G., Angus, D. C., Linde-Zwirble, W. T. *et al.* (1998). Measuring resource use in the ICU with computerized Therapeutic Intervention Scoring System-based data. *Chest*, **113**, 434–442.

Cohen, I. L., Bari, N., Strosberg, M. A. *et al.* (1991). Reduction of duration and cost of mechanical ventilation in an intensive care unit by use of a ventilatory management team. *Crit. Care Med.*, **19**, 1278–1284.

Cullen, D. J., Civetta, J. M., Briggs, B. A., Ferrara, L. C. (1974). Therapeutic Intervention Scoring System: a method of quantitative comparison of patient care. *Crit. Care Med.*, **2**, 57–60.

de Clercq, H., De Decker, G., Alexander, J. P., Huyghens, L. (1983). Cost evaluation of infections in intensive care. *Acta Anaesthesiol. Belg.*, **34**, 179–189.

Department of Health. (1989). *Working for Patients.* HMSO Publications Centre.

Diaz Molina, C., Garcia Martin, M., Bueno Cavanillas, A. *et al.* (1993). The estimation of the cost of nosocomial infection in an intensive care unit. *Med. Clin. (Barc.)*, **100**, 329–332.

Drummond, M. F., Stoddart, G. L., Torrance G. W. (1987). *Methods for the Economic Evaluation of Health Care Programmes*. Oxford University Press.

Edbrooke, D. L., Ridley, S. A., Hibbert, C. L., Corcoran, M. C. *et al.* (2001). Variations in expenditure between adult general intensive care units. *Anaesthesia*, **56**, 208–216.

Edbrooke, D. L., Wilson, A. J., Gerrish, S. P. *et al.* (1995). The Sheffield Costing System for Intensive Care. *Care Crit. Ill*, **11**, 106–110.

Edbrooke, D. L., Stevens, V. G., Hibbert, C. L. *et al.* (1997). A new method of accurately identifying the costs of individual patients in intensive care: the initial results. *Intensive Care Med.*, **23**, 645–650.

Edbrooke, D. L., Hibbert, C. L., Ridley, S. A. *et al.* (1999a). The development of a method for comparative costing of individual intensive care units. Intensive Care National Working Group on Costing. *Anaesthesia*, **54**, 110–120.

Edbrooke, D. L., Hibbert, C. L., Kingsley, J. M. *et al.* (1999b). The patient-related costs of sepsis patients in a UK adult general intensive care unit. *Crit. Care Med.*, **27**, 1760–1767.

Folland, S., Goodman, A. C., Stano, M. (1997). *The Economics of Health and Health Care*, 2nd edn. Prentice-Hall Inc.

Gapen, P. (1983). Intensive care units: they save lives, but physicians argue whether their high cost justifies use. *Am. Med. News*, **26**, 7–8.

Gilbertson, A. A., Smith, J. M., Mostafa, S. M. (1991). The cost of an intensive care unit: a prospective study. *Intensive Care Med.*, **17**, 204–208.

Glance, L. G., Osler, T., Shinozaki, T. (1998). Intensive care unit prognostic scoring systems to predict death: a cost-effectiveness analysis. *Crit. Care Med.*, **26**, 1842–1849.

Gyldmark, M. (1995). A review of cost studies of intensive care units: problems with the cost concept. *Crit. Care Med.*, **23**, 964–972.

Halpern, N. A., Bettes, L., Greenstein, R. (1994). Federal and nationwide intensive care units and health care costs: 1986–1992. *Crit. Care Med.*, **22**, 2201–2207.

Havill, J. H., Caspari, M., McConnell, H. *et al.* (1997). Charging for intensive care using direct nursing hours as the cost marker. *Anaesth. Intensive Care*, **25**, 372–377.

Heyland, D. K., Kernerman, P., Gafni, A. *et al.* (1996). Economic evaluations in the critical care literature: Do they help us improve the efficiency of our unit? *Crit.Care Med.*, **24**, 1591–1598.

Hibbert, C. L., Edbrooke, D. L., Corcoran, M. (1999). Is organ support the answer to costing care in the ICU? *Intensive Care Med.*, **25**, S170.

Holt, A. W., Bersten, A. D., Fuller, S. *et al.* (1994). Intensive care costing methodology: cost benefit analysis of mask continuous positive airway pressure for severe cardiogenic pulmonary oedema. *Anaesth. Intensive Care*, **22**, 170–174.

Jacobs, P., Noseworthy, T. W. (1990). National estimates of intensive care utilization and costs: Canada and United States. *Crit. Care Med.*, **18**, 1282–1286.

Jefferson, T., Demicheli, V., Mugford M. (2000). *Elementary Economic Evaluation in Health Care*, 2nd edn. BMJ Books, BMJ Publishing Group.

Keene, A. R., Cullen, D. J. (1983). Therapeutic Intervention Scoring System: Update 1983. *Crit. Care Med.*, **11**, 1–3.

Knaus, W. A. (1987). Too sick and old for intensive care. *Br. J. Hosp. Med.*, **37**, 381.

Loes, O., Smith-Erichsen, N., Lind, B. (1987). Intensive care: cost and benefit. *Acta Anaesthesiol. Scand.*, **84**, S3–19.

Martin, L. E. (1972). Cost and management: problems of intensive care units. *Mod. Hosp.*, **11**, 97–99.

McGuire, A., Henderson, J., Mooney, G. (1998). *The Economics of Health Care, an Introductory Text*. Routledge.

Medical Economics and Research Centre, Sheffield. (2000). *Cost Block Report.* Medical Economics and Research Centre.

Nedey, R. (1980). Attempted cost analysis for the intensive care service at the Hopital Foch carried out by the computer service. *Ann. Anesthesiol. Fr.*, **21**, 330–334.

Noseworthy, T. W., Konopad, E., Shustack, A. *et al.* (1996). Cost accounting of adult intensive care: methods and human and capital inputs. *Crit. Care Med.*, **24**, 1168–1172.

Organisation for Economic Cooperation and Development. (1989). *Health Care Expenditure and Other Data: an International Compendium from the OECD. Health care financing review 1989. Annual Supplement* pp 111–194, Organisation for Economic Cooperation and Development.

Patrick, D. L., Erickson, P. (1996). Applications of health status assessment to health policy. In: *Quality of Life and Pharmacoeconomics in Clinical Trials*, 2nd edn. (B. Spilker, ed.) pp 717–727, Lippincott-Raven.

Phillips, G. D. (1977). Life support systems in intensive care: a review of history, ethics, cost, benefit and rational use. *Anaesth. Intensive Care*, **5**, 251–257.

Reis Miranda, D. (1986). ICUs in Europe. In*: The ICU, a cost-benefit analysis* (D. Reis Miranda, D. Langrehr, eds). International Congress Series No. 709. Excerpta Medica.

Reis Miranda, D., de Rijk, A., Schaufeli, W. (1996). Simplified Therapeutic Intervention Scoring System: the TISS–28 items-results from a multicenter study. *Crit. Care Med.*, **24**, 64–73.

Ridley, S., Biggam, M., Stone, P. (1991). Cost of intensive therapy: A description of methodology and initial results. *Anaesthesia*, **46**, 523–530.

Ridley, S., Biggam, M., Stone. P. (1993). A cost-benefit analysis of intensive therapy. *Anaesthesia*, **48**, 14–19.

Rittenhouse, B. (1996). Designing and conducting cost-minimization and cost-effectiveness analyses. In: *Quality of Life and Pharmacoeconomics in Clinical Trials*, 2nd edn. (B. Spilker, ed.) pp 1093–1105, Lippincott-Raven.

Royal College of Anaesthetists and Royal College of Surgeons. (1996). *Report of the Joint Working Party on Graduated Patient Care.* Royal College of Anaesthetists and Royal College of Surgeons.

Rubenfeld, G. D. (1998). Cost-effectiveness considerations in critical care. *New Horiz.*, **6**, 33–40.

Schapira, D. V., Studnicki, J., Bradham, D. D. *et al.* (1993). Intensive care, survival, and expense of treating critically ill cancer patients. *JAMA*, **269**, 783–786.

Singer, M., Myers, S., Hall, G. *et al.* (1994). The cost of intensive care: a comparison on one unit between 1988 and 1991. *Intensive Care Med.*, **20**, 542–549.

Slatyer, M. A., James, O. F., Moore, P. G., Leeder, S. R. (1986). Costs, severity of illness and outcome in intensive care. *Anaesth. Intensive Care*, **14**, 381–389.

Stevens, V. G., Hibbert, C. L., Edbrooke, D. L. (1998). Evaluation of proposed case-mix criteria as a basis for costing patients in the adult general intensive care unit. *Anaesthesia*, **53**, 944–950.

Swart, E. L., van Schijndel, R. J., van Loenen, A. C., Thijs, L. G. (1999). Continuous infusion of lorazepam versus midazolam in patients in the intensive care unit: sedation with lorazepam is easier to manage and is more cost-effective. *Crit. Care Med.*, **27**, 1461–1465.

Sznajder, M., Leleu, G., Buonamico, G. *et al.* (1998). Estimation of direct cost and resource allocation in intensive care: correlation with Omega system. *Intensive Care Med.*, **24**, 582–589.

Torrance, G. W. (1996). Designing and conducting cost-utility analyses. In: *Quality of Life and Pharmacoeconomics in Clinical Trials*, 2nd edn. (B. Spilker, ed.) pp 1105–1111, Lippincott-Raven.

Wachter, R. M., Luce, J. M., Safrin, S. *et al.* (1995). Cost and outcome of intensive care for patients with AIDS, Pneumocystis carinii pneumonia, and severe respiratory failure. *JAMA*, **273**, 230–235.

Wagner, D. P., Wineland, T. D., Knaus, W. A. (1983). The hidden costs of treating severely ill patients: Charges and resource consumption in an intensive care unit. *Health Care Financ. Rev.*, **5**, 81–86.

Chapter 11

Ethics issues in critical care outcome

Malcolm Booth

Introduction

Intensive care is becoming ever more complex and expensive. Our ability to keep a patient alive in the face of a poor prognosis now exceeds all previous expectations. However, the cost of intensive care is enormous and a number of patients admitted to intensive care will have no chance of recovery. Ideally, these patients should be identified prior to their admission to intensive care. This requires methods of predicting intensive care outcome for different groups of patients with varying disease processes and co-morbidities.

The collection and interpretation of data to facilitate outcome prediction in the critically ill has been discussed in previous chapters. There are, however, a number of ethical issues pertaining to the use of prognostic scoring systems, especially when they may affect not only how, but also which, patients are treated. Before discussing these it would be useful to review the main principles of medical ethics and how they guide our actions.

Principles of medical ethics

Medical ethics is a set of moral principles that doctors and other healthcare professionals use to guide their actions. These principles also underpin our actions in society in general.

There are two main schools of philosophical thought. The first is utilitarianism, which aims to maximize good, while the second is deontology where one acts in accordance with perceived duties. Although often conflicting, these principles can be unified using the four principles of medical ethics described by

Table 11.1 Principles of medical ethics

- Autonomy
  The principle of self-rule or self-determination

- Non-maleficence
  'primum non nocere' – first do no harm

- Beneficence
  Attempt to benefit one's patients

- Justice
  The fair and equitable distribution of healthcare resources

---

Beauchamp and Childress (1989). These principles are respect for autonomy, non-maleficence, beneficence and justice (Table 11.1).

The principle of respect for autonomy

Autonomy is self-rule and entails an individual having control over his or her life, free from outside influence. The principle of respect for autonomy developed during the latter half of the twentieth century with the advance of various rights movements. In medicine, autonomy applies primarily, but not exclusively, to the right to consent to or refuse any medical intervention. With the right to act autonomously comes the responsibility not to act in a way that would conflict with the autonomy of another. Therefore, and most importantly, an autonomous patient cannot demand treatment that an autonomous doctor does not consider indicated (Brett and McCullough, 1986; Luce, 1995).

The requirement that autonomous actions be free from the undue influence or control of others would appear to preclude any form of authority being allowed to influence an individual's thoughts or actions. This is not strictly true. Provided that the person freely accepts an authority's powers as legitimate and chooses to act in accordance with rules or regulations laid down by that authority, then the individual would still be seen to be acting autonomously. Thus a patient may say 'doctor, do what you think necessary' and, provided this was done willingly and without coercion, this is an autonomous decision. A second oft-quoted example is a Jehovah's Witness who chooses to follow his church's teaching precluding the administration of blood or blood products. Such individuals make an autonomous decision not to accept blood products even if this results in complications or death.

In order to make an autonomous decision, however, the individual must receive the necessary information required to make that decision. It must also be presented in such a way that the patient can comprehend, assimilate and interpret. Interestingly, it is usually only when a person refuses recommended treatment that the patient's competence to make decisions is questioned; rarely does a doctor question a person's ability to consent to suggested therapy.

Information describing potential outcomes is exactly the sort of data required for making decisions about treatment including critical care. When deciding to undergo any proposed therapy regimen, the benefits need to be weighed against the possible burdens involved including the long-term consequences.

Non-maleficence and beneficence

Non-maleficence is summed up by the phrase 'primum non nocere' – first do no harm. Despite appearing an intuitively simple maxim to follow, it can be difficult to know when harm may occur. Indeed every medical intervention involves some element of risk. With the drive for evidence-based medicine, more clinical practice is becoming 'evidence led' and this should help eliminate ineffective therapies and reduce the risk of harm occurring.

Conversely, beneficence is the duty to attempt to do good and benefit one's patients. Although initially appearing to be similar to non-maleficence, beneficence is a distinct and separate obligation. Beauchamp and Childress (1989) distinguish the two principles by separating them into four hierarchical elements:

Non-maleficence:
1. One ought not to inflict evil or harm

Beneficence:
2. One ought to prevent evil or harm
3. One ought to remove evil or harm
4. One ought to do or promote good.

While the three elements of beneficence entail positive actions (i.e. preventing or removing harm and promoting good), non-maleficence requires avoiding a negative action (i.e. inflicting harm). Arranged in this way it is easy to see that the first element (non-maleficence) takes moral precedence over the others (beneficence).

Justice

Justice in healthcare implies the fair distribution of resources, according to need and to those most able to benefit from them. But what is fair? In an ideal world the resources would be available so that everyone could receive the healthcare that they need. Unfortunately, this does not describe most healthcare systems in the 21st century. Resources are finite and therefore some method of distributing these justly is of paramount importance.

The doctor's obligation to society at large is to use the scarce health resources justly and fairly. This includes an obligation not to squander resources. Assessing the efficacy of treatment and using only that which has evidence to support its effectiveness is one way to use resources efficiently. Consequently, evidence-based medicine is an expanding discipline, guiding many areas of medicine.

Evidence-based medicine

In recent years there has been an explosion in the use of evidence-based medicine where, ideally, care decisions are based on the 'conscientious, explicit and judicious use of current best evidence' (Sackett *et al.*, 1996). Properly applied evidence-based medicine should help underpin the ethical principles discussed above. Evidence-based decision making supports the clinician's obligation to be honest with patients about treatments, risks and prognoses. Sharing such information with the patient empowers the patient to reach a well informed, autonomous decision. Using evidence-based medicine should also ensure that risks are minimized (non-maleficence), the potential for benefit maximized (beneficence) and the principle of justice upheld by concentrating resources on effective therapies.

Prognostic scoring systems with the emphasis on outcome are forms of evidence-based medicine. By measuring physiological disturbance, patients can be grouped according to severity of illness and then treatments compared. This helps in deciding if new evidence about treatment efficacy is applicable to present patients. The fact that these scoring systems address groups of patients and generally cannot be applied to the individual must always be remembered.

A criticism is that, although evidence-based medicine claims to reject the influence of the 'expert opinion' and attempts objectively to assess the evidence from research and trials, it is still the experts who determine the research objectives, interpret the results and implement the findings. There is a need for the other stakeholders, such as patient groups, to be encouraged to influence the research priorities (Kerridge *et al.*, 1998).

Medical decision making involves much more than purely scientific factors. Personal experiences, values and biases affect the decision making process along with local, national, political and economic pressures. Ethical considerations must also be included. Exactly how all these factors are integrated into the final decision making process is unclear. Because many are difficult to quantify, it would be virtually impossible to include them all in some form of evidence-based decision making model. The ability to integrate all these factors depends largely on the physician's skill and clinical judgement.

Clinical judgement and outcome scoring

The role of the doctor is to apply his knowledge and experience to interpret medical history, clinical examination and investigations to arrive at a diagnosis. Based on this, a treatment schedule can then be recommended together with a probable prognosis. This process is partly scientific, supported by the knowledge base available, and partly an art of interpreting that particular patient's signs and symptoms.

Presenting an accurate prognosis helps a patient to decide whether the burdens and discomforts of treatment are worth enduring. This becomes all the more important as the burdens increase and the probable benefits decline. For every patient there will come a point at which any benefit is overshadowed by the risks or outcome associated with the intervention. Prognostic scoring systems can aid clinical judgement by objectively assessing the probability of survival. They can provide a quantitative method to enhance clinical judgement but it should be remembered that any outcome score applies to a population of patients and not to any one individual. Although the scoring system will calculate a score and predicted outcome, what the patient really wants to know is what will his or her outcome actually be! Answering this honestly requires experience and judgement in order to interpret all the facts, not just the prognostic score.

The question as to whether it is ethical to use outcome scoring to aid making clinical decisions is easily answered. If it is ethical for a doctor to use his clinical judgement when making a decision and a prognostic scoring system can assist this process (in a similar way to laboratory or radiological investigations) then it is appropriate to make use of it. The important issue is not whether outcome prediction should assist medical decision making but how accurate the prediction of survival or death is in practice.

Limitations of scoring systems

Severity of illness models calculate an estimated hospital mortality for a critically ill patient and have now become indispensable in clinical practice in several ways. They compare outcomes of intensive care units (ICUs) with differing patient populations; examples include audit such as those undertaken by Intensive Care National Audit and Research Centre and the Scottish Intensive Care Audit Group. They also provide severity of illness measures for intensive care research. One of the most widely used scores is the APACHE (Acute Physiologic And Chronic Health Evaluation) system, which calculates a severity of illness score and predicted mortality (Knaus *et al.*, 1985). However, just how well do the outcome prediction models compare to the clinical judgement of the experienced clinician?

The APACHE II score has been rigorously assessed since its inception and has been shown to be accurate when applied to patient populations. Clinicians, however, are better at predicting the outcome of individual patients (Brannen *et al.*, 1989; McClish and Powell, 1989; Marks *et al.*, 1991). This is perhaps not surprising as a scoring system is developed on current knowledge over a relatively short time frame. In contrast, the knowledge and experience of a clinician evolves continuously. Indeed, major changes in treatment may make it necessary to adapt and retest a scoring system to maintain accuracy (Zoch *et al.*,

1992). Another limitation of all scoring systems, including the APACHE II system, is that they are developed on a particular patient population that may or may not resemble the local intensive care population. Thus its applicability to individual ICUs has to be assessed and on occasion some re-calibration undertaken (Patel and Grant, 1999; Livingston et al., 2000).

Scoring systems such as the APACHE II are static systems that take a snapshot of the first 24 h of ICU stay to predict outcome. Critical illness and the associated intensive care is a dynamic process with the disease process evolving, possibly over days, and the intensive care management responding accordingly. The onset of new organ failures, such as acute renal failure, can have a major effect on the probable outcome and this may be completely missed by a single point scoring system applied at, or shortly after, admission. The other limitation already alluded to is the need for an accurate diagnosis to allow the APACHE II risk of death to be estimated. Often the primary diagnosis is unclear; for example, is cardiovascular failure a consequence of pneumonia or a predisposing factor in developing a pneumonia?

Theoretically, dynamic scoring systems should adjust the outcome prediction over time with changes in the severity of the critical illness and more accurately predict the prognosis for an individual patient. The Riyadh Intensive Care Program (Table 11.2) is a predictive model that uses trends in daily analysis of organ failure scores (Chang et al., 1989).

The purpose of the program is to predict which patients will not survive intensive care and so assist in the clinical decision to withdraw life support. When assessed in the hospital where it was developed, the Riyadh Intensive Care Program performed very well. The predictions were superior to those made by the doctors and there were no false positive predictions (predicting death in a patient who ultimately survived). False positive predictions are dangerous as they could lead to the inappropriate withdrawal of support and potentially the avoidable death of a patient. In the original study by Chang, doctors and nurses incorrectly predicted death in 9 to 16% of cases. In another study of 617 critically ill patients, 119 were predicted to die of whom 24 recovered sufficiently to be discharged home. This is a false positive rate of 5.2%, which is probably unacceptable (Hope and Plenderleith, 1995). Whether the false positive rate might improve if the algorithm used could be modified to the local hospital population is unknown. Assessing the accuracy of clinician judgement cannot be determined because once the decision to alter the aims of intensive care is made and acted upon, the predicted death almost certainly follows.

Futility prediction

Every severity of illness model has a score above which survival is unprecedented and inevitably a number of patients who cannot survive will be identified. For these patients continuing treatment could be deemed futile. Using

Table 11.2 Riyadh Intensive Care Program algorithm

Daily trend analysis using organ failure scores (OFS)
OFS = APACHE II × (1 + organ failure coefficient)
$Score_n$ = OSF on day n

Organ failure coefficients

Days of failure	1 organ	2 organs	≥3 organs
1	0.022	0.052	0.080
2	0.031	0.067	0.095
3	0.034	0.066	0.093
4	0.035	0.062	0.096
5	0.040	0.056	0.1
6	0.042	0.064	0.1
≥7	0.041	0.68	0.1

Patients were predicted to die if:

1 $score_1$ > 35
2 $score_1$ > 31 ≤ 35 and on day 2 $score_1$ − $score_2$ ≤ 2
3 $score_n$ increased by > 2.5 over the previous day and absolute score > 27
4 those who deteriorated gradually increasing their score by only 1 or 2 points per day if $score_n$ > 35

Modified from Chang, R. W. S., Lee, B., Jacobs, S., Lee, B. (1989). Accuracy of decisions to withdraw therapy in critically ill patients: clinical judgement versus a computer model. *Crit. Care Med.*, **17**, 1091–1097

scoring systems as the sole guide to deciding if further support or treatment is futile is currently unacceptable (Danis *et al.*, 1997). Most importantly, the patient's values and realistic treatment goals must be considered in any decision. For example, continuing to support a patient with metastatic colonic carcinoma who develops respiratory failure would seem futile from the purely pathological viewpoint. However, the patient may have very good reasons, such as the opportunity to say goodbye to family and friends, to want a brief period of intensive care support.

Futility is a difficult concept that must be broached with caution as once a treatment limiting decision is made it is highly likely that the patient will succumb. There is a danger that the diagnosis of futility becomes a self-fulfilling prophecy. There is also the danger of stifling progress. Consciously, or not, once treatment is considered futile the doctor may feel under pressure because of lack of resources, economic constraints or managerial demands to discontinue treatment and maintain comfort measures only. It is only by revisiting what is considered futile that progress can be made as medicine advances.

Public fears concerning futility

Modern medicine has transformed the common perception of death from a biological and natural event into a sign of failure. The family of a deceased patient often shares this view. The public concept of what medicine can actually achieve is often woefully optimistic. This is partly the fault of a profession that over the last 40 years has encouraged the belief that medical technology can conquer all disease. The public perception of medicine also stems from its portrayal in the media. Medical dramas make compulsive viewing for some and they influence the public understanding of what medicine can achieve. Their accuracy, especially around end of life events such as cardiac arrest, is highly questionable.

Diem and colleagues (1996) reviewed the outcome of victims following cardiac arrest on American medical dramas (most of which are also popular in the UK) and found that 75% survived the immediate arrest and 67% left hospital. Compared to reality, where survival is at best 27%, this is unrealistically optimistic and may influence expectations amongst the public (Parish *et al.*, 1999). A similar study based on UK medical dramas found the overall success rate slightly more realistic (Gordon *et al.*, 1998). Based on these findings, it is not suprising that patients and their families are often dismayed when confronted by the limitations of modern medicine.

The pronouncement that further treatment is futile will be profoundly traumatic for a patient and family. Until that moment the fact that treatment continues suggests that there is still some, albeit remote, hope. Doctors are fallible and make mistakes including those estimating prognosis. How sure can the family be that treatment is really futile? After all, doctors cannot say recovery will never happen, just that the possibility is so remote that to continue would be futile. Such concerns can only be overcome by good communication between all parties involved.

The patient or family may also question whether the motives behind the decision that further treatment is futile are purely clinical. Everyone is aware of the current financial constraints affecting healthcare provision. Is the treatment being withheld or stopped for purely financial reasons? In the case of Child B, a second bone marrow transplantation after the first failed was refused funding on the basis that prognosis was so poor that the costs (physical and financial) outweighed any benefit. The Court of Appeal eventually upheld this view. In this case, the courts took the view that resources are finite and that they have to be distributed responsibly. This obligation includes not spending time and money on therapy which clinicians perceive as ineffective (Ham, 1999).

Is intensive care being withheld or withdrawn in order to save money? While it is irresponsible to waste resources, only small savings would be generated by withholding or withdrawing futile care. In the USA, 27–30% of annual Medicare costs are expended on the 5–6% of patients who die that year. This equals $13 316 per person for those that die, compared to $1924 for survivors, giving a ratio of healthcare dollars of 6.9:1 in favour of those that die. Over 40% of costs are incurred in the last month of life. However, it has been estimated that encouraging the use of advance directives to limit heroic and ineffective interventions would save only 3.3% of total costs (Emmanuel and Emmanuel, 1994).

Another study from the USA of financial savings made by withdrawing treatment from those cases deemed futile suggests little reduction in costs. The definition of futility, defined as the chances of 2 months survival being less than 1%, was fulfilled by 115 of 4302 patients in the study. A total of $224 M was spent, with the futile group costing $8.9 M. Stopping treatment when futility was first recognized would only have saved $1.08 M or 0.48% of the total (Capron, 1994). A similar study in the UK produced comparable results (Atkinson et al., 1994).

Is intensive care being stopped to enable another patient, considered more deserving, to be treated instead? Again the evidence would not appear to support this contention. When surveyed about reasons to withhold or withdraw therapy, intensive care specialists put 'irreversibility of the acute process' and 'patient unlikely to survive hospital' as the most important reasons. The possibility of other patients being more likely to benefit and that finite resources existed were ranked 14th and 16th respectively (McLean and Booth, 1998).

Predicting morbidity

Mere physiological survival is not the only outcome of importance to the critically ill patient, their families and carers. Intensive care is burdensome, undignified and often unpleasant, so the potential quality of life afterwards is of crucial importance. Undoubtedly the degree of remaining disability each individual is willing to accept in order to survive will vary enormously. Predictive scoring systems, by and large, do not anticipate the quality of a survivor's life but merely group patients into survivors and non-survivors.

The failure of most outcome scoring systems to predict morbidity arises because they are designed for heterogeneous patient populations. The Glasgow outcome score (GOS), however, was designed specifically to predict the sequelae of head injuries and classifies survivors according to social outcome and their requirement for social support (Jennett and Bond, 1975). Even so, in a recent study of mild head injuries, it still failed to predict accurately moderate dysfunction in approximately a third of survivors (Thornhill et al., 2000).

When the incompetent patient cannot be questioned, deciding what quality of life would be acceptable to the patient is, at best, guesswork. While the relatives may give some insight into the views of the patient there is no evidence that they can accurately predict what the patient would actually desire. Their capacity to predict the wishes of the patient may be tempered by conflicting emotions. Feelings of guilt about treatment being stopped may result in an insistence that it be continued for far longer than the patient would have found acceptable. Alternatively, they may underestimate what disability the patient would accept to survive in a desire to avoid inflicting further suffering. Some record of patients' wishes, should they become incompetent, would be useful.

Advance directives

Central to the principle of respecting autonomy is that a person is able to make healthcare decisions for himself. A person may grant or withhold consent for treatment or even decide at some point that they do not wish to continue with a course of therapy. Many of the patients in the ICU are mentally incompetent, either as a consequence of their illness or its treatment, and therefore lack decision making capacity. Unlike the USA where legal proxies may act on behalf of the incompetent individual, in the UK no one has such authority. In Scotland this changed in 2001 when the Adults with Incapacity (Scotland) Act introduced the reality of consent by proxy. One way a patient may prepare for such an eventuality, and so retain autonomy, is to prepare an advance directive (Table 11.3).

An advance directive or 'living will' documents a patient's wishes and treatment preferences in the event of becoming incompetent in the future and are probably most widely known for setting limits on the treatments likely to be instituted. Kutner (1969) proposed the concept in 1969, as a mechanism of the patient protecting himself from unwanted aggressive life-sustaining treatment. Initially advance directives were envisaged as being of most use to people with chronic debilitating diseases, such as senile dementia. Preparing an advance directive would enable the individual to influence treatment decisions even once incompetent. The most common example of an advance directive is the card carried by many Jehovah's Witnesses stating their refusal of blood or blood products.

The use of advance directives is supported, even encouraged, by a number of charities campaigning and caring for people with chronic debilitating diseases. Singer (1994) has even suggested developing disease specific advance directives for those with chronic disease. The major advantage in preparing an advance directive is that the writer retains control even when incompetent; such directives support the principle of autonomy and self-determination. Knowing the wishes of the patient helps the doctor avoid undesired treatments and introduce only those that would be acceptable. In this way an advance directive may be seen to support all the principles of medical ethics outlined above. Advance directives have also been supported by most major religions. However, some individuals regard life as sacrosanct and object on the grounds that it is not for the person but God to decide when life should end.

Advance directives are still uncommon in the UK, which is in contrast to the USA where the Patient Self-Determination Act 1991 obliges all hospitals to explain to patients their right to write a living will and refuse treatment. The Act also made complying with the directive mandatory subject to state law. In the UK there is no specific legislation dealing with advance directives but their legal authority has recently become clearer. In Re C (1994), the court upheld as competent the decision of a man diagnosed with paranoid schizophrenia to refuse, when he was lucid, life-saving surgery now and in the future. The right of a Jehovah's Witness to refuse blood has also been supported (Re T, 1993) and most recently the right of a woman to refuse medical intervention even if that

Table 11.3 An example of an advanced directive

To my family, my doctor and my solicitor

This declaration is made by me _____
(full name and address)

at a time when I am of sound mind and after careful consideration

I the said _____ in the event of my being unable to take part in decisions concerning my medical care due to my physical or mental incapacity, and in the event that I develop one or more of the medical conditions listed in clause (3) below and in the event that two independent physicians conclude that there is no reasonable prospect of my making a substantial recovery, do hereby **declare** that my wishes are as follows:

(1) I request that my life shall not be sustained by artificial means such as: life support systems, intravenous fluids and/or drugs, intravenous or tube feeding.
(2) I request that distressing symptoms caused by either the illness or by lack of food or fluid should be controlled by appropriate sedative treatment even though such treatment may have the incidental and secondary effect of shortening my life.
(3) The said medical conditions are:
  1. Severe and lasting brain damage sustained as a result of accident or injury.
  2. Advanced disseminated malignant disease.
  3. Advanced degenerative disease of the nervous and/or muscular systems with severe limitations of independent mobility, and no satisfactory response to treatment.
  4. Stroke with extensive persisting paralysis.
  5. Pre-senile, senile or Alzheimer type dementia.
  6. Other conditions of comparable gravity.
(4) I request that, in the event of my becoming incapable of giving or withholding consent to any medical treatment or procedures proposed to me, the Court of Session be petitioned to appoint as my proxy the following person: _____
  whom failing:
  _____
  whom failing: such person as deemed by the Court to be a fit person. It is my specific request that in exercising his or her powers to consent or withhold consent on my behalf to any medical treatment or procedures, my tutor shall take into account, in any determination of what is my best interests, the requests laid out in clauses (1) and (2) of this document.

And I declare that I hereby absolve my medical attendants of all legal liability arising from action taken in response to and in terms of this declaration.

I reserve the right to revoke this declaration at any time, before witnesses, in writing or orally.

_____   _____   _____
(Signature)   (Town/Place)   (Day/Month/Year)

Clause (4) refers to the appointment of a tutor – who has the power under Scots law to make decisions relating to the person of an incapax. During 2001 the Adults with Incapacity (Scotland) Bill will recognise the use of a proxy to act on behalf of the incapax.

From Mason, J. K., McCall Smith, R. A. (1994). *Law and Medical Ethics* (4th edn), pp 439–440, Butterworths refusal put the life of her fetus at risk as well as her own (St George's Healthcare NHS Trust v S, 1998). These appear to demonstrate the law's desire to support the individual's right to self-determination even once incompetent.

There are potential limitations to the value of an advance directive, not least the information and instructions contained within it. Some are written in such a general manner as to be of little use in determining the person's wishes, while others are so restrictive that they could potentially act against the patient. An oft-quoted example is a patient's advance directive declining renal dialysis. This could be interpreted as even excluding short-term renal support needed during a period of reversible renal failure such as may occur during critical illness.

The durability of an opinion expressed in the advance directive is a concern. Will the patient still hold the same opinion when the envisaged set of circumstances occurs? Lord Goff stated 'the same principle (respect of a patient's wishes) applies where the patient's refusal to give his consent has been expressed at an earlier date, before he became unconscious or otherwise incapable of communicating it; though in such circumstances special care may be necessary to ensure that the prior refusal of consent is still properly to be regarded as applicable in the circumstances which have subsequently occurred' (Airedale NHS Trust v Bland, 1993). This introduces the problem of how a clinician is to know if the directive still applies in the current circumstances. He or she cannot question the patient as to what they wish. Providing some effort is made to speak to relatives or the general practitioner and the doctor acts in good faith then little criticism can be levelled. Conversely, clinicians choosing, even with the best intentions, to go against the patient's wishes as laid out in the advance directive, have been found guilty of assault (Malette v Shulman, 1990).

Incorporating a life values statement into the advance directive could reduce the problem of deciding if the circumstances envisaged have occurred (Table 11.4). Rather than specifying what treatments are acceptable, a life values statement describes the quality of life that the person would accept as a result of surviving the illness. Thus, depending on the expected outcome, a particular therapy might be appropriate under one set of circumstances but not another.

Several hurdles have arisen in relation to implementing advance directives in the USA. Knowing of the directive's existence and its whereabouts are probably the most important of these. The anger and anxiety resulting from ignoring an advance directive are well described by a physician whose mother suffered needlessly when her advance directive was not invoked (Hansot, 1996). This problem has been addressed in Denmark where a Living Will Register has been established. Its success has been limited because the register is not reliably consulted to ascertain whether a patient has lodged a directive (Dolley, 1993).

A number of organizations now publish advance directive forms and guidance on their use. Some of the most useful are produced by the Voluntary Euthanasia Society and the Terence Higgins Trust. The Voluntary Euthanasia Society of Scotland, which advocates a life values guided statement, publishes its directive on the internet (www.euthanasia.org/vh.html). The British Medical Association has published a Code of Practice to advise doctors and the public on drawing up and implementing advance directives

Table 11.4 Example of a life values statement of the type sometimes used in advance directives to help guide decision making

Circle the number on the scale of one to five that most closely indicates your feelings about each of the situations described.	Much worse than death: I would definitely not want life sustaining treatment	Somewhat worse than death: I would probably not want life sustaining treatment	Neither better nor worse than death: I'm not sure whether I want life sustaining treatment	Somewhat better than death: I would probably want life sustaining treatment	Much better than death: I would definitely want life sustaining treatment
(a) Permanently paralysed. You are unable to walk but can move around in a wheelchair. You can talk and interact with other people.	1	2	3	4	5
(b) Permanently unable to speak meaningfully. You are unable to speak to others. You can walk on your own, feed yourself and take care of daily needs such as bathing and dressing yourself.	1	2	3	4	5
(c) Completely unable to care for yourself. You are bedridden, unable to wash, feed or dress yourself. You are totally cared for by others.	1	2	3	4	5
(d) Permanently in pain. You are in severe bodily pain that cannot be totally controlled or completely eliminated by medications.	1	2	3	4	5
(e) Permanently mildly demented. You often cannot remember things, such as where you are, not reason clearly. You are capable of speaking, but not capable of remembering the conversations; you are capable of washing, feeding and dressing yourself and are in no pain.	1	2	3	4	5
(f) Being in a short-term coma. You have suffered brain damage and are not conscious and are not aware of your environment in any way. You cannot feel pain. You are cared for by others. These mental impairments may be reversed in about 1 week leaving mild forgetfulness and loss of memory as a consequence.	1	2	3	4	5

Reproduced with permission © 1996 from a *Living Will document* by C. G. Docker, Living Will and Values History project, BM 718 London WC1N 3XX (all rights reserved)

(web.bma.org.uk/ethics.nsf.webguidelines?openview). It emphasizes that in order for the statement to have maximal authority then:

1. the signatory must be competent and understand the implications of the document
2. the directive needs to be signed
3. the document must be available when required.

Despite all the emotion that living wills may invoke, many people still have no knowledge of them. A recent study found that a majority of elderly people (a group of potential beneficiaries of advance directives) had not heard of them. However, most would be interested in preparing one (Schiff *et al.*, 2000). Interestingly 92% of study participants indicated that they would not want their lives prolonged by medical interventions. Over half those indicating an interest in preparing an advance directive felt it would allow their views to be known and remove the responsibility for decision making from their family.

When faced with an incompetent patient the only alternative method of discovering their opinion about treatment is to speak with family or close friends. This allows a substituted judgement to be made on behalf of the patient. Unfortunately, few people discuss end of life issues, either within the family or with their family doctor. The accuracy of substituted judgements is open to question. Seckler *et al.* (1991) found an accuracy rate of 58 to 81% when investigating patient preferences, surrogates' predictions and the extent of agreement between the two. This research was performed before the Self-determination Act was passed and interestingly 7 years later little had changed with surrogates' average accuracy remaining at 66% (Sulmasy *et al.*, 1998).

The role of ethics committees

Several professional bodies such as the British Medical Association Ethics Committee, General Medical Council, various Royal Colleges and the Nuffield Council on Bioethics give guidance on healthcare ethical issues. Ethics committees in UK hospitals are largely Local Research Ethics Committees (LRECs) and are limited to a role in reviewing research applications. Unlike the situation in the USA, they have no role in the resolution of ethical conflicts. Since the 1970s clinical ethics consultation committees have been an integral part of many US institutions. Their role is to assist staff, residents and families with the resolution of ethical concerns and typically engage in policy review and development, case review and education (Chichin and Olsen, 1995).

The situation in the UK is slowly changing with clinical, as opposed to research, ethics committees developing in a number of trusts (Slowther and Hope, 2000). There are several reasons for this. Medical ethics is now part of the core medical curriculum. Ethical issues often receive a high profile in the media (Phillips, 2000) and clinical governance will, undoubtedly, have to include an ethics component. Clinical ethics support is also developing in other countries, either as part of the research ethics committee or as a separate entity (Macneill *et al.*, 1994). To date there have been no rigorous evaluations of the value or effectiveness of these committees in resolving ethical conflicts, even in the USA. Their effectiveness will need to be demonstrated if the time and effort of running a committee is to be justified.

Futile therapy – treating the patient and the family

The advances made by medicine since the inception of intensive care medicine have been staggering. It is now possible with better resuscitation, greater understanding of the disease processes and more invasive monitoring and support to keep people alive when previously they would certainly have died. Unfortunately, in some circumstances life may be supported artificially for prolonged periods without any realistic hope of recovery. If the re-establishing of a person's autonomy and quality of life is the primary function of medicine then it must be accepted that prolongation of life does not mean a mere suspension of the act of dying, but contemplates, at the very least, a remission of symptoms enabling a return towards a normal, functioning integrated existence. There often comes a point at which it is necessary for physicians, nurses and relatives to face the difficult question of when to stop life-sustaining therapy for someone who cannot recover.

The critically ill patient is exposed to both the benefits and potential side effects of therapy. When the negative aspects outweigh any possible benefit the competent patient is at liberty to decide that his current or expected quality of life is unacceptable and may, therefore, decide to refuse further interventions, even if this results in death. Elizabeth Bouvia exemplified this when a Californian court upheld her decision to refuse nutritional support imposed by her physicians. The court ruled that feeding could be stopped as Bouvia had a right to refuse life-sustaining therapy and that 'no criminal or civil liability attaches to honouring a competent informed patient's refusal of medical treatment' (Bouvia v Superior Court, 1986). Courts in the UK have also upheld this principle. Lord Scarman called the right of a patient to make his own decision concerning treatment 'a basic human right protected by the common law' (Sidaway v Board of Bethlem Royal Hospital). The competent patient has the right and the ability to refuse potentially life-saving therapy should he or she so wish. The incompetent patient also has this right but has no method by which to exercise it.

When intensive care is unable to alleviate the underlying disease process, the needs of the patient change. It is not unusual for patients or their family to request that active treatment be stopped and only comfort measures be continued. Assessing that treatment has become futile requires frequent reappraisal of the patient and the response to therapy. The diagnosis may become obvious quite quickly, for example during the resuscitation of a cardiac arrest victim, or more slowly over days or weeks. Once the clinician considers that recovery is not possible and death inevitable then his or her duties change, from those of aggressive therapy with the intention to cure, to providing comfort care and minimizing discomfort.

Defining what is futile therapy has been the cause of much discussion and confusion. Simply stating that futile therapy is therapy that is 'never successful' has been extremely difficult as doctors are, in general, unhappy to use the word 'never'. Schneiderman and Jecker (1995) suggested an alternative definition whereby a treatment would be considered futile if it had not worked in the last 100 cases, or if it failed to restore consciousness or alleviate total dependence on intensive care support.

The obvious limitation with this definition is the requirement to have experience of 100 similar cases; this may not be possible because of the heterogeneous nature of critical illness. An alternative definition is that treatment is futile when it 'cannot within a reasonable probability cure, ameliorate, improve, or restore a quality of life that would be satisfactory to the patient' (Quinn, 1994). Using this definition, treatment that is extremely unlikely to benefit the patient, extremely costly (both to the patient and society) or of marginal benefit might be considered inappropriate and hence inadvisable and so could be withheld or withdrawn (Parish *et al.*, 1999).

There are few patient groups that fulfil the criteria of futility in advance of their admission to intensive care. One such group might be those with haematological malignancy developing multiple organ failure. Well designed prospective studies have demonstrated a survival of less than 1% even in centres treating large numbers of these patients (Rubenfeld and Crawford, 1996). The limited ability of outcome scoring systems to identify those patients who will not survive intensive care support has already been alluded to. It is more usual for the diagnosis of futility to develop over time as the disease process evolves and fails to respond to therapy.

Recognizing and accepting that therapy, in a particular instance, is futile has three important benefits:

1. Stopping otherwise distressing treatment when all hope of benefit has gone permits pain and suffering to be minimized. This is simple humanity.
2. Recognizing futility allows patients and their family to come to terms with the fact. This may allow the patient to prepare themselves and their affairs.
3. The principle of justice requires that resources are not squandered on those unable to benefit from them.

The moral basis of the doctor–patient relationship is the doctor's obligation to attempt to do the patient some good. Any action that does not contribute to this is not morally required. This was addressed in the case of Bland, a victim of the Hillsborough disaster who survived in a persistent vegetative state and whose family wanted treatment, in the form of continued nutrition and hydration, stopped so that he could be allowed to die. In the context of the incompetent patient, the doctor's licence to treat that person is based upon an obligation to act in the patient's 'best interests'. When treatment is no longer in the best interests of the patient the licence to continue treatment ends and such care must cease (Airedale NHS Trust v Bland, 1993).

Rather than viewing the diagnosis of futility nihilistically, it is important to accept that some patients are unable to recover. 'To presume that the incompetent person must always be subjected to what many rational and intelligent persons may decline, is to downgrade the status of the incompetent person by placing a lesser value on his intrinsic worth and vitality . . .' (Belchertown State School Superintendent v Saikewicz, 1997). The crux of the issue is that death or total dependence on intensive care support is inevitable even if maximal treatment is continued.

The decision that further active therapy is not in the interests of the patient is just the beginning of the final phase of care. The quality of end-of-life care, as it is termed, is becoming recognized as an ethical obligation on healthcare providers. Indeed, in the USA, there are several major initiatives underway, such as the American Medical Association's Education for Physicians on End-of-Life Care project, to improve the quality of end-of-life care. Although several expert groups have published frameworks for ensuring good care at the end of life, none of these viewed the issue from the perspective of the patient. It is, after all, the patient who is to be the recipient of any end-of-life care.

When interviewed, 126 participants from three patient groups identified five main areas of concern in terminal care. These were adequate pain relief and symptom control, avoiding inappropriate prolongation of dying, maintaining a sense of control if possible, relieving the burden on their family and strengthening relationships with loved ones (Singer *et al.*, 1999). None of these desires are surprising. The increasing importance of end-of-life care in North America reflects a difference in the provision of palliative care and hospice support compared to the UK.

Once a decision is taken that further treatment is not in the best interests of the patient it should be discussed with the patient or, more commonly, his family. In most cases the family agree with the decision to withhold or withdraw therapy. But what if they disagree? Can they demand that treatment considered inappropriate be continued? Some ethicists believe that they can. Veatch and Spicer (1992) maintain that a doctor is obliged to persevere even if the request 'deviated intolerably' from accepted practice. This opinion and others like it have so influenced doctors' thinking in the USA that Paris discovered that physicians almost always continue with futile treatment if requested. They do this under the (false) impression that patient autonomy carries with it the right to demand whatever treatment the patient wishes (Paris *et al.*, 1993).

This suggests putting the autonomy of the patient above that of the physician or other carer. Undoubtedly the balance of the doctor–patient relationship has shifted in favour of the patient in recent times but this does not mean that the doctor can forgo his responsibilities and delegate all decision making to the patient. The appropriate response is to bring the patient, or proxy, fully into the decision making process. Clinical ethics committees can also play an important role in resolving dilemmas such as this.

If the treatment cannot achieve the underlying goal of improving the condition of the patient then it loses its justification and should be withdrawn (President's Commission for the Study of Ethical Problems in Medicine and Biomedical

Research, 1993). The Courts in the UK have supported this approach and do not require a doctor to act against his clinical judgement (Re J, 1992). In fact, the doctor probably has a duty not to provide such treatment.

If the demand for inappropriate treatment is sustained then persuading the family of its futility can be very difficult. There is no easy solution to the situation but good communication and support for the family is essential. This may involve help from clergy or counsellors. Other options are to obtain a second opinion or review of the case. In the USA, an 'ethics consult' often allows the different parties to negotiate successfully.

Rationing and resource allocation

The fourth principle of medical ethics is that of justice. In the context of daily healthcare decision making, this refers to the just allocation of resources or rationing. The demand for healthcare outstrips supply in the public healthcare system of every developed country in the world. Consequently, rationing occurs under a variety of guises.

Decisions concerning resource distribution occur at three levels. Macroallocations of resources are made at national level, mesoallocations at the health authority or hospital level and microallocations concern the individual patient (McKneally *et al.*, 1997). All three are interrelated but it is those decisions that affect individual patients that cause clinicians most concern.

Aristotle's principle of distributive justice states that equals should be treated equally and those who are unequal should be treated unequally. Unequal treatment is justified only when resources are distributed in response to morally relevant differences such as need or likely benefit (Doyal, 1994). Unfortunately, there is no theory of justice that can balance all competing claims, so publicly accountable methods of resource allocation procedures are important.

The need for resources to be distributed across a population is leading some ethicists to consider that the traditional fiduciary duty of the doctor towards the patient is changing. Traditionally the doctor had to do everything they believed to benefit a patient without consideration of cost or other societal factors (Levinsky, 1984). The Hippocratic Oath, the Declaration of Geneva and the International Code of Medical Ethics all charge the doctor with putting the well-being of the patient first (British Medical Association, 1993). More recently Morreim (1995) has suggested that the clinician must also consider the competing interests of other patients and society which pays for healthcare.

Principles of rationing

Several rationing principles have been described, each of which attempts to distribute resources equitably. Essentially they can be described as needs principles, maximizing principles and egalitarian principles (Cookson and Dolan, 2000).

Needs based distribution allocates healthcare in proportion to apparent need. Need, however, must be defined. Is it the need to avoid an immediate life-threatening event or the need to be relieved of pain and suffering? In the former, diseases such as cancer or heart disease would gain high priority. But if the latter definition is implemented, then many chronic and debilitating, but not life-threatening, diseases such as rheumatoid arthritis, would merit consideration. These two definitions are often amalgamated under the heading of 'the rule of rescue' implying that society has a duty to rescue those whose well-being is in immediate peril. With the 'rule of rescue' there is no necessity for the benefit gained to be sustained. Thus preventing the immediate death of an octogenarian could possibly take precedence over providing long-term support to younger patients whose illnesses are not immediately fatal, for example human immunodeficiency virus victims.

This fairly narrow interpretation of need includes distributing resources on the basis of lifetime ill health (potentially favouring the young as they are generally fitter with less chronic ill health), immediate ability to benefit (the less ill would gain) and the potential lifetime benefit (again favouring the young with their greater life expectancy).

Maximizing theories are utilitarian in outlook and aim to maximize health throughout society. Treatments are supplied depending on the anticipated consequences and whose lifetime health gain was likely to be the greatest. Again this might favour the young and fit and discriminate against the old or disabled. Maximal health gain might also be achieved by preventing ill health in the first place so public health programmes such as immunization would be prioritized over many other interventions.

An egalitarian approach would attempt to reduce inequalities in health. Using the 'fair innings' argument everyone is entitled to an equally long and healthy life (Williams, 1997). Healthcare resources are distributed to even out inequalities. This theory would also tend to discriminate in favour of the young. Unlike some other rationing schemes, this bias would remain even when the expected health gain was low, such as a child with cancer.

Equalizing the opportunity that everyone has for health is an alternative egalitarian theory. It allows the individual to make choices that may influence his or her health for better or worse. An assessment of blame (drug use or smoking) may accompany any resultant ill health and be taken into account before treatment is sanctioned.

Quality Adjusted Life Years (QALYs)

A completely different approach is to quantify the economic and opportunity costs of medical interventions. The quality adjusted life year or QALY attempts this. It judges to what extent and for how long a treatment will improve quality of life and how much this will cost. In this way different treatments at different costs may be compared. If the improvement in health is large and long lasting then it scores a high quality of life rating. If it is also inexpensive then the cost per unit of quality of life is low. QALYs theory favours treatments that achieve large increases in the quality of life for the longest period and the least cost (Newdick, 1995).

Using renal support therapy as an example the costs of different treatments can be compared. Continuous ambulatory peritoneal dialysis is inexpensive but with a health gain of only 4 years costs £13 434 per QALY. Haemodialysis (8 years gained) costs £9075 per QALY, while transplantation, although the most expensive initially, gives 10 years of health gain and is ultimately the cheapest option at £1413 per QALY.

The disadvantage of QALYs, like many other distributive theories, is that it discriminates against the elderly who have the fewest years to gain and the disabled whose health gain is not as large.

None of the theories discussed solve the quandary of how to distribute healthcare resources most fairly. However, they are a basis from which the problem can be answered. Rationing by one method or another already occurs. In the UK, the National Institute for Clinical Effectiveness will probably be at the forefront of a formal rationing policy as it is charged with assessing the efficacy of new treatments and deciding if the cost benefit ratio favours introduction or not. To ensure acceptance of whatever method of distribution is used the decision making process must be transparent and fair. The public must be involved in setting priorities. This has not yet happened in the UK to any extent. One small study found that the public supports a combination policy amalgamating aspects of the needs, maximizing and egalitarian principles in a way that has not been previously proposed (Cookson and Dolan, 1999).

The Oregon plan

Deciding how to distribute limited resources will not be easy but the state of Oregon in the USA has already tried. In response to rising healthcare costs, many states in the USA sought ways to reduce their Medicaid budgets. In Oregon the legislature approached the problem in a novel way. Following a 3-year discussion period with multiple community meetings to access public opinion, the Oregon Health Plan was published. This was a prioritized list of diagnoses and treatments.

The commission charged with establishing the list defined seventeen categories of health problem such as the potentially fatal but treatable, chronic conditions unlikely to be fatal, maternity services, etc. All diagnoses and their treatment were assigned to one of these categories and were then ranked according to criteria including life expectancy, quality of life and cost effectiveness. Treatments preventing death with a full recovery were ranked top, maternity care next and those preventing death without a full recovery were third. Any treatment resulting in minimal or no improvement in the quality of life was ranked at the bottom. Once prioritized all treatments were costed and a line was drawn below which treatment would not be provided by Medicaid (Bodenheimer, 1997).

Approximately 700 diagnosis/treatment pairs were assessed and the line drawn, initially, at pair 606 but it has since moved to pair 574 (Table 11.5). Most of the treatments below the cut-off line have little effectiveness. The top items include the treatment of moderate or severe head injury, insulin dependent diabetes mellitus, peritonitis and acute glomerulonephritis (including dialysis therapy).

The Oregon plan has been a brave experiment in healthcare planning, utilizing public consultation in a way not previously employed. Overall it would appear to have been successful as both the public and the medical profession seem happy. It has also succeeded in extending Medicaid cover to an extra 100 000 people.

So far no other authority has been tempted to emulate Oregon's approach. 'Muddling through' would tend to describe the situation in many other countries, including the UK. Here resource allocation may be likened to a circus juggler trying to juggle too many balls at once. Every time a ball falls to the ground the audience shouts until the juggler picks it up only to drop another. Just as the juggler will eventually decide how many balls can be coped with, every healthcare system will need to make similar decisions about healthcare provision.

In practice it is the duty of the doctor to provide the best care possible within the restrictions imposed by the resources provided. The following guidelines may prove helpful in this respect (McKneally *et al.*, 1997):

1. Base intervention on evidence of effectiveness
2. Avoid interventions or tests of marginal benefit
3. Advocate for one's patients but avoid manipulating the system to gain unfair advantage for them
4. Resolve conflicting claims on the basis of morally relevant criteria such as need and benefit.

Even with an Oregon-like policy it is unlikely that all allocation decisions will go unchallenged. Indeed there have already been a number of cases where healthcare provision has been challenged in the courts. Administrative law, the body of rules by which courts examine the legality of bureaucratic decisions, is now impacting on medicine in a way not previously seen. The types of medical decision that may be reviewed include those that discriminate between patients, policies not to provide certain treatment and decisions not to provide certain promised services. Decisions not to provide services based upon purely clinical or financial grounds are presently beyond the power of the court's review (Stewart, 2000). This is another area where data on outcome and prognosis may be of great importance, both to decide what resources should be financed and to help defend those decisions once made.

Conclusion

Prognostic outcome scoring systems have an important role to play in healthcare decision making despite their reservations. Prognosis scoring can bolster but not

Table 11.5 An illustrative example of the priorities in health care set by Oregon

---

Top five diagnosis/treatment pairs
1   Severe/moderate head injury: haematoma/edema with loss of consciousness
    Medical and surgical treatment
2   Insulin dependent diabetes mellitus
    Medical therapy
3   Peritonitis
    Medical and surgical treatment
4   Acute glomerulonephritis
    Medical therapy including dialysis
5   Pneumothorax and hemothorax
    Tube thoracostomy/thoracotomy, medical therapy

Diagnosis/treatment pairs around cut-off at pair 574
572 Internal derangement of the knee, ligamentous disruption of the knee grade II & III
    Surgical repair and medical therapy
573 Dysfunction of the nasolacrymal system
    Medical and surgical treatment
574 Venereal warts excluding cervical condyloma
    Medical therapy
                                                      Cut-off at 1st October 2000
575 Chronic anal fissure and fistula
    Sphincterotomy, fissurectomy, medical therapy
576 Dental service (broken appliances)
    Complex prosthetics
577 Impulse disorders
    Medical and psychotherapy

Bottom five diagnosis/treatment pairs
739 Dental services (orthodontics)
    Cosmetic
740 Tubal dysfunction and other cause of infertility
    IVF, GIFT
741 Hepatorenal syndrome
    Medical therapy
742 Spastic dysphonia
    Medical therapy
743 Disorders of refraction and accommodation
    Radial keratotomy

Adapted from The Office of Oregon Health Plan Policy and Research Prioritized List of Health Services effective from 1 October 2000 (http://216.218.233.168/ohppr/)

replace clinical judgement, including deciding who may or may not benefit from admission to intensive care and for how long life support measures should be employed. Their other main function is to provide a mechanism for auditing the activity and effectiveness of ICUs. This will allow units to compare their outcomes with others and, in time, will probably have a role in clinical governance and the setting of clinical standards.

In the future as scoring systems become more 'real-time' and their accuracy improves, they will influence decision making more, including decisions to withhold or withdraw therapy. This could include informing patients, enabling them to make decisions based on their potential for recovery. Increased use and knowledge of advanced directives would enable the patient's wishes to be followed even when incapacitated by illness. The accurate identification of patients who cannot benefit from intensive care could not only allow resources to be targeted at those who could gain but, more importantly, prevent a patient unnecessarily suffering the indignities and discomfort associated with intensive care.

The other major area yet to be addressed is that of resource allocation. Apart from Oregon, no other legislature has had the courage to tackle this problem. Accurate knowledge of outcome is vital for any attempt at fair resource distribution. Public education and discussion will be a prerequisite for implementing any Oregon-like plan. Only by the use of accurate and non-politicized data can funding be directed towards those areas where it can be most effective.

Predicting outcome in the intensive care setting is a developing science that will become more important over time. Although not perfect, its future importance cannot be underestimated and acknowledging its limitations will prepare the way for future development.

References

Airedale NHS Trust v Bland 1. (1993). All England Reports, 821.

Atkinson, S., Bihari, D., Smithies, M., Daly, K., Mason, R., McColl, I. (1994). Identification of futility in intensive care. *Lancet*, **334**, 1203–1206.

Beauchamp, T. L., Childress, J. F. (1989). *Principles of Biomedical Ethics*, 3rd edn. pp 67–306, 122–123, Oxford University Press.

Belchertown State School Superintendent v Saikewicz 373. (1997). Massachusetts Supreme Judicial Court Reports, 728.

Bodenheimer, T. (1997). The Oregon health plan – lessons for the nation (first of two parts). *N. Engl. J. Med.*, **337**, 651–655.

Bouvia v Superior Court 225. (1986). Californian Reporter, 297.

Brannen, A. L., Godfrey, L. J., Goetter, W. E. (1989). Prediction of outcome from critical illness. A comparison of clinical judgement with a prediction rule. *Arch. Int. Med.*, **149**, 1083–1086.

Brett, A. S., McCullough, L. B. (1986). When patients request specific interventions. *N. Engl. J. Med.*, **315**, 1347–1351.

British Medical Association (1993*). Medical Ethics Today.* BMJ Publishing Group.

Capron, A. M. (1994). Medical futility: strike two. *Hastings Centre Report*, **5**, 42–43.

Chang, R. W. S., Lee, B., Jacobs, S., Lee, B. (1989). Accuracy of decisions to withdraw therapy in critically ill patients: Clinical judgement versus a computer model. *Crit. Care Med.*, **17**, 1091–1097.

Chichin, E. R., Olsen, E. (1995). An ethics consult team in geriatric long-term care. *Cambridge Quarterly of Healthcare Ethics*, **4**, 178–184.

Cookson, R., Dolan, P. (1999). Public views on health care rationing: a group discussion study. *Health Policy*, **49**, 63–74.

Cookson, R., Dolan, P. (2000). Principles of justice in health care rationing. *J. Med. Ethics*, **26**, 323–329.

Danis, M., Devita, M., Baily, M. A. *et al.* (1997). Consensus statement of the Society of Critical Care Medicine's Ethics Committee regarding futile and other possibly inadvisable treatments. *Crit. Care Med.*, **25**, 887–891.

Diem, S. J., Lantos, J. D., Tulsky, J. A. (1996). Cardiopulmonary resuscitation on television – miracles and misinformation. *N. Engl. J. Med.*, **334**, 1578–1582.

Dolley, M. (1993). Public uses Denmark's living will. *Br. Med. J.*, **306**, 414.

Doyal, L. (1994). Needs, rights and the moral duties of clinicians. In: *Principles of Health Care Ethics* (R. Gillon, A. Lloyd, eds) pp 2217–2230, Wiley and Sons.

Emmanuel, E. J., Emmanuel, L. L. (1994). The economics of dying. *N. Engl. J. Med.*, **330**, 540–544.

Gordon, P. N., Williamson, S., Lawler, P. G. (1998). As seen on TV: observational study of cardiopulmonary resuscitation in British television medical dramas. *Br. Med. J.*, **317**, 780–783.

Ham, C. (1999). Tragic choices in health care: lessons from the Child B case. *Br. Med. J.*, **319**, 1258–1261.

Hansot, E. (1996). A letter from a patient's daughter. *Ann. Int. Med.*, **125**, 149–151.

Hope, A. T., Plenderleith, J. L. (1995). The Riyadh Intensive Care Program mortality prediction algorithm assessed in 617 intensive care patients in Glasgow. *Anaesthesia*, **50**, 103–107.

Jennett, B., Bond, M. (1975). Assessment of outcome after severe brain damage. A practical scale. *Lancet*, **152**, 480–484.

Kerridge, I., Lowe, M., Henry, D. (1998). Ethics and evidence based medicine. *Br. Med. J.*, **316**, 1151–1153.

Knaus, W. A., Draper, E. A., Wagner, D. P., Zimmerman, J. E. (1985). APACHE II. A severity of disease classification. *Crit. Care Med.*, **13**, 818–829.

Kutner, L. (1969). Due process of euthanasia: the living will, a proposal. *Indiana Law Journal*, **44**, 539–554.

Levinsky, N. G. (1984). The doctor's master. *N. Engl. J. Med.*, **311**, 1573–1575.

Livingston, B. M., MacKirdy, F. N., Howie, J. C., Jones, R., Norrie, J. D. (2000). Assessment of the performance of five intensive care scoring models within a large Scottish database. *Crit. Care Med.*, **28**, 1820–1827.

Luce, J. M. (1995). Physicians do not have a responsibility to provide futile or unreasonable care if a patient or family insists. *Crit. Care Med.*, **23**, 760–766.

Macneill, P. M., Walters, J., Webster, I. W. (1994). Ethics decision making in Australian hospitals. *Med. J. Aus.*, **160**, 63–65.

Malette v Shulman 67. (1990). Dominion Law Reoprts, 4th edn. 321.

Marks, R. J., Simons, R. S., Blizzard, R. A., Browne, D. R. G. (1991). Predicting outcome in intensive therapy units – a comparison of APACHE II with subjective assessments. *Intensive Care Med.*, **17**, 159–163.

McClish, D. K., Powell, S. H. (1989). How well can physicians estimate mortality in a medical intensive care unit? *Med. Dec. Making*, **9**, 125–132.

McKneally, M. F., Dickens, B. M., Meslin, E. M., Singer, P. A. (1997). Bioethics for clinicians: 13. Resource allocation. *Can. Med. Ass. J.*, **157**, 163–167.

McLean, S. A. M., Booth, M. (1998). Withholding and withdrawing life-prolonging treatment. *Med. Law Int.*, **3**, 169–182.

Morreim, E. H. (1995). *Balancing Act: the New Medical Ethics of Medicine's New Economics*, p. 2, Georgetown University Press.

Newdick, C. (1995). Resources in the NHS. In: *Who Should We Treat? Law, Patients and Resources in the N.H.S.* pp 22–30, Oxford University Press.

Paris, J. J., Schreiber, M. D., Statter, M., Arensman, R., Siegler, M. (1993). Beyond autonomy – the physicians refusal to use life-prolonging extracorporeal membrane oxygenation. *N. Engl. J. Med.*, **329**, 345–357.

Parish, D. C., Dane, F. C., Montgomery, M., Wynn, L. J., Durham, M. D. (1999). Resuscitation in the hospital: differential relationships between age and survival across rhythms. *Crit. Care Med.*, **27**, 2137–2141.

Patel, P. A., Grant, B. J. B. (1999). Application of mortality prediction systems to individual intensive care units. *Intensive Care Med.*, **25**, 977–982.

Phillips, M. (2000). The law cannot be a killer – it must save one twin. *Sunday Times,* 10 September 2000, p. 17, Times Newspaper Ltd.

President's Commission for the Study of Ethical Problems in Medicine and Biomedical Research. (1993). Deciding to forego life sustaining treatment: a report on the ethical, medical and legal issues in treatment decisions (President's Commission 1993). Government Printing Office.

Quinn, J. B. (1994). Taking back their health care. *Newsweek*, 27 June 1994, p. 36, Newsweek Inc.

Re C (Adult: refusal of treatment) 1. (1994). *Weekly Law Reports*, 290.

Re J (A minor) (Child in care: Medical treatment) 3. (1992). *Weekly Law Reports*, 507.

Re T (Adult: refusal of treatment). (1993). *Family Court*, 95.

Rubenfeld, G. D., Crawford, S. W. (1996). Withdrawing life support from mechanically ventilated recipients of bone marrow transplants: a case for evidence based guidelines. *Ann. Int. Med.*, **125**, 625–633.

Sackett, D. L., Rosenberg, W. M. C., Gray, J. A. M., Hayes, R. B., Richardson, W. S. (1996). Evidence based medicine: what it is and what it isn't. *Br. Med. J.*, **312**, 71–72.

Schiff, R., Rajkumar, C., Bulpitt, C. (2000). Views of elderly people on living wills: interview study. *Br. Med. J.*, **320**, 1640–1641.

Schneiderman, L. J., Jecker, N. S. (1995). Ethical implications of medical futility. In: *Wrong Medicine*, pp 97–118, Johns Hopkins University Press.

Seckler, A. B., Meier, D. E., Mulvihill, M., Paris, B. E. C. (1991). Substituted judgement: how accurate are proxy predictions? *Ann. Int. Med.*, **115**, 92–98.

Sidaway v Board of Bethlem Royal Hospital. (1985). Appeal Court, 882.

Singer, P. A. (1994). Disease-specific advance directives. *Lancet*, **344**, 594–596.

Singer, P. A., Martin, D. K., Kelner, M. (1999). Quality end-of-life care. Patients' perspectives. *JAMA*, **281**, 163–168.

Slowther, A. M., Hope, T. (2000). Clinical ethics committees. *Br. Med. J.*, **321**, 649–650.

St George's Healthcare NHS Trust v S; R v Collins exp S 3. (1998). *Weekly Law Reports*, 936.

Stewart, C. (2000). Tragic choices and the role of administrative law. *Br. Med. J.*, **321**, 105–107.

Sulmasy, D. P., Terry, P. B., Weisman, C. S. *et al.* (1998). The accuracy of substituted judgements in patients with terminal diagnoses. *Ann. Int. Med.*, **128**, 621–629.

Thornhill, S., Teasdale, G. M., Murray, G. D. *et al*. (2000). Disability in young people and adults one year after head injury: prospective cohort study. *Br. Med. J.*, **320**, 1631–1635.

Veatch, R. M., Spicer, C. M. (1992). Medically futile care: the role of the physician in setting limits. *Am. J. Law Med.*, **18**, 15–36.

Williams, A. N. (1997). Intergenerational equity: an exploration of the 'fair innings' argument. *Hlth Econ.*, **6**, 117–132.

Zoch, G., Schemper, M., Kyral, E., Meissl, G. (1992). Comparison of prognostic indices for burns and assessment of their accuracy. *Burns*, **18**, 109–112.

Index